Dynamics of

New Dynamics of Disability and Rehabilitation

Ivan Harsløf • Ingrid Poulsen
Kristian Larsen
Editors

New Dynamics of Disability and Rehabilitation

Interdisciplinary Perspectives

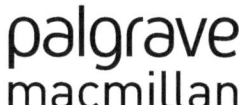

Editors
Ivan Harsløf
Department of Social Work, Child Welfare
and Social Policy
Oslo Metropolitan University
Oslo, Norway

Ingrid Poulsen
Department of Neurorehabilitation
Rigshospitalet, University of Copenhagen
Copenhagen, Denmark

Kristian Larsen
Department of Learning and Philosophy
Aalborg University Copenhagen
Copenhagen, Denmark

ISBN 978-981-13-7345-9   ISBN 978-981-13-7346-6   (eBook)
https://doi.org/10.1007/978-981-13-7346-6

This Palgrave Macmillan imprint is published by the registered company Springer Nature Singapore Pte Ltd.
The registered company address is: 152 Beach Road, #21-01/04 Gateway East, Singapore 189721,
Singapore

Preface

This book combines scholarship from various social science and health disciplines relevant to medical or vocational rehabilitation or derived fields. Most of the contributors are Danish or Norwegian, but Sweden, the United Kingdom, Germany, Switzerland, and Australia are also represented.

Most of the research presented in this book is the product of a common research network called Phlegethon, initiated in 2011 (www. phlegethon.net). Fully titled 'Professions, legitimacy and evidence in transforming health and welfare organizations', Phlegethon was conceived as part of a successful application to the Research Council of Norway (RCN) to allow Professor Jaber Gubrium a one-year stay as guest researcher at the then Oslo University College (now OsloMet—Oslo Metropolitan University). In borrowing the name of a river of fire in the infernal regions of the underworld in Greek mythology, we allude to the critical undercurrents in modern society (Bourdieu's 'structural homologies'), cutting across and hence affecting diverse areas of society.

This book has received support from numerous sources. The RCN project *Transitions in rehabilitation: Biographical reconstruction, experiential knowledge and professional expertise* (Grant No. 229082) has allowed for seminars, as has OsloMet's interfaculty Care, Health, and Welfare programme. We are also grateful for support from the Danish-Norwegian

Cooperation Fund, the Danish Victims' Foundation, and the University of Aalborg.

We wish to thank the commissioning editor Joshua Pitt for a fruitful collaboration, and the publisher's external reviewers for critical and constructive advice. In addition, we wish to thank the following persons for their general support and/or comments on the book's chapters: Rune Halvorsen, Helene Lundgaard Søberg, Niels Sandholm Larsen, Grace Inga Romsland, Unni Sveen, and Bjørg Christiansen.

Oslo, Norway   Ivan Harsløf
Copenhagen, Denmark   Ingrid Poulsen
                                                                        Kristian Larsen

January 2019

Contents

Notes on Contributors

Tone Alm Andreassen is a sociologist and professor at the Centre for the Study of Professions, Oslo Metropolitan University, and head of the interdisciplinary and inter-institutional core research group INTEGRATE. Together with Jaber Gubrium and Per Koren Solvang she has edited the volume *Reimagining the Human Service Relationship'* (2016).

Clare Bambra (PhD, FAcSS) is Professor of Public Health, Newcastle University, UK. She is an interdisciplinary social scientist with expertise across health politics & policy, medical sociology, and health geography. She has authored over 175 publications including *Work, Worklessness and the Political Economy of Health* (Oxford University Press, 2011).

Jerome Bickenbach is a health scientist and lawyer, head of the Disability Policy Group at Swiss Paraplegic Research and a professor at the Department of Health Science and Health Policy, Lucern University, Switzerland. His research focuses on disability epidemiology, law and policy, and rehabilitation and health systems research.

Ingo Bode is a professor at the Institute of Social Work and Social Welfare, University of Kassel. He has had positions in Wuppertal, Edinburgh and Nancy. His research explores developments and problems in the design and infrastructure of current welfare states, addressing both institutional logics and organizational arrangements. Current research projects concentrate on manifestations and outcomes of increasingly hybrid and partially marketized systems of welfare provision, from a local, national, and international perspective.

Inge Storgaard Bonfils is an associate professor at the Department of Social Work, University College Copenhagen, Denmark. She holds a PhD in Political Science from the University of Copenhagen and has worked for several years as a researcher in the field of applied science focusing on social work and welfare services, disability, rehabilitation, and new forms of governance.

Mette Ryssel Bystrup is a PhD student at the Department of Learning and Philosophy, Aalborg University Copenhagen, Denmark and Hammel Neurorehabilitation and Research Centre, Denmark. She is a member of the Phlegethon research network. Her PhD research topic concerns inequalities in the rehabilitation process after a severe acquired brain injury of adolescents.

Berth Danermark is Professor (Emeritus) of Sociology at The Swedish Institute for Disability Research, School of Health Sciences, Örebro University. He is the co-author of *Interdisciplinarity and Wellbeing: A Critical Realist General Theory of Interdisciplinarity* and co-editor of *The Experience of Hearing Loss: Journey Through Aural Rehabilitation*.

Ingrid Egerod RN, MSN, PHD, is professor of clinical nursing, Intensive Care Unit, Rigshospitalet, University of Copenhagen. She is a qualified critical care nurse. She has worked in Copenhagen, Honolulu and San Francisco. She is co-founder of the Nordic Association for Intensive Care Nursing Research (NOFI), author of 115 peer reviewed publications, 32 professional publications, and 27 book contributions.

Marte Feiring is Associate Professor at the Faculty of Health, Oslo Metropolitan University, Norway, where she teaches at the Master's Programme on Rehabilitation and Habilitation. She holds a PhD in

Sociology from the University of Oslo on the history of rehabilitation. Her research projects cover historical and critical perspectives on health policies, welfare services, professional and inter-professional knowledge, rehabilitation practices, and civil movements.

Ivan Harsløf is an associate professor at the Department of Social Work, Child Welfare and Social Policy, Oslo Metropolitan University. He has co-edited *The Dynamics of Poverty* (in Norwegian, 2008) and *Inclusive Consumption* (2019) for Scandinavian University Press, and *Changing Social Risks and Social Policy Responses in the Nordic Welfare States* for Palgrave Macmillan (2013).

Anette Lykke Hindhede is an associate professor at the Department of Learning and Philosophy, Aalborg University Copenhagen. She holds a MA in Education from the University of Copenhagen and a PhD in Educational Sociology from Aarhus University. She has 20 years of research experience within the field of the sociology of the body and work.

Karin Højbjerg is an associate professor, PhD, at the Department of Learning and Philosophy, Aalborg University Copenhagen.

Kristian Larsen is a full professor at the Department of Learning and Philosophy, Aalborg University Copenhagen. Furthermore, he holds an adjunct position at the Faculty of Health Sciences, Oslo Metropolitan University. He sits in the editorial committee for the Nordic language journal, *Praktiske grunde* (Practical reasons) and is chair of the board for the *HEXIS—Nordic forum for culture and social science.* Larsen has been editor of several edited collections, most recently *Kritiske perspektiver i helsefagene: Utdanning, yrkespraksis og forskning* (Critical perspectives in the health sciences).

Lene Odgaard PhD, MHS, is a nurse, and datamanager for the Danish Head Trauma Database at Hammel Neurorehabilitation and Research Center, Aarhus University, Hammel, Denmark. Her dissertation investigated survivors of severe traumatic brain injury in Denmark in terms of incidence, inpatient rehabilitation, and return to work prognosis.

Ingrid Poulsen is educated as a nurse and holds a PhD in Geriatric Rehabilitation from Lund University in Sweden. Since 2005, she has had a position as post-doctoral researcher and since 2009 as research manager at the Department of Neurorehabilitation, Rigshospitalet, University of Copenhagen. She also holds the position of an associate professor at Section of Nursing Science, Aarhus University. She conducts research in clinical areas relevant for patients with severe brain injury, for example, pain assessment, dysphagia, and prevention of pressure ulcers.

Anne-Stine B. Røberg is a nurse specialist and researcher at TRS National Resource Center for Rare Disorders. She holds a master's degree in Nursing Science, Oslo University, and PhD in Health Sciences, Oslo Metropolitan University. Her research includes nursing and traumatic brain injuries, and critical perspectives on disability and rehabilitation practices related to health policies and welfare state development.

Per Koren Solvang is a sociologist and Professor of Rehabilitation at the Department of Physiotherapy, Oslo Metropolitan University. Solvang has published studies on a wide variety of themes related to disability and rehabilitation. Among these are strategies applied by professionals assisting disabled people, transnational meeting places for deaf people, disability art, and controversies on the medicalization of dyslexia.

Peter W. Stubbs is a physiotherapist and lecturer at the Graduate School of Health, Discipline of Physiotherapy, University of Technology Sydney. He graduated with a BSc in Sport and Exercise Science from Auckland University in 2005, a master's degree in Physiotherapy from Sydney University in 2008, and a PhD in Clinical Neurophysiology and Neurorehabilitation from Aalborg University and Hammel Neurorehabilitation Centre in 2011. He has done post-doctoral research at Neuroscience Research Australia and Hammel Neurorehabilitation Centre, where he remains affiliated.

List of Figures

List of Tables

List of Boxes

1

Introduction: New Dynamics of Disability and Rehabilitation

Ivan Harsløf, Ingrid Poulsen, and Kristian Larsen

Medical and vocational rehabilitation concerns human beings undergoing critical transitions. These transitions include the dramatic changes from living an everyday life to experiencing a sudden, disabling accident or illness, and subsequent efforts, underpinned by health and social services, to restore health and independent living. Under these circumstances, the persons are also likely to experience critical status transitions,

I. Harsløf (✉)
Department of Social Work, Child Welfare and Social Policy, Oslo Metropolitan University, Oslo, Norway
e-mail: ivan.harslof@oslomet.no

I. Poulsen
Department of Neurorehabilitation, Rigshospitalet, University of Copenhagen, Copenhagen, Denmark
e-mail: Ingrid.Poulsen@regionh.dk

K. Larsen
Department of Learning and Philosophy, Aalborg University Copenhagen, Copenhagen, Denmark
e-mail: kl@learning.aau.dk

© The Author(s) 2019
I. Harsløf et al. (eds.), *New Dynamics of Disability and Rehabilitation*,
https://Doi.org/10.1007/978-981-13-7346-6_1

changing type of occupation, financial situation, or family situation. More concretely, persons undergoing rehabilitation encounter transitions, as they are sent from specialized health services to general health services, as well as between different branches of the public sector (e.g. from the healthcare sector to the work and welfare sector), although these processes seldom occur in a linear fashion.

According to the British philosopher Roy Bhaskar, 'in periods of transitions or crisis, generative structures, previously opaque, become more visible' (Bhaskar, quoted in Danermark et al. 2002, p. 104). Hence, by studying the transitions undertaken by rehabilitation patients (life transitions, status transitions, and the mundane transfers across agencies and sectors), one may learn a lot about individuals' and families' abilities to respond to the cumulative crises (loss of health, loss of identity, loss of job, loss of income, etc.), about society's apparatus to support the individuals and families in these efforts, and more generally about the inclusive and excluding mechanisms operating in organizations, in health systems, and in labour markets.

Prompted by this rationale, this book aims to bring the study of transitions within rehabilitation into the wider context of the welfare state's changing role. The notion of universalism is central to discussions of medical and vocational rehabilitation services and how they have evolved along the course of the welfare state's development. To introduce this book, this chapter considers the notion of universalism, including the debates it has engendered, and relates it to the provision of medical and vocational rehabilitation services in Northern European welfare states. To set the stage for case studies on rehabilitation for survivors of traumatic brain injury (TBI), which is the topic of five contributions in this volume, this chapter discusses the composition and developments of TBI patient groups. It considers persons with TBI to be characterized by not only physical/neurological but also biographical and social disruptions. It further discusses the potential for extrapolating TBI research findings to other areas of rehabilitation and healthcare. This excursus is followed by a summary of the book's chapters and a general conclusion.

1.1   Rehabilitation Services in the Universal Welfare State

In his deeply touching postscript to his very last book on social policy (published posthumously in 1974), Richard M. Titmuss describes his stay at the then Westminster Hospital, where he was being treated for terminal cancer. With great enthusiasm, he describes the other patient who shares his room, Bill, a war veteran of working-class background. For several decades, Titmuss learns, Bill has received top-quality rehabilitation since sustaining injuries during World War II. The two men even attempt to calculate the total value of health services he has received throughout his life.

For Titmuss, public health services, as the ones provided for him and Bill, are the prime example of universalism, as a domain where citizens of all social classes meet one another and enjoy equal standards. He also notices that, for most middle-class persons, health services are the welfare state's prime interface, allowing them to appreciate what their taxes fund. Hence, universalism is the constituent factor of community (Bauman 1998). Accommodating everybody across social class, who are characterised by a given need, universal services are less stigmatizing than targeted measures. For Titmuss, universal welfare state institutions serve to alleviate the 'social costs' of modern society, that is, the externalities generated by the capitalist market, from air pollution to workplace accidents (Titmuss 1974, p. 72). The welfare state was supposed to support the victims 'who in time of product and process innovation become the price of economic growth', as Reisman summarizes it (Reisman 2001 [1977], p. 159).

In essence, rehabilitation services are delivered for the purpose of restoring and reconstructing individuals' capacities, invoking notions of normalizing and standardizing, but also—as increasingly acknowledged—for adopting changes in affected individuals' social context for their own mechanisms to function again (cf. Brante 2011, p. 17). Indeed, rehabilitation services across medicine and social services became a cornerstone of the post-war, universal welfare state in Northern Europe.

Peaking around 1960, universalism was soon attacked from quite different political positions. First, criticism was raised against one material manifestation of universalism: the set of 'people-changing' organizations, where citizens were to be treated and normalized (Hasenfeld 1972). Liberalists saw the organizations, such as mental hospitals, residential drug abuse clinics, and rehabilitation institutions, as representing a statist, costly, and outmoded 'one-size-fits-all' way of thinking. The progressive left, inspired by sociological research (such as Goffman's (1961) fieldwork in asylums) and even popular culture (such as Forman's (1975) *One Flew Over the Cuckoo's Nest*), saw them as overtly oppressive (Kaukonen and Stenius 2005).

Universalism has faced new pressure in recent decades, broadly related to societal transformations since the mid-1970s, with the service economy becoming increasingly dominant and the growing internationalization and interdependence of national economies (termed 'globalization' from around the 1990s). These deep-seated developments displaced and obscured processes of externalization, making it increasingly difficult to grasp the relation between those who produced and those who bore Titmuss' 'social costs'. In effect, people on the receiving end of this chain of externalities were increasingly blamed for their own misery and considered less deserving of benefits and services (Harsløf and Ulmestig 2013).

Under conditions of austerity, the liberalist argument against universalism—that targeted benefits and services are more cost-efficient—has gained momentum. As the apt title of a book discussing the increasing emphasis on targeting and 'tailoring' of services sums it up: 'Now it's personal' (Ben-Galim and Sachradja 2010). The European Union, with its recent initiatives in the social domain, including the *Platform against poverty* and the *Social Investment Package*, strongly advices member states to better target the provision of cash benefits and social services, in order to increase efficiency and effectiveness (Gómez-Barroso et al. 2017).

Meanwhile, the progressive left is increasingly concerned with ethnocentric and excluding features of universalism, a critical position that has gained a stronghold in recent welfare state research and disability studies (Anttonen et al. 2012). The new progressive left's position tends to downplay that rehabilitation services are part of a universal safety net, stretched beneath all citizens. Instead, subscribing to Foucault's (2003, p. 15) notion that 'politics is war by other means' (inverting Clausewitz's classic dictum), they consider the welfare state's repertoire of 'active' measures, including rehabilitation programmes, as 'governance technologies' to instil a new subjectivity concomitant with the prevailing social order. Accordingly, this position advocates redesigning rehabilitation systems to accommodate diversity across groups that differ in levels of functioning, and a host of gender and social identities. In these efforts, among both academics and social activists, such as the disability movement, language has been a major site of struggle. Their criticism of terms such as 'patient' or 'victim' illustrates the linguistic turn in the field of rehabilitation: in this context, 'patient' is considered pejorative, given its etymological association with passive suffering (McPherson et al. 2015, p. vii), while 'victim' is allegedly inappropriate (and should be replaced with 'survivor') as also this term, it is argued, misconstrues the person's level of agency. The criticism of peoples' choice of words is often indifferent to their intentions or the context in which they apply them.

Whilst the case made for replacing a word with another is often convincing in itself, this obsession with language, and eagerness to correct and sanction those who cling to outmoded terminology, may challenge the tenets of universalism, by depriving ordinary people a 'valid' language to take part in discussions on disability and rehabilitation. Having an updated vocabulary for engaging in discourses on disability and rehabilitation becomes, in a Bourdieusian sense, a critical part of one's cultural capital.[1]

As Chap. 2 will detail, rehabilitation services have had to adapt to major changes in the overarching contexts in which they are organized, delivered, and consumed. Paradigmatic shifts in the field of medicine, resulting from advancements in medical technologies and service organization, alongside new conceptions of health and work, have greatly affected rehabilitation services. It has also been significantly influenced by shifts in the organization and management of the state. Finally, the labour market, in which rehabilitated patients are to be (re)integrated, is a third relevant context that has undergone dramatic changes.

---

[1] In a recent book in the field, the authors go as far as making reservations as to the terms and concepts they apply, anticipating that chances are that even the terms they have chosen exquisitely may in the future be considered pejorative (Leplège et al. 2015, p. 22n).

Responding to these shifts and pressures, the field of vocational rehabilitation has seen general retrenchments, prioritizing shorter-term measures ('work-first') at the expense of long-term retraining ('human capital investment') (Harsløf 2008). Aligning with this trend, one has also seen a process of de-institutionalization (Bollingmo 1997). Another trend has been the introduction of measures to instil better responsiveness to individual users and a general juridification equipping the user with more rights to services. Seemingly, the trends of cost-cutting and the trend of enhancing user rights and involvement are contradictory. Observers have pointed out how dilemmas about how to cope with such contradictions are 'decentralized' to lower levels of governance and eventually the service professionals (Vike 2018). From a welfare state perspective, these changes may have created new winners and losers. For example, as concrete healthcare and social services are enshrined as statutory rights, service users are empowered vis-à-vis the health and social authorities and their professional representatives. Yet, as welfare state scholars have pointed out, the formalization of social rights does not guarantee that required services are actually delivered, and there is the possibility that more privileged groups (e.g. better educated) are best suited to know about and hence exercise their social rights (Hatland 2011; Bærøe and Bringedal 2014, p. 158).

Consequently, new divisions within the group of users may emerge, leaving those with less education or less access to various forms of favourable social networks increasingly marginalized.[2] Such divides may also surface in differences between specific patient groups: for example, those disabled due to chronic diseases (constituting the majority of the disabled population) are characterized by having lower education, and may find it more difficult to take upon themselves the active role increasingly required to realize their rights (Geyer 2016; Strand and Madsen 2016).

This book presents analyses of medical and vocational rehabilitation services within the changing context of the Northern European welfare

---

[2] By favourable networks, we mean interpersonal support systems that may, among other benefits, be advantageous in matters of personal health and social welfare, through mainly two types of support: *informational* (providing advice, guidance, or information relevant to the situation) and *instrumental* (providing concrete aid or assistance). Through personal contacts, for example, one may be advised on one's social rights and how to realise them (Gele and Harsløf 2010).

state. Medical rehabilitation services entail a range of health services pro-vided by professionals such as physicians, psychologists, nurses, physio-therapists, and occupational therapists, whether in specialized hospitals and clinics, or in people's homes. Vocational rehabilitation services are those performed by social workers, labour market consultants, counsel-lors, and related professionals. The field is intersected, and the provision of services is not cumulative. The vocational ('return-to-work'-oriented) part of rehabilitation may begin in the hospital and heavily involve health personnel. Hospitals also employ social workers to attend to patients' social situation (such as income maintenance, contact with current/previ-ous employer, etc.), just as social work offices or public employment ser-vices employ physicians and psychologists to advise on medical aspects. As a supplement or alternative to medical and vocational rehabilitation services, social rehabilitation services may be provided.

This book adopts a broad notion of Northern Europe that includes the United Kingdom (UK) and Germany, that is, the predominantly Protestant parts of Europe (Cunningham and Grell 1997). As we shall discuss further in Chap. 2, there is considerable variance even within this region in approaches to providing health and social services.

The various studies presented in the book focus on discerning how changes in overall policies, institutions, and organizations affect various groups of users and their relatives. Hence, this volume aims to investigate how such changes affect patients, caregivers, professionals, and organiza-tions, and how the changes have manifested themselves in different Northern European welfare states, representing different welfare models. The contributions cut across the seldom-connected scientific areas of health sciences, medical sociology, disability studies, and welfare state research (Rosqvist et al. 2017).

We believe it is necessary to subject the field of rehabilitation to such multidisciplinary analyses. As the Bhaskar quotation in the opening part of this chapter suggests, by studying transitions such as those involved in individual rehabilitation processes, one may learn about critical mecha-nisms that are only latent under normal conditions. It is during times of crisis that individuals will tend to mobilize the full capacity of their accu-mulated resources, whether financial, cognitive, or embedded in their social networks.

Five chapters in this volume (Chaps. 7, 8, 9, 10, and 11) use traumatic brain injuries (TBIs) as an instrumental case for understanding healthcare and social practices more generally. In the following section, we present the area of TBI rehabilitation and advocate the usefulness of its study to gain broader understanding of the changing context of rehabilitation services in the welfare state.

1.2   The Case of Traumatic Brain Injury Rehabilitation

TBIs are a global public health problem that (depending on the injury's severity) can cause varying levels of disability and potentially lead to death (Nguyen et al. 2016). A TBI is defined as an alteration in brain function, or other brain pathology, caused by an external force (Menon et al. 2010). Alteration in brain function implies one of the following clinical signs: any period of loss (or decreased level) of consciousness; any loss of memory relating to events immediately before or after the injury; neurological deficits (weakness, loss of balance, change in vision, dyspraxia paresis/plegia, paralysis, sensory loss, aphasia, etc.); or any alteration in mental state at the time of the injury (confusion, disorientation, slowed thinking, etc.) (Menon et al. 2010).

TBI survivors exhibit a wide range of complex and potentially profound disabilities and deficits spanning medical, physical, cognitive, psychological, emotional, and social domains; they often need extensive specialized rehabilitation services (Stocchetti and Zanier 2016). Moreover, the physical disabilities can be long lasting, and the complex neurobehavioural abnormalities often reduce the quality of life. Patients find that cognitive and behavioural changes, difficulties maintaining personal relationships, and problems coping with school and work are more disabling than their residual physical deficits (Khan et al. 2003). The consequences of TBIs are also serious for the families of survivors, who have to take on new roles as caregivers (Olesen et al. 2012).

The mean patient age for all levels of TBI severity is about 50 years for men and 60 years for women. Across countries, a greater proportion of males than females (irrespective of age, severity, and injury mechanism) suffer from TBIs. In Europe, the proportion of males ranges from 55% (Sweden) to 80% (Ireland) (Brazinova et al. 2016). Historically, traffic accidents have been the most common cause of injury, but this pattern may be changing due to improved traffic safety, and following the demographic trend of population aging, more TBIs can be attributed to falls (Brazinova et al. 2016). Only a few studies have examined the epidemiological causes of immediate injury events; however, alcohol is considered a possible risk factor for traffic or personal violence incidents (Brazinova et al. 2016).

1.2.1 Rehabilitation Services for TBI Patients

The World Health Organization (WHO) defines rehabilitation as:

> a process aimed at enabling [disabled people] to reach and maintain their optimal physical, sensory, intellectual, psychological and social functional levels. Rehabilitation provides disabled people with the tools they need to attain independence and self-determination. (Quoted in Sjölund 2013, p. 1634)

The WHO's definition outlines an objective for achieving and maintaining functioning in a broad sense, and entails a process for attaining independence and self-determination. The WHO has also created the *International Classification of Functioning, Disability and Health* (ICF) for assessing people's health status in relation to rehabilitation. The ICF is based on the biopsychosocial model, whose components include functioning, contextual, and personal factors.

The care and rehabilitation of TBI patients has evolved substantially in recent decades, and the need for specialized rehabilitation is widely accepted (Ashley 2012). Thirty years ago, there were only a few types of interventions, which mostly comprised conservative observations, treatments, and prophylactic activities. Since then, technological and medical innovations in all phases and types of clinical treatment have produced much more successful quality- and length-of-life outcomes for TBI patients. Specialized clinical and research institutions have been established and new areas of professional expertise have developed, including networks related to research (e.g. scientific journals on rehabilitation), education, and clinical practice. As specialized knowledge, technologies, professions, and research increasingly support rehabilitation as a clinical practice, stroke has been rising significantly in the otherwise relatively stable hierarchy of disease prestige (Album et al. 2017).

In general, patients who survive moderate and severe TBIs have complex rehabilitation needs due to the complexity of disease presentation. In Denmark, the National Health Authority recommend that these patients receive specialized rehabilitation in regional and highly specialized rehabilitation departments/centres providing an interdisciplinary approach to rehabilitation, with staff comprising neurologists, nurses, physiotherapists, occupational therapists, neuropsychologists, and speech language pathologists.

Access to rehabilitation services after severe TBI varies between countries. In Denmark, 84% of patients were admitted to highly specialized rehabilitation. Studies find that women, older people, and people with non-working status prior to the injury are less likely to be admitted to specialized treatment, but this is likely explained by the injury's severity and cause, as, for example, young males tend to endure more severe injuries that necessitate specialized treatment (Odgaard et al. 2015).

Across European countries, there is substantial structural and process variation in inpatient acute rehabilitation and referral to post-acute rehabilitation for patients with moderate and severe TBIs (Cnossen et al. 2017). In a study of 70 neurotrauma centres across 20 European countries, only 41% of intensive care units and 49% of wards were found to have a multidisciplinary rehabilitation team. Moreover, only 13 of the 70 participating centres used rehabilitation guidelines or protocols for the rehabilitation of TBI patients, and most of the guidelines were based on expert knowledge, rather than evidence-based knowledge. In about half of the centres, age was reported as a major determinant of patient referral: younger patients were usually referred to specialized rehabilitation units, whereas patients aged 65 or older tended to be referred to nursing homes or local hospitals (Cnossen et al. 2017).

Access to various forms of rehabilitation after a TBI has also been examined in a sociological context, offering a wider perspective on healthcare professionals' referral decisions. Foster and Tilse (2003) provide a conceptual model grounded in social problems theory. Their model has three main components that describe the different aspects influencing the decision-making process: the *characteristics of the individual with TBI*; the *activities of healthcare professionals and the processes of referral*; and the *context of care*. The *characteristics of the individual with TBI* include the initial severity of the injury, and thus the potential capacity to regain function, independence, and (if of working age) employment. Moreover, non-clinical characteristics such as social identity and the individual's value in society are considered. *Activities of healthcare professionals and the processes of referral* concern how these professionals select and interpret information and determine referrals in their capacity as 'gatekeepers' for healthcare resources. Finally, the *context of care* refers to how the health professionals engage with external resources and the policies that define the field of rehabilitation. For example, policymakers value evidence and 'value for money', and the latter criterion may favour patients with obvious potential for rehabilitation, including return-to-work prospects.

To summarize, the field of rehabilitation for TBI patients is a suitable 'observatory' for understanding the wider transformations of institutions, technology, knowledge, and the roles of patients, caregivers, professionals. TBIs occur in a wide range of activities and affect a diverse population across social strata. They can also involve long-term ailments with both medically objective findings and symptoms of a more diffuse nature. Thus, in their trajectories through 'people-changing organizations' (hospitals) and 'people-processing organizations' (work and welfare institutions), patients depend on having the right status conferred on them at every point in time, requiring intricate negotiations and 'stigma management' (Hasenfeld 1972; Goffman 1963).

1.3   Overview of the Book's Contents

This book's chapters fall into different clusters. Chapter 2 outlines the overall theoretical framework for the presented studies on medical and vocational rehabilitation services. While each chapter adopts its own specific theoretical lens, this framework represents the overall approach that motivates and guides the book. The aim of the chapter is to show connections between the levels of analysis—individual, organizational, national, and transnational—investigated in the various chapters. The chapter argues that rehabilitation programmes at the intersection of health and social services were an integral and important part of early initiatives to establish a comprehensive welfare state. Hence, these programmes played an important role in larger projects of nation building and efforts to create a well-functioning labour market. However, in a post-national and post-industrial context, rehabilitation programmes no longer serve the same purpose. Rather, vocational rehabilitation has become immersed in the general field of 'active' social and labour market policies with the purpose of enhancing labour market flexibility and countering structural unemployment. Moreover, such programmes are now operating within a political context in which the industrial rationale has been almost inverted. Whilst the old rationale saw work as exhausting and as a source of exclusion (what we term the 'deficit model'), work is now considered health-promoting and the world of work is conceived as an arena for inclusion, in line with an emerging 'asset model'. The chapter also argues that the type of welfare state—whether social democratic, conservative-corporative, or liberal—strongly influences the manner in which rehabilitation services have been organized in different Northern European countries. However, some convergence can now be observed (due to policy diffusion, supranational regulation, and international integration of markets), causing countries to leave their traditional orbit.

The theoretical chapter sets the stage for a cluster of chapters (Chaps. 3, 4, 5 and 6), presenting country cases or comparative studies. In Chap. 3, Bode portrays the institutional and organizational context of rehabilitation in Germany, drawing attention to apparent paradoxes and recent dynamics of change. He argues that rehabilitation in Germany exhibits a rather holistic orientation taking shape in a specialized professional field outside acute healthcare and community care—although the infrastructure of both the funding and supply side appears disintegrated in various respects. Furthermore, Bode depicts how recent shifts in the governance of the rehabilitation system tend to exacerbate extant fragmentation—irrespective of parallel efforts to endorse the aforementioned holistic orientation. Given both a subtle influence of the New Public Management mantra and a growing importance of capitalistic businesses in that system, Bode argues, the onus increasingly lies on individual users when it comes to ensure an integrated service trajectory—which proves a high burden for people in need of more sophisticated, case-specific support.

In Chap. 4, Bambra situates rehabilitation services in the UK within a wider welfare and social policy context. She traces significant changes from the 'passive welfare' of the 1970s (characterized by compulsory employment quotas and unconditional benefits), through the 'active welfare' of the 1990s and 2000s (combining antidiscrimination legislation with welfare to work and active welfare benefits), to the workfare approach entrenched in the present system (typified by benefit sanctions and compulsory work-for-benefit). Bambra examines the effects of these policy shifts on the employment of people with a disability or chronic condition and on social inequalities. She identifies a radical shift in the perception of rehabilitation service beneficiaries, from 'deserving' to 'undeserving', as indicated by the gradual abolition of unconditional support to people with disabilities or chronic conditions.

The next two chapters concern the Scandinavian case, represented by Denmark and Norway. In Chap. 5, studying recent governance reforms of health and rehabilitation services in these countries, Feiring and Bonfils identify trends that are comparable to, but yet distinct from, developments in Germany and the UK. Stressing Gibbons' perspective on the so-called Mode 2 logic of knowledge production, they observe how the types of knowledge adopted to regulate rehabilitation services increasingly combine legal argumentation (focusing on users' rights) with evidence-based argumentation (focusing on documented effects). This mixing of rationales is reflected in the manner that various regulating documents refer to one another for mutual justification. Due to these *interdiscursive* and *intertextual* exercises, it is difficult to establish whether arrangements to facilitate cohesive patient trajectory are instituted because users are entitled to them or because they have been scientifically demonstrated to produce desired outcomes. The underlying issue is that producing hard evidence on medical and vocational rehabilitation is notoriously difficult, given the composite and interdisciplinary character of interventions and service chains, as well as the distinctiveness of individual cases.

Posing questions about power relations and governmental rationalities, Røberg focuses in Chap. 6 on ongoing changes in the Norwegian welfare system. She applies a critical discourse framework to analyse public documents and interviews with rehabilitation professionals. Røberg demonstrates how rehabilitation is articulated as a reactive clinical practice, responding to individuals' physical or mental condition. A second nodal discourse emerging from her analysis construes rehabilitation as a management practice, framed as mercantile tasks and approaches. The chapter discusses how Norwegian authorities govern by political rationales and programmes intended to reduce the use of costly services, through downscaling clinical practices and increasing both the efficiency of rehabilitation professionals and the activation and self-realization of individuals.

As a bridge between the country-level chapters and those investigating the TBI case, the contribution by Odgaard, Harsløf, and Stubbs in Chap. 7 considers studies on TBI patients' return-to-work rates in different countries. TBI patients' cognitive impairments may particularly hamper their chances of meeting the requirements of the post-industrial labour market. This fact, they argue, makes the TBI patient group an important case to study in countries spearheading the development towards the post-industrial society. They draw on data from Northern European countries representing social democratic (Denmark, Norway) and conservative–corporatist models (France, and the Netherlands), as well as available data from a liberal welfare state (USA). This comparison reveals that the Nordic countries (Denmark and Norway) exhibit relatively low success in returning people to work; the relatively good general employment situation in these countries, by the time the studies were conducted, makes the low return-to-work rate especially conspicuous. Potential explanations suggested by the authors include low legal obligations for previous employers to reemploy (a feature that is deeply rooted in the Nordic welfare state model, as it aims to secure employers high levels of flexibility), few part-time work opportunities, and the availability of generous disability benefits, which may disincentivize a return-to-work trajectory, because embarking on such a trajectory may undermine eligibility for benefits, should the return-to-work process not be successful.

Based on the concept of boundary work, Hindhede focuses in Chap. 8 on how survivors of severe TBIs construe themselves in relation to society, and how enacting boundaries is especially important for these individuals' constitution of self. The qualitative study features in-depth interviews with working-age people from across Denmark five years post injury. The data suggest two diverse age-related constructions of boundary work. The older respondents reinforced collective norms of the typical brain-injured individual, thus manifesting strong symbolic boundaries at the levels of individual and collective identity. However, the younger respondents, who had more at stake, sought to challenge the predominant stereotype of being unable to work and thus transform their collective identity. Hindhede concludes that boundary work for survivors of severe TBIs is a continuous process even many years after their accident; these individuals must negotiate the official categories into which they are placed, along with the types of discourse that sustain them, despite being relatively well rehabilitated.

In Chap. 9, Bystrup and Hindhede explore how different network resources (theorized as social capital) are invested and converted by the relatives of young people with severe TBI during the rehabilitation process. They base their study on direct observations of hospital discharge meetings, and in-depth interviews with and questionnaire surveys of families six months after discharge. They find that families with a 'strong closed family structure' are most successful in transforming their resources during the rehabilitation process, compared to a 'small and weak family structure'. Those with a 'split family structure' struggled the most in this regard. The benefits obtained by mobilising network resources include advantages such as preferential treatment, or additional services and a general 'smoothness' and 'continuity' in the rehabilitation process.

Andreassen presents in Chap. 10 an institutional and organizational analysis of complex and critical transitions, focusing on TBI patient trajectories and the organization of this field in Norway. She argues that the rehabilitation processes of working-age citizens involve several organizations and professions, requiring interorganizational and interprofessional coordination and collaboration across hospitals, community healthcare, and employment services. Because the services seemingly belong to a joint organizational field of rehabilitation, an expectation that involved agencies are collaborating with each other on the coordination of services is justified. However, infrastructure deficits, knowledge transfer from hospitals that does not meet the needs of frontline professionals, and 'pure' forms of professionalism all seem to hinder knowledge-sharing and joint action. Connective and collaborative forms of professionalism, including boundary-spanning tasks, seem necessary to ensure smooth transitions, undisrupted pathways, and coordinated services to injured citizens.

In Chap. 11, Højbjerg, Egerod, and Poulsen explore TBI patients' transitions between different health organizations involved in their rehabilitation. Their aim is to identify how healthcare organizations and their professionals contribute to producing and reproducing inequality in health. Their ethnographic fieldwork and interviews show declining specialization and financial resources in the course of patient trajectories, as well as changing patterns of decision-making practices affecting transfer. Many resources are available to save patients' lives during the acute stage, but resources dwindle as the patient approaches long-term rehabilitation. This form of prioritizing resources may perpetuate inequality in healthcare, as in particular, weaker groups of patients are in need of the general rehabilitation services.

The two final chapters explore the changing epistemology of the rehabilitation field. Both adopt an international perspective, either comparative or transnational.

In Chap. 12, Solvang and Feiring argue that rehabilitation is a contested interdisciplinary field, torn between medical dominance and psychosocial challenges. Higher education is an important arena for epistemological work. Solvang and Feiring's chapter elucidates the scholarly profile outlined in educational programmes where rehabilitation is a core component in Scandinavia, the UK, and Germany. In discussing the diversity of programmes, Solvang and Feiring refer to Bourdieusian perspectives on field struggles in academic settings, the Mode 2 type of knowledge production at the intersection between clinical practice and academia, and even the interest in animality and disability intersections in recent post-humanist writing.

Finally, in Chap. 13, Bickenbach and Danermark take point of departure in the growing interest in promoting interdisciplinary research across health and social sciences. Perhaps no other area of health research more obviously benefits from interdisciplinary research than rehabilitation. Besides biomedical and clinical practice-oriented research, interdisciplinary research is needed for rehabilitation management within health systems. After clarifying the notion of interdisciplinarity in general, the authors argue that rehabilitation—understood as a health strategy whose primary aim is to optimize human functioning across (simple to complex) domains of action—is ideally suited to the interdisciplinary research paradigm. This is partly because rehabilitation practice is fundamentally about 'functioning' (as understood in the ICF).

1.4   Conclusions

Taken together, the chapters in this volume point at new dynamics in disability and rehabilitation. On the positive side, an orientation towards the social aspects of rehabilitation has gained momentum in Northern European welfare states. One has come to realize how peoples' own mechanisms, severely debilitated by an accident or illness, may be allowed to function if accommodations are made in their social context—in the family, in the workplace, in the manner services are provided and coordinated and so on. Internationally, this orientation is reflected in and stimulated by the World Health Organization's interdisciplinary framework for approaching peoples' functioning, as discussed in Bichenbach and Danermark's chapter. In the Northern European countries, we see how the authorities, following this new orientation, aim to build bridges across sectors, and stimulate collaboration between service providers. In Germany, for example, as Bode discusses it, the authorities aim at bringing about a holistic approach. This approach entails that the different involved actors and institutions align in a network-based and 'all-inclusive' fashion to account for the patient's impairment, and the multiplicity of identified needs. Likewise, in Scandinavia, as Feiring and Bonfils demonstrate, authorities put great emphasis on making service providers and service professionals to take responsibility for the case in its entirety. In particular, one aims at attuning services to the specific user—the patient or client—aiming to give the individual a much stronger say in taking decisions about the case.

However, despite these clear intentions, and the organizational reforms that have aimed at realising them, as Alm Andreassen demonstrates in her chapter, patients are still striving to muddle their way through the field. The system still appears to be fragmented. One may also question if the value of the social aspects of rehabilitation, that is, the emphasis on social services vis-à-vis health services, have been fully acknowledged in the manner priorities are set and resources allocated. Højbjerg, Egerod, and Poulsen show that across institutions involved in the rehabilitation process, from the acute over the post-acute to the general rehabilitation, one can observe a clear hierarchy reflected in the resources invested to treat patients; whilst enormous resources are invested in medical equipment and staff in the acute stage, they find a relatively meagre spending on the general rehabilitation in the phase where people are in need of social services to get on their feet again and attain an independent living. Through the comparative approach adopted in this volume, we further note that the degree of acknowledging the social (or societal) aspect of rehabilitation differs between countries. Koren and Feiring's analysis of curricula, show that social science perspectives feature most strongly in educational programmes on rehabilitation in the Nordic countries.

The stronger responsibility placed on the user is a common trait across the countries considered in this volume, even if it is most conspicuous in the UK case, where, as Bambra accounts for, users are even considered responsible for the initial health condition triggering the need for rehabilitation. Indeed, as Røberg shows, articulating user responsibility is a clear tendency in recent policy documents introducing and motivating reforms in the field. As Bystrup and Hindhede show, considering the case of adolescents, users who are embedded in a strong family structure and can mobilize their social network, obtain better and smoother passages through the rehabilitation system. Hence, there is a clear risk that social inequalities in health are reinforced by these recent trends. The 'job' as patient, in the post-industrial society is, as Hindhede shows in her analysis of Danish TBI patients, not confined to the practical issues of accessing the necessary health and social services, and the general restoring of a disrupted biography; through 'boundary work' patients also find themselves in need of negotiating various systems of classification, in order to develop a sustainable social identity. In a context where good physical and mental health is increasingly considered a necessary competence across the spheres of work and leisure, it is important for rehabilitation patients to demonstrate that they are fit for taking upon themselves active roles in the labour market and civil society.

Does medical and vocational rehabilitation still feature as a strong 'universal' service in Northern European welfare states? In certain respects, one can argue that it has actually been strengthened. Advancements in rehabilitation medicine have significantly improved the healthcare services provided. Certainly, statutory rights of patients have been strengthened. To a certain extent, efforts by policymakers to enhance user involvement and coordinate across sectors and service providers reflect an interest in reinforcing this welfare state service. On the other hand, we also observe tendencies of polarization and fragmentation. Part of vocational rehabilitation's domain is now supplanted with more short-term and less generous workfare programmes. The active line is increasingly dominating rehabilitation medicine and return-to-work services entail the risk of marginalizing weaker group of patients. In this sense, rehabilitation, as a shared 'community', may be declining. Rehabilitation services have been decoupled from larger projects of nation building, and the state is increasingly reluctant to pick up the bill to cover the 'social costs' created by a rampant, transnational economy.

References

Album, D., Johannessen, L. E. F., & Rasmussen, E. B. (2017). Stability and change in disease prestige: A comparative analysis of three surveys spanning a quarter of a century. *Social Science & Medicine, 180*, 45–51.

Anttonen, A., Häikiö, L., & Stefánsson, K. (2012). *Welfare state, universalism and diversity.* Cheltenham: Edward Elgar.

Ashley, M. J. (2012). Repairing the injured brain: Why proper rehabilitation is essential to recovering function. *Cerebrum, 8.*

Bærøe, K., & Bringedal, B. (2014). Professionalism, discretion and juridification: Social inequality in health and social citizenship. In H. S. Aasen, S. Gloppen, A.-M. Magnussen, & E. Nilssen (Eds.), *Juridification and social citizenship* (pp. 146–161). Cheltenham: Edward Elgar Publishing.

Bauman, Z. (1998). *Work, consumerism and the new poor. Issues in society.* Buckingham: Open University Press.

Ben-Galim, D., & Sachradja, A. (2010). *Now it's personal: Learning from welfare-to-work approaches around the world.* London: Institute for public policy research.

Bollingmo, G. (1997). Survey of employment services and vocational outcomes for individuals with mental retardation in Norway. *Journal of Vocational Rehabilitation, 8,* 269–283.

Brante, T. (2011). Professions as science-based occupations. *Professions and Professionalism, 1*(1), 4–20.

Brazinova, A., Rehorcikova, V., Taylor, M. S., Buckova, V., Majdan, M., Psota, M., et al. (2016). Epidemiology of traumatic brain injury in Europe: A living systematic review. *Journal of Neurotrauma, 33,* 1–30.

Cnossen, M. C., Lingsma, H. F., Tenovuo, O., Maas, A. I. R., Menon, D., Steyerberg, E. W., et al. (2017). Rehabilitation after traumatic brain injury: A survey in 70 European neurotrauma centers participating in the CENTER-TBI study. *Journal of Rehabilitation Medicine, 49*(5), 395–401.

Cunningham, A., & Grell, O. P. (1997). *Health care and poor relief in Protestant Europe 1500–1700.* London: Routledge.

Danermark, B., Ekström, M., Jakobsen, L., & Karlsson, J. C. (2002). *Explaining society: Critical realism in the social sciences.* London/New York: Routledge.

Foster, M., & Tilse, C. (2003). Referral to rehabilitation following traumatic brain injury: a model for understanding inequities in access. *Social Science and Medicine, 56*(10), 2201–2210.

Foucault, M. (2003). *"Society must be defended": Lectures at the Collège de France.* New York: Picador.

Gele, A., & Harsløf, I. (2010). Types of social capital resources and self-rated health among the Norwegian adult population. *International Journal of Equity in Health, 9,* 8.

Geyer, S. (2016). Soziale Ungleichheiten beim Auftreten chronischer Krankheiten [Social inequalities in chronic diseases]. *Bundesgesundheitsblatt, Gesundheitsforschung, Gesundheitsschutz, 59*(2), 181–187.

Goffman, E. (1961). *Asylums: Essays on the social situation of mental patients and other inmates.* New York: Anchor Books.

Goffman, E. (1963). *Stigma: Notes on the management of spoiled identity.* Harmondsworth: Penguin Books.

Gómez-Barroso, J., Barillà, S., & Harsløf, I. (2017). The European Union policy framework for social services. Agendas, regulations and discourses. In F. Martinelli, A. Anttonen, & M. Mätzke (Eds.), *Social services disrupted. Implications and challenges for Europe in a time of austerity* (pp. 49–70). Cheltenham: Edward Elgar Publishing.

Harsløf, I. (2008). Conditionality in Norwegian welfare policies. In L. Kay & O. Hartwich (Eds.), *When hassle means help: The international lessons of conditional welfare* (pp. 47–58). London: Policy Exchange.

Harsløf, I., & Ulmestig, R. (2013). *Changing social risks and social policy responses in the Nordic welfare states.* Basingstoke: Palgrave Macmillan.

Hasenfeld, Y. (1972). People processing organizations: An exchange approach. *American Sociological Review, 37*(3), 256–263.

Hatland, A. (2011). Rettsliggjøringen av velferdspolitikken [The juridification of welfare policies]. In A. Hatland (Ed.), *Veivalg i velferdspolitikken* [Choosing which path to take in welfare policies] (pp. 153–172). Bergen: Fagbokforlaget.

Kaukonen, O., & Stenius, K. (2005). Universalism under re-construction: From administrative coercion to professional subordination of substance misusers. In N. Kildal & S. Kuhnle (Eds.), *Normative foundations of the welfare state: The Nordic experience* (pp. 130–148). London: Routledge.

Khan, F., Baguley, I., & Cameron, I. (2003). Rehabilitation after traumatic brain injury. *Medical Journal of Australia, 178*(6), 290–297.

Leplège, A., Barral, C., & McPherson, K. (2015). Conceptualizing disability to inform rehabilitation: Historical and epistemological perspectives. In K. McPherson, B. E. Gibson, & A. Leplège (Eds.), *Rethinking rehabilitation: Theory and practice.* Boca Raton: CRC Press.

McPherson, K., Gibson, B. E., & Leplège, A. (2015). *Rethinking rehabilitation: Theory and practice.* Boca Raton: CRC Press.

Menon, D. K., Schwab, K., Wright, D. W., & Maas, D. I. (2010). Position Statement: Definition of Traumatic Brain Injury. *Archives of Physical Medicine and Rehabilitation, 91*(11), 1637–1640.

Nguyen, R., Fiest, K. M., McChesney, J., Kwon, C. S., Jette, N., Frolkis, A. D., et al. (2016). The international incidence of traumatic brain injury: A systematic review and meta-analysis. *Canadian Journal of Neurological Sciences, 43*(6), 774–785.

Odgaard, L., Poulsen, I., Kammersgaard, L. P., Johnsen, S. P., Nielsen, A. R., & Feldbæk, J. (2015). Surviving severe traumatic brain injury in Denmark: incidence and predictors of highly specialized rehabilitation. *Clinical epidemiology, 7*, 225–34.

Olesen, J., Gustavsson, A., Svensson, M., Wittchen, H. U., & Jönsson, B. (2012). The economic cost of brain disorders in Europe. *European Journal of Neurology, 19*(1), 155–162.

Reisman, D. (2001 [1977]). *Richard Titmuss: Welfare and society*. Basingstoke: Palgrave Macmillan.

Rosqvist, H. B., Katsui, H., & McLaughlin, J. (2017). (Dis)abling practices and theories?: exploring chronic illness in disability studies. *Scandinavian Journal of Disability Research, 19*(1), 1–6.

Sjölund, B. H. (2013). Rehabilitation. In M. D. Gellman & J. R. Turner (Eds.), *Encyclopedia of behavioral medicine* (pp. 1634–1638). New York: Springer.

Stocchetti, N., & Zanier, E. R. (2016). Chronic impact of traumatic brain injury on outcome and quality of life: A narrative review. *Critical Care, 20*(1), 148.

Strand, B. H., & Madsen, C. (2016). *Social inequalities in health*. Oslo: Norwegian Institute of Public Health. https://www.fhi.no/en/op/hin/groups/social-inequalities/?term=chronic&h=1. Accessed 14 Dec 2018.

Titmuss, R. (1974). What is social policy? In B. Abel-Smith & K. Titmuss (Eds.), *Social policy: An introduction* (pp. 23–32). New York: Pantheon Books.

Vike, H. (2018). *Politics and bureaucracy in the Norwegian welfare state: An anthropological approach*. Basingstoke: Palgrave Macmillan.

2

Northern European Rehabilitation Services in the Context of Changing Healthcare, Welfare, and Labour Market Institutions: A Theoretical Framework

Ivan Harsløf, Ingrid Poulsen, and Kristian Larsen

2.1 Introduction

This chapter outlines an overall theoretical framework for the studies on medical and vocational rehabilitation services presented in this volume. The aim is to show connections between the levels of analysis of the various studies. The chapter first describes the critical role of rehabilitation services as a cornerstone of the welfare state, particularly in its heyday and

I. Harsløf (✉)
Department of Social Work, Child Welfare and Social Policy, Oslo Metropolitan University, Oslo, Norway
e-mail: ivan.harslof@oslomet.no

I. Poulsen
Department of Neurorehabilitation, Rigshospitalet, University of Copenhagen, Copenhagen, Denmark
e-mail: Ingrid.Poulsen@regionh.dk

K. Larsen
Department of Learning and Philosophy, Aalborg University Copenhagen, Copenhagen, Denmark
e-mail: kl@learning.aau.dk

© The Author(s) 2019
I. Harsløf et al. (eds.), *New Dynamics of Disability and Rehabilitation*,
https://doi.org/10.1007/978-981-13-7346-6_2

early period of maturation. It then addresses critical changes in medicine, state governance structures, and the labour market, as contexts for the production and consumption of medical and vocational rehabilitation services. Against this background, the chapter sets out to formulate an integrative theoretical framework for analysing the rehabilitation field.

2.2   Rehabilitation, Nation Building, and Mobilizing Labour Power

Access to rehabilitation services was a critical part of the social contract between citizens and the state as European welfare states developed in the twentieth century. As Dean (2018, p. 108) argues, this was a time 'in which the status and identity of the "worker" under industrial capitalism's wage labour system was forged in conjunction with the creation of the sovereign nation-state'. In particular, the two world wars invigorated the role of rehabilitation services in wider projects of nation building and mobilizing labour power (Hendriks 2005, p. 189). Hence, in response to the grave needs of survivors of the First World War battlefields, the 1920s saw several countries begin to implement extensive physical rehabilitation services (Bonfiglioli Stagni et al. 2015). An important component of these efforts was returning the disabled to work. In the aftermath of the Second World War, inventions in medicine, surgery, and prosthetics, as well as the need for labour to rebuild societal infrastructure, reinforced this work orientation (Leplège et al. 2015).

In the European countries with extensive direct involvement in the two world wars, the expansion of rehabilitation services aligned with Heraclitus' old contention that 'war is the father of all things'. In the Scandinavian countries, less affected by the wars, rehabilitation efforts focused particularly on survivors of infectious diseases (polio and tuberculosis). Whereas vocational rehabilitation was a state project from the outset in Continental Europe, the Scandinavian countries saw early initiatives grow from popular movements, particularly guild- or union-run sick-benefit associations (Lindqvist 1990; Schmid 1995). Nevertheless, also in Scandinavia, a strong focus on medical and vocational rehabilitation emerged to become a hallmark of early social welfare efforts (Bengtsson 2013, p. 52). Accordingly, rehabilitation featured prominently in the Active Labour Market Policy toolbox prescribed in the Swedish Rehn–Meidner model, developed in the 1950s to increase the value of labour (Andersson 2013). During the 1960s, Norway, Sweden, and Denmark instituted encompassing and long-term programmes combining elements of treatment, work capacity assessment, education, and job placement. The new rehabilitation programmes coincided with the introduction of more generous disability benefit programmes (Drøpping et al. 2000). Indeed, vocational rehabilitation programmes can be regarded as a 'gate keeping' intervention to counter the costly inflow into permanent disability benefit programmes (Lindqvist 2000).

This interconnection of generous benefits and active rehabilitation measures was emphasized in the 1942 Beveridge Report, which became an important guide to social reforms across Europe (Whiteside 2014):

> It is a logical corollary to the payment of high benefits in disability that determined efforts should be made by the State to reduce the number of cases for which benefit is needed. (Beveridge 1942, p. 426)

In many countries, medical and vocational rehabilitation has been emphasized as a central instrument for curbing sickness and disability pension rates and for mobilizing marginal labour power. For instance, when the Norwegian Government instituted its 'Work Approach' ethos in the early 1990s, declaring that all benefits and services should encourage participation in employment, it was launched with a white paper on vocational rehabilitation. The white paper stated that

> ... it is important to counter tendencies of social or, more generally, life-problems, being ... 'medicalized'. Social security provisions have to be designed so that the *Work Approach* becomes the first choice for all involved parties. (Ministry of Labour 1992, pp. 8–9; authors' translation; emphasis in original)

Although not pertaining to medical rehabilitation, initiatives from the 1951 European Coal and Steel Community, the EU's predecessor, merit attention. The community initiated and financed comprehensive redeployment programmes that were similar to vocational rehabilitation services, aiming to channel extensive numbers of superfluous coal and steel workers into other sectors (Hantrais 2000). Several European countries subsequently adopted this occupational retraining into their regular social and labour market policies (*Le Monde* 1970, May 9). We cite this historical example to illustrate the connection between micro-level efforts to amend and enhance the value of labour power through rehabilitation programmes, or other institutional equivalents, and wider, macro-level efforts towards nation and community building.

Today, the EU strongly encourages member states to develop strategies for enhancing disabled persons' labour market participation (Gobelet and Franchignoni 2006). However, translating this commitment into concrete and enforceable rights has proved difficult. Administrative definitions of disability—whose uses include allocating public funding for workplace adaptations—differ across member states (Mabbett 2005, p. 112). Indeed, such definitions are often anchored in local practices, and ultimately developed at the discretion of street-level bureaucrats, that is, the professionals (medical doctors, physiotherapists, social caseworkers, etc.), who work directly with patients. On the one hand are national- and international-level regulation, public management, and policy orientations and discourses; on the other are local practices, organization, and the experiences and outcomes of rehabilitation services. The multifarious interplay between them is a central theme of this volume.

2.3   Rehabilitation Services in Different Models of Welfare

In this section, we aim to situate the role of rehabilitation services in a theoretical framework of the wider welfare state. Comparative welfare research considers different models of welfare provision according to the extent and manner of the state's direct or indirect intervention in the labour market. Such interventions may come in the form of benefits and services that mediates the supply and demand mechanisms of the market, or through regulations. Esping-Andersen's (1990, 1999) influential typology labels welfare states according to dominant political ideologies, distinguishing between a liberal, a conservative–corporatist, and a social democratic model, each representing markedly different approaches to welfare provision. The liberal model, he contends, embraces private market solutions; the conservative–corporatist model prefers arrangements that preserve a patriarchal family status hierarchy, underpinned by performance- and occupation-related insurance programmes; and the social democratic model prioritizes universal, state-run welfare programmes allocated on the basis of citizenship.

National patterns in health services do not seem to parallel Esping-Andersen's welfare state typology (Jensen 2008). Hence, whilst the USA's health system does fit the typology, incarnating the ideal-type liberal health system with little public health services, the liberal and otherwise market-oriented UK has maintained the publicly financed and comprehensive National Health Service. Likewise, the healthcare systems of the Nordic countries do not, for the most part, differ significantly from other countries' systems. Although there are some special Nordic features, they are not typical of social democratic ideology (Haave 2006).

However, at the intersection between the health and the work-and-welfare sectors, rehabilitation services exhibit patterns that are somewhat congruent with Esping-Andersen's typology. Thus, the German vocational rehabilitation system has had strong corporatist features. Among other features, the German (and largely the Continental European) system is distinguished by operating a quota system, requiring employers to maintain a certain percentage of disabled people in their workforce or otherwise pay a fee (Waddington 1996). In this tradition of placing extensive social responsibilities on the employer, one finds examples, as in Italy, of strict regulation on recruitment and dismissals, based on such criteria as the person's obligations as family provider (Jensen 1999).

In contrast, Scandinavian countries have largely abstained from such overt regulations, preferring to use state-run and relatively generous supply-side measures (Waddington 2001, p. 148). These measures are regarded as 'social investments', aiming to stimulate the economy, and enhancing the tax-base by securing citizens' active participation in the labour market (Kvist 2015). Arguably, this approach is concomitant with a business structure, dominated by small and medium-sized enterprises, whose strong exposure to international competition necessitates lax regulation. Their relatively small size is considered to preclude bearing major social responsibility. However, the security element of this 'flexicurity' approach has been moderated since the 1990s: Following Organisation for Economic Co-operation and Development (OECD) recommendations, the Nordic countries have reduced benefit generosity and strengthened return-to-work services (Scharle and Váradi 2013).

In the UK, which represents the liberal model, compulsory employment regulation to promote the labour market inclusion of people with disabilities was introduced during the Second World War. However, according to observers, this regulation had limited practical significance prior to its abandonment in 1995 (Barnes 2000, p. 43; Waddington 2001, p. 151). The quota system was replaced by a reasonable adjustment law, instructing employers to remove barriers that employees with disabilities may face. Critical observers contend that this form of legislation essentially privatizes what should be a public responsibility (Lawson 2008, pp. 258–266). The ineffective implementation and ultimate repeal of the quota system, followed by the later 'privatization' of responsibility, is consistent with the UK's adherence to a liberal welfare model.

Welfare state typologies are intrinsically static. Indeed the 'three worlds of welfare capitalism' have moved on since their 1990 'discovery' by Esping-Andersen. The 1990s brought a strong wave of globalization, sparked by the end of the Cold War and the collapse of communism. With accelerating market integration, increasing cultural interconnectedness, and growing international migration, national welfare systems came under considerable pressures. Recent decades have also seen supranational regulation imposing critical frameworks that limit national governments' room for manoeuvre.

We next examine the derived changes, and the new context they constitute for rehabilitation services.

2.4   A New Context for Medical and Vocational Rehabilitation Services

Having been established as fully-fledged programmes in the golden age of the welfare state, rehabilitation services now operate in a rather different context, shaped by deep-seated societal developments. As suggested above, we may loosely associate these developments with transnational processes, that is, those external to the given society, but internal structural changes in the economy and society are also important. In particular, one should consider developments in the field of medicine, the state's governance structures, and the labour market.

Throughout its long history, the field of medicine has undergone a process of differentiation, manifesting in ever more specialized medical fields and ever more specific health professional groups (Højbjerg and Larsen 2018; Pinell 2011). These changes have not necessarily originated from developments in medicine itself, but from developments in other areas of society, expressed in needs and rationalities such as growth and planning, division of labour, productivity, and cost-containment (Vallgårda 1999).

National health policies can be analysed as part of a broader and transnational medical and healthcare field, where intergovernmental organizations (such as the UN and EU), multinational corporations, and transnational interest groups all have an impact (Collyer 2018). A key organization affecting national health policies is the OECD, which has been a strong agitator for work-oriented health policies, arguing that '[w]ork needs to be put at the heart of sickness and disability policies' (OECD 2008, p. 12). It has also called for more private players in the field of rehabilitation and a system of outcome-based funding to motivate these players to deliver (OECD 2008).

In general, a new active and 'asset-based' approach has gained a strong foothold in the field of medicine. The focus on activity is partly rooted in new medical discoveries. In the area of traumatic brain injuries, for example, it is now recognized as important for patients to engage in motion exercises in the first days following the injury, so as to strengthen their impaired limbs; even unconscious patients should be helped to move through therapist-assistance (Nudo 2013). We also note how the trend towards active approaches in medicine, is encapsulated in the now ubiquitous calls for 'early onset' of intensive treatments and interventions (e.g. Danish Directorate for Health 2011). Also, in the later stages of rehabilitation, modern medicine and nursing now prescribes high levels of activity for the patient to maintain and improve functioning (WHO 2011).

The strong impulse towards activity resonates with larger societal trends. A new social order is manifesting in notions such as 'active ageing', 'active citizenship', 'active learning', 'active civil society', and 'active welfare', implying the 'activation' of various groups of benefit recipients. In the field of medicine, these new dynamics entail an altered perspective on patient subjectivity. The new dynamic patient perspective, is for example reflected in viewpoints such the Chair of OECD's Health Committee, Olivia Wigzell's statement that 'patients should no longer just consume care but help to produce better health and wellness too' (Wigzell 2017, p. 23). One can observe a changing 'contract' between patient and health system. Patients are now considered active, knowledge-seeking individuals that not only possess rights, but also exercise and, if successful, actualize them. Thus, as have other patients, rehabilitation patients have, to some degree, changed from objects into subjects, requiring goals to be attuned through systematic involvement (on individual as well as overall levels, where users are represented through various associations), meetings, coordination devices (such as individual care plans), and so on. The level of activity expected on the part of the patient extends to the general population. As Rose (2006) argues, today people increasingly take on roles as 'pre-patients', acting proactively through training, diet, and the monitoring of their bodies to prevent illnesses from occurring.

Furthermore, new regimens of knowledge (imposing standardized and 'evidence-based' practice) and changing structures of healthcare organizations (with accelerated turnover in hospitalized patients and more specialized interventions) contribute to transforming rehabilitation processes. Such changes are also affecting the role of health professionals. Whereas authority and prestige were previously rooted in accumulated experience and classic professional hierarchies (Freidson 1988), established hierarchies are currently challenged by new types of institutional management, demands for evidence, standardization, and accelerated innovations in medical technology. Hierarchies in the overall medical field are well consolidated, as relations of dominance are built into hierarchies of diagnoses (Album et al. 2017; Hindhede and Larsen 2018).

Recent changes in the state and its institutions across the healthcare and work-and-welfare sectors imply a transition from *government* to *governance*. As part of this change, network forms of organization have partly supplanted traditional hierarchal government. Although power has not disappeared, as networks also contain stronger and weaker members, and a certain 'pecking order', arguably it has now become less visible (Pollitt and Bouckaert 2017, pp. 20–22). The transition from government to governance, and its network orientation, is also characterized by a change towards participatory and collaborative governance, the former advocating extensive user involvement (individually or through user associations), and the latter urging increased private-public and interagency collaboration. Finally, the change has entailed focusing on 'management by objectives' and related financial incentive structures from the New Public Management toolbox, rather than 'hard law' (Bellamy and Palumbo 2010). To illustrate, the change towards participatory governance can be observed in the 2001 German Social Security Code IX, representing a paradigmatic shift 'from the welfare and passive care given to the disabled … through to participation and active self-determination' (Schian 2006, p. 309). These changes in public management have been influenced by the situation of unremitting austerity prevailing in Northern Europe, which has called for measures to improve efficiency and curb inflows into welfare transfer programmes (Pollitt and Bouckaert 2017, pp. 23–25).

Indeed, the asset-based approach—that is, focus on possibilities rather than obstacles—has also been adopted in vocational rehabilitation services (Håvold et al. 2018). For example, in the UK, the government encourages GPs to issue 'fit notes' instead of 'sick notes' (Brijnath et al. 2013). Rather than seeing the glass as half empty, it seems the GPs are encouraged to see it as half full. Likewise, in Denmark, a 'resource profile' has been adopted to identify the capacities of people at the crossroads of rehabilitation or disability pension, abandoning the previous focus on incapacities (OECD 2008). The asset-based approach entails a radical reconceptualization of work and health. Previously regarded as exhausting and stressful—incompatible with recovery and restitution (and conceptualized as the 'deficit approach')—work activities are now increasingly conceived as health promoting. Consider, for example, the explanatory memorandum from the 2012 Danish law proposal L 53 that significantly restricted access to disability pension: 'For many people, working is a part of the way to recovery. This goes for both somatic and psychological illnesses' (Minister of Employment 2012, p. 25; authors' translation). Of course, such paradigmatic changes are strongly associated with actual changes in the world of work (to which we shall turn below), but it also seems that changes in the conceptions of work are being actively constructed by social agents. In this volume, Chaps. 6 and 7 especially interrogate such processes at the discursive level with reference to the rehabilitation policy field. To understand the subtle processes of manufacturing the 'asset-oriented' work conception, one should also look for what perspectives and actors are omitted. For example, the absence of the National Institute of Occupational Health (representing a type of expertise arguably related to the 'deficit approach') in the newly established Norwegian Council for Work and Health.

Finally, the labour market—the 'target' for vocational rehabilitation—is transforming at an increasing pace. Digitalization, robotic process automation, lean management strategies, specialization of production, and outsourcing to low-cost countries are changing the face of Northern European labour markets. These developments are reducing incidences of fatal injuries in Northern European workplaces, as most dangerous work has been made either safer or relocated to other nodes in global value chains (Loomis 2015). The work hazards related to the production of smartphones (the prime artefact of the postindustrial worker and citizen), for example, are faced by workers very far away from Northern European health and safety authorities. Few rehabilitation measures are put in place for the African mine workers involved in the dangerous extraction of chemicals for the phone battery, and there is little in terms of social safety net for the Chinese assembly workers putting the phones together, whereas in some factories, a physical net may be installed around the building to prevent workers from committing suicide by jumping out of the window (Ngai and Chan 2012).

Northern European labour markets are becoming heavily dynamic, requiring numeric and functional flexibility of workers and turning stable jobs into temporary roles or positions, such as contractor or freelancer. They are also becoming increasingly internationalized, with many jobs requiring physical mobility for shorter or longer-term job assignments, intercultural competencies, and adaption to changing international management cultures and strategies (Gustafson 2006; Hampson and Junor 2010). Finally, these labour markets are becoming increasingly knowledge intensive, requiring high levels of education and frequent renewal of skills (Harsløf et al. 2013). Research has demonstrated how de-industrialization is associated with a growing polarization of employment, with chronically ill and disabled people becoming increasingly marginalized. This development is most pronounced in the liberal UK, but also present in the social democratic Nordic countries (Holland et al. 2011). The strong requirements for up-to-date formal and informal skills prompt a reorientation of vocational rehabilitation services towards de-institutionalized, on-the-job retraining (the so-called 'place, then train' model) to replace previous, more segregated models ('train, then place') (Corrigan and McCracken 2005; Harsløf 2004). However, these dramatic changes in the world of work do not necessarily imply reduced employment chances for people in vocational rehabilitation. In fact, some argue that the new 'gig economy' opens up new opportunities, such as flexible work, working from home, and working reduced hours (Dobson 2017).

2.5   Integrating Theoretical Perspectives

This volume investigates rehabilitation services at different analytical levels, including the international (transnational), national, institutional, and individual agent level (the latter concerning patients, relatives, and professionals). This multi-level orientation requires an integration of theoretical perspectives.

To understand welfare state benefits and services, and how they impact disabled citizens' life chances, the theoretical concept of de-commodification is suitable (Esping-Andersen 1990). This concept maintains that generous and encompassing benefits and services, allocated on the basis of citizenship, relieve people of their structural status as 'commodities' in the market; they have autonomy to withdraw fully or partly from the labour market according to aspirations and capacities. However, there is some confusion regarding the concept. In a context where the importance of labour market participation for disabled people is increasingly acknowledged, it has been argued that this group should fight to become commodified, rather than de-commodified (Drøpping 1996; Barnes 2000, p. 34). This perspective, which has also been advanced for other groups with low attachment to the labour market, may rest on misconstruing the concept. In essence, being commodified entails becoming *dependent* on selling one's labour power; of course, it is perfectly possible to participate in the labour market without being dependent on doing so (cf. Jensen 1996, pp. 30–31). Empirically, the Nordic countries were the most de-commodifying in Esping-Andersen's analysis and also display the highest labour market participation rates (OECD 2017). Even after accounting for employment-to-population ratios and average annual working hours, the Nordic countries exhibit labour mobilization levels that outperform less de-commodifying Continental European countries (Ganssman 2003).

In research on the institutions and the interaction between their professions and patients, several studies of the mesolevel mobilize literature from the tradition of new institutionalism. They particularly focus on work concerning 'institutional logics', namely the overarching symbolic systems and material practices that institutional actors are subjected to and draw upon (Thornton and Ocasio 2008). Different groups of professionals operate according to different institutional logics, depending on their anchoring in larger organizational systems. These differences in prevailing institutional logics can be related to different perspectives on ailments, captured in the terms disease, sickness, and illness (Twaddle 1979). The *disease perspective*, with a medically grounded focus on physical malfunctioning, is predominant in healthcare services, with health service professionals guided by this logic. The *sickness perspective*, with its socio-legal focus on social role capacity, dominates the work-and-welfare services and professionals working in this sector. As individual rehabilitation trajectories cut across these sectors, requiring collaboration, coordination, and transfers of knowledge, resources and so on, these two logics sometimes collide (Håvold et al. 2018; Harsløf et al. 2017). Patients and their relatives bring to bear the institutional logic of the family and community, which involves affections and subjectivity, that is, 'loyalty to its members and their reproductive needs' (Friedland and Alford 1991, p. 248). The *illness perspective* accommodates patients' subjective interpretations of their own state of health.

Inspired by the sociology of Bourdieu's (1977, 1984) concepts of social space, field, capital and position, disposition (habitus), and positioning, our ambition is to integrate macro-, meso-, and micro-levels. These concepts help us to understand the genesis (development) and structure of the field of rehabilitation as part of a broader medical field, which is itself part of a national and a transnational field. Nested within one another like Russian dolls, they have relative autonomy. For example, a field may 'protect' its borders by reference to professional autonomy and certain forms of field-specific and credited/authorized knowledge and technologies. Fields are contexts of on-going struggle to define the 'rules of the game', whether explicit guidelines or informal, taken-for-granted principles (what Bourdieu calls 'doxa'). Some agents in the field occupy dominant positions, giving them great influence in defining and interpreting the rules.

Bourdieusian concepts are also helpful to understand inequalities related to different classes of patients and relatives, and how their dispositions match the implicit rules of the field, and how they go along with the incentives build into institutions. Specifically, the notion of capital, designating various assets that individuals possess, is important for understanding inequalities in rehabilitation outcomes. As a means to integrate different analytical perspectives, we shall consider rehabilitation services as a process through which the patient's 'health capital' is reconstructed. This concept regards the physical, surgical, nutritional, chemical, and mental work with, on, and in the body as forms of investments by agents to reestablish, maintain, or optimize their social position—activities that rehabilitation patients, through the assistance of health and social professionals, engage in in order to reacquire their previous position. The term 'health capital' is not new. Grossman (1972) used it in proposing that an individual's 'stock of health' should be considered a resource that can be exhausted but also renewed through medical care, diet, and other reproductive activities. However, in contrast to this substantialist perspective, which reduces health capital to the individual's biological processes, we draw on Bourdieu's (1977, 1984, 1986) relational perspective on the forms of capital. In this perspective, the effect of capital endowments 'cannot be reduced to the set of properties individually possessed by a given agent' (Bourdieu 1986, p. 109n). Rather, there is a dialectic between agents of different class background, where those with low health assets make those with high endowments 'look good', emphasizing their good qualities (Bourdieu 1984, p. 179).

Hence, expanded from Bourdieu's theoretical apparatus, the concept of health capital is meant to capture how certain health assets are not only embodied (as biological processes and physical/mental constitution) or present as objects (possessions that signify one's state of health) but ultimately validated (or disproved and repressed) through their relations with wider societal institutions (cf. Larsen et al. 2013). Explained thus, the concept aligns well with the bio-psychosocial model of rehabilitation described above. Interrogating the importance of different patient groups' dispositions and assets in their rehabilitation process, Guldager et al. (2018) identifies a form of capital specific to the field of medical rehabilitation, including the persons' abilities to meet recognized standards of behaviour (be 'a good patient'), display proactivity, be 'self-initiating', and adhere to prescribed training programmes and so on. This capital, she finds, gives its possessor advantages in the form of more or better services, such as extra CAT-scans (a special X-ray test), specialist referrals, exercises, and extended hospital stays.

We regard health capital as an 'integrative concept' to stimulate effective interdisciplinary research (Kessel et al. 2008, p. 6). It relates simultaneously to the fields of health sciences—the physical and mental body—and social sciences, in terms of the institutional setting comprising various 'fields' to be negotiated by rehabilitation patients, as well as the larger commodifying and de-commodifying structures provided by the welfare state. Accordingly, the concept is well suited for interdisciplinary collaboration.

2.6 Conclusion

This chapter has presented a rough outline of the background to interdisciplinary studies of medical and vocational rehabilitation services in Northern European welfare states. We emphasized the critical role of such services in the early development of welfare state arrangements, closely tied to efforts to build cohesive nation states and cater for industrial labour markets. Understanding this historical background is important for recognizing how these services are functioning under the current postnational and postindustrial conditions. In establishing a compromise between capital and labour, such services played an instrumental role in mitigating social conflicts. Workers knew they had access to wide-ranging health and vocational services, including assistance for longer-term retraining—provided as statutory citizenship rights—should they ever need it. Comprehensive rehabilitation services, along with general encompassing national healthcare services, instituted health and return-to-work processes as a state responsibility.

In the current postnational and post-industrial context, where rehabilitation services no longer constitute the proud flagship of the welfare state, it seems that the state is in a sense abdicating responsibilities. Increasing emphasis on governance networks involving non-state actors, public-private partnerships, hyper-efficient hospital services, and place-then-train reemployment models seems to be leading to the individualization of responsibility for health and employability. Are we witnessing a recommodification of the physical and mental body, where the individual surviving an injury or struggling with a severe health condition must nurture health as a personal capital to regain employability in the post-industrial labour market? These are the overall themes that this book sets out to explore.

References

Album, D., Johannessen, L. E. F., & Rasmussen, E. B. (2017). Stability and change in disease prestige: A comparative analysis of three surveys spanning a quarter of a century. *Social Science & Medicine, 180,* 45–51.

Andersson, J. (2013). *Between growth and security: Swedish social democracy from a strong society to a third way* (Critical labour movement studies). Manchester: Manchester University Press.

Barnes, H. (2000). *Working for a living: Employment, benefits and the living standards of disabled people.* Bristol: Policy Press.

Bellamy, R., & Palumbo, A. (2010). *From government to governance.* Farnham: Ashgate.

Bengtsson, S. (2013). Sådan produceres ligebehandling [This is how equal treatment is produced]. In S. Bengtsson, I. S. Bonfils, & L. Olsen (Eds.), *Handicap og ligebehandling i praksis* [Disability and equal treatment] (pp. 41–60). Copenhagen: SFI.

Beveridge, W. (1942). *Social insurance and allied services.* New York: Macmillan.

Bonfiglioli Stagni, S., Tomba, P., Viganò, A., Zati, A., & Benedetti, M. G. (2015). The first world war drives rehabilitation toward the modern concepts of disability and participation. *European Journal of Physical Rehabilitation Medicine, 51*(3), 331–336.

Bourdieu, P. (1977). *Outline of a theory of practice.* Cambridge: Cambridge University Press.

Bourdieu, P. (1984). *Distinction: A social critique of the Judgement of taste.* London: Routledge & Kegan Paul.

Bourdieu, P. (1986). The forms of capital. In J. G. Richardson (Ed.), *Handbook of theory and research for the sociology of education* (pp. 241–258). New York: Greenwood Press.

Brijnath, B., Mazza, D., & Singh, N. (2013). *A process evaluation of the new certificate of capacity for compensation claims.* Report number 1213-082-R2A, Institute for Safety Compensation and Recovery Research.

Collyer, F. (2018). Envisaging the healthcare sector as a field: Moving from Talcott Parsons to Pierre Bourdieu. *Social Theory & Health, 16*(2), 111–126.

Corrigan, P. W., & McCracken, S. G. (2005). Place first, then train: An alternative to the medical model of psychiatric rehabilitation. *Social Work, 50*(1), 31–39.

Danish Directorate for Health. (2011). *Hjerneskaderehabilitering—en medicinsk teknologivurdering* [Brain injury—A medical technology assessment]. Copenhagen.

Dean, H. (2018). EU citizenship and 'work': Tensions between formal and substantive equality. In S. Seubert, O. Eberl, & F. van Waarden (Eds.), *Reconsidering EU citizenship: Contradictions and constrains* (pp. 108–132). Cheltenham: Edward Elgar Publishing.

Dobson, B. (2017). *Gainful gigging: Employment services for the platform economy*. London: Reform.

Drøpping, J. A. (1996). *The other side of de-commodification: Postwar Norwegian and British disability policies*. Trondheim: NTNU.

Drøpping, J. A., Hvinden, B., & Van Oorschot, W. (2000). Reconstruction and reorientation: Changing disability policies in the Netherlands and Norway. *European Journal of Social Security, 2*(1), 35–68.

Esping-Andersen, G. (1990). *The three worlds of welfare capitalism*. Cambridge: Polity Press.

Esping-Andersen, G. (1999). *Social foundations of postindustrial economies*. Oxford/New York: Oxford University Press.

Freidson, E. (1988). *Profession of medicine: A study of the sociology of applied knowledge*. Chicago: University of Chicago Press.

Friedland, R., & Alford, R. R. (1991). Bringing society back in: Symbols, practices, and institutional contradictions. In W. W. Powell & P. J. DiMaggio (Eds.), *The new institutionalism in organizational analysis* (pp. 232–266). Chicago: University of Chicago Press.

Ganssman, H. (2003). *Labor force mobilization and the feasibility of comprehensive welfare states*. Paper presented at ESPAnet Conference, Copenhagen, 2003.

Gobelet, C., & Franchignoni, F. (2006). *Vocational Rehabilitation*. Paris: Springer.

Grossman, M. (1972). On the concept of health capital and the demand for health. *Journal of Political Economy, 80*(2), 223–255.

Guldager, R., Poulsen, I., Egerod, I., Mathiesen, L. L., & Larsen, K. (2018). Rehabilitation capital: A new form of capital to understand rehabilitation in a Nordic welfare state. *Health Sociology Review, 27*(2), 199–213.

Gustafson, P. (2006). Work-related travel and family obligations. *Work, Employment and Society, 20*(3), 513–530.

Haave, P. (2006). The hospital sector: A four-country comparison of organisational and political development. In N. F. Christiansen, K. Petersen, N. Edling, & P. Haave (Eds.), *The Nordic model of welfare: A historical reappraisal* (pp. 215–242). Copenhagen: Museum Tusculanum Press.

Hampson, I., & Junor, A. (2010). Putting the process back in: Rethinking service sector skill. *Work, Employment and Society, 24*(3), 526–545.

Hantrais, L. (2000). *Social policy in the European Union* (2nd ed.). London: Macmillan Press.

Harsløf, I. (2004, June). *Enterprise rehabilitation: Involving enterprises in the vocational rehabilitation efforts in Denmark*. Paper presented at the 20th World Congress of Rehabilitation International, Lillestrøm.

Harsløf, I., Scarpa, S., & Andersen, S. N. (2013). Changing population profiles and social risk structures in the Nordic countries. In I. Harsløf & R. Ulmestig (Eds.), *Changing social risks and social policy responses in the Nordic welfare states* (pp. 25–49). Basingstoke: Palgrave Macmillan.

Harsløf, I., Søbjerg Nielsen, U., & Feiring, M. (2017). Danish and Norwegian hospital social workers' cross-institutional work amidst inter-sectoral restructuring of health and social welfare. *European Journal of Social Work, 20*(4), 584–595.

Hendriks, A. (2005). Promoting disability equality after the treaty of Amsterdam: New legal directions and practical expansion strategies. In A. Lawson & C. Gooding (Eds.), *Disability rights in Europe from theory to practice: Essays in European law* (pp. 187–198). Oxford: Hart Publishing.

Hindhede, A. L., & Larsen, K. (2018). Prestige hierarchies of diseases and specialities in a field perspective. *Social Theory & Health*, 1–18. https://doi.org/10.1057/s41285-018-0074-5.

Holland, P., Burström, B., Whitehead, M., Diderichsen, F., Dahl, E., Barr, B., et al. (2011). How do macro-level contexts and policies affect the employment chances of chronically ill and disabled people? Part I: The impact of recession and deindustrialization. *International Journal of Health Services, 41*(3), 395–413.

Højbjerg, K., & Larsen, K. (2018). At lære at agere i et sundhedsvæsen under forandring [Learning to act in a changing healthcare system]. In S. Hundborg (Ed.), *Sundhedsvæsenet under forandring* [The changes of the healthcare system] (pp. 9–33). Copenhagen: Munksgaards Forlag.

Håvold, O. K., Harsløf, I., & Andreassen, T. A. (2018). Externalizing an 'asset model' of activation: Creative institutional work by frontline workers in the Norwegian labour and welfare service. *Social Policy and Administration, 52*(1), 178–196.

Jensen, P. H. (1996). *Komparative velfærdssystemer: Kvinders reproduktionsstrategier mellem familien, velfærdsstaten og arbejdsmarkedet* [Comparative welfare systems]. København: Nyt fra Samfundsvidenskaberne.

Jensen, P. H. (1999). Velfærdsstatens politiske ideologi: En kritik af Esping-Andersen [The political ideology of the welfare state: A critique of Esping-Andersen]. *Grus, 20*, 84–100.

Jensen, C. (2008). Worlds of welfare services and transfers. *Journal of European Social Policy, 18*(2), 151–162.

Kessel, P., Rosenfield, L., & Anderson, N. B. (2008). *Expanding the boundaries of health and social science: Case studies in interdisciplinary innovation.* Oxford: Oxford University Press.

Kvist, J. (2015). *ESPN thematic report on social investment–Denmark*. Brussels: European Commission, Directorate-General for Employment, Social Affairs and Inclusion.

Larsen, K., Cutchin, M., & Harsløf, I. (2013). Health capital: New health risks and personal investments in the body in the context of changing Nordic welfare states. In I. Harsløf & R. Ulmestig (Eds.), *Changing social risks and social policy responses in the Nordic welfare states* (pp. 165–188). Basingstoke: Palgrave Macmillan.

Lawson, A. (2008). *Disability and equality law in Britain: The role of reasonable adjustment*. Oxford: Hart Publishing.

Le Monde. (1970, May 9). Dans l'histoire de la CECA, du rose et du gris [The history of the ECSC: Good times and bad], p. 6.

Leplège, A., Barral, C., & McPherson, K. (2015). Conceptualizing disability to inform rehabilitation: Historical and epistemological perspectives. In K. McPherson, B. E. Gibson, & A. Leplège (Eds.), *Rethinking rehabilitation: Theory and practice*. Boca Raton: CRC Press.

Lindqvist, R. (1990). *Från folkrörelse till välfärdsbyråkrati: Det svenska sjukförsäkringssystemets utveckling 1900–1990* [The popular movement to welfare bureaucracy]. Lund: Arkiv.

Lindqvist, R. (2000). *Att sätta gränser: Organisationer och reformer i arbetsrehabilitering* [Organizations and reforms in vocational rehabilitation]. Umeå: Boréa.

Loomis, E. (2015). *Out of sight: The long and disturbing story of corporations outsourcing catastrophe*. New York: The New Press.

Mabbett, D. (2005). The development of rights-based social policy in the European Union: The example of disability rights. *Journal of Common Market Studies, 43*(1), 97–120.

Ministry of Employment. (2012). *Lov om ændring af lov om en aktiv beskæftigelsesindsats, lov om aktiv socialpolitik, lov om social pension og forskellige andre love* (L 53) [Amendments to the Law on active employment].

Ministry of Labour. (1992). *Attføring og arbeid for yrkeshemmede. Sykepenger og uførepensjon, St.meld. nr. 39 1991–1992* [Vocational rehabilitation and work for people with disabilities]. Oslo.

Ngai, P., & Chan, J. (2012). Global Capital, the State, and Chinese Workers: The Foxconn Experience. *Modern China, 38*(4), 383–410.

Nudo, R. J. (2013). Recovery after brain injury: Mechanisms and principles. *Frontiers in Human Neuroscience, 7*, 887.

OECD. (2008). *Sickness, disability and work: Breaking the barriers*. Paris: OECD.

OECD. (2017). *Employment outlook.* Paris: OECD.

Pinell, P. (2011). The genesis of the medical field: France, 1795–1870. *Revue Française de Sociologie, 52*(5), 117–151.

Pollitt, C., & Bouckaert, G. (2017). *Public management reform: A comparative analysis into the age of austerity* (4th ed.). Oxford: Oxford University Press.

Rose, N. (2006). *The politics of life itself: Biomedicine, power, and subjectivity in the twenty-first century.* Princeton: Princeton University Press.

Scharle, Á., & Váradi, B. (2013). *Identifying barriers to institutional change in disability services.* WWW for Europe Working Paper 41.

Schian, H. M. (2006). Vocational rehabilitation and participation in working life: The German model. In C. Gobelet & F. Franchignoni (Eds.), *Vocational rehabilitation* (pp. 309–328). Paris: Springer.

Schmid, H. (1995). Velfærdsstatens solidaritetsformer [Forms of solidarity of the welfare state]. *Dansk Sociologi, 6*(3), 38.

Thornton, P. H., & Ocasio, W. (2008). *Institutional logics. The SAGE handbook of organizational institutionalism.* London: SAGE.

Twaddle, A. C. (1979). *Sickness behavior and the sick role.* Boston: Hall.

Vallgårda, S. (1999). The rise, heyday, and incipient decline of specialization: Hospitals in Denmark, 1930–1990. *International Journal of Health Services, 29*(2), 431–457.

Waddington, L. (1996). Reassessing the employment of people with disabilities in Europe: From quotas to anti-discrimination laws. *Comparative Labor Law Journal, 18*(1), 62–101.

Waddington, L. (2001). Evolving disability policies: From social-welfare to human rights: An international trend from a European perspective. *Netherlands Quarterly of Human Rights, 19*(2), 141–165.

Whiteside, N. (2014). The Beveridge report and its implementation: A revolutionary project? *Histoire@Politique, 24*(3), 24–37.

WHO. (2011). *World report on disability.* Geneva: WHO.

Wigzell, O. (2017). People-centred healthcare: What empowering policies are needed. *OECD Observer, 309*(Q1), 23.

3

The Post-corporatist Rehabilitation System in Germany: High Potential, Critical Moments

Ingo Bode

3.1 Introduction

Contemporary Western welfare states have created institutions and organizations with a remit to improve, or re-establish, human capacities to cope with health problems and various sorts of impairments, beyond mere medical care. At a global scale, a generic term to label these institutions and organizations is 'rehabilitation', referring to a wide 'infrastructure of legal, medical, and social service resources' (Meinert and Yuen 2014, p. 1) orchestrated by the welfare state and run by various agencies. From a socio-scientific perspective, it is crucial to understand the regulatory mechanisms underpinning this infrastructure. These mechanisms are multi-faceted and include, for instance, the behaviour of relevant actors (professions, users) at street-level and the meaning systems underlying social life in general (see Safilios-Rothschild 1970). Importantly, however, these driving forces mostly become effective through public regulation, which institutionalizes such behaviour and meaning systems.

I. Bode (✉)
Institute of Social Work and Social Welfare, Kassel, Germany
e-mail: ibode@uni-kassel.de

© The Author(s) 2019
I. Harsløf et al. (eds.), *New Dynamics of Disability and Rehabilitation*,
https://doi.org/10.1007/978-981-13-7346-6_3

More generally, regulatory mechanisms *reflect* how a given society confronts problems related to chronic disease, impairment, and disabilities. They embody the 'societal steering' or, in more popular terms, the 'governance' of rehabilitative endeavour. Therefore they deserve particular attention in seeking to elucidate the dynamics of rehabilitation systems as a whole.

It is through this 'governance' lens that this chapter portrays the recent developments in contemporary Germany's rehabilitation system. By examining a distinctive institutional approach to 'handling' the (global) challenge of meeting increasing rehabilitative needs, it illustrates how the stunning paradox inherent in rehabilitative endeavour—the coexistence of *holistic* concepts and a *fragmented* organization of relevant interventions—plays out in the special context of a (post-)corporatist governance model. Holism denotes an approach to rehabilitation in which relevant actors and institutions account for all personal circumstances of a given impairment, the multiplicity of identified needs, and the complex dynamics inherent in a reintegration trajectory, with major interventions being processed in *specialized* clinical settings. Fragmentation is the 'contraindication', namely, a state in which such actors and institutions become engaged only with isolated elements of given circumstances, needs, and trajectories, which often implies dispersed interventions.

This chapter's analysis differs slightly from the perspective adopted by much of the scholarship on rehabilitation (see, e.g. Meinert and Yuen 2014) as it emphasizes *socio-medical intervention*, including for citizens with no 'disability status' or long-lasting impairment. It, therefore, glosses over some important issues concerning institutional support to disabled people, for example, assisted living, specialized education, or sheltered employment. Given its focus on the *governance* of rehabilitative endeavour, this chapter pays particular attention to evolving patterns of coordination and administration, including managerial control and market influences, both of which have become highly relevant to human service provision internationally (see Klenk and Pavolini 2015).

The chapter's key message is twofold. On the one hand, it shows that a holistic orientation and network-based governance are entrenched features of Germany's contemporary rehabilitation system, with some of these features having even been strengthened in recent times; this is why this system exhibits high potential. On the other hand, it argues that changes in the system's governance—including enhanced space for market-like coordination and formalized performance control—have introduced new challenges and tend to bolster fragmentation. As these movements deepen the paradox of holism and disintegration, the German rehabilitation system confronts critical moments concerning its wider future.

This chapter's argument is based on a literature review and on analysis of the wider debate among experts regarding rehabilitation in Germany, as detailed in reports, media communication, and practice papers. It also draws on several interviews conducted with industry specialists during 2016 and 2017. The next section overviews the German approach to rehabilitation, elucidating its holistic orientation, complex infrastructure, and historical fragmentation. The third section portrays the evolving orchestration of the German rehabilitation system, illuminating recent tendencies towards 'post-corporatist governance' throughout. Finally, the chapter's conclusion elaborates on the wider prospects of that system, outlining lessons for other Western welfare states from experiences in Germany.

3.2   The 'German Way' of Rehabilitation: A Holistic Approach Within a Jungle of Institutions

3.2.1   A Holistic Orientation Overall

Germany is often deemed a pioneer in orchestrating rehabilitation as a multi-professional intervention in clinical settings. In general terms, the German welfare state provides various benefits to users in need and exhibits strong commitment to specialized service provision, combining social, medical, and work-related interventions. This also applies to activities concerning brain-injured patients, which other chapters of this book consider more extensively. For example, concepts developed in Germany have been cited as good practice by the Danish National Board of Health, drawing on German experience when discussing reform options in the late 1990s.

Such *holistic orientation* is manifested in different dimensions. First, various welfare schemes grant financial benefits meant to compensate for health-related impediments (in a large sense); allowances depend on the nature of the impairment and how far a given impediment is acknowledged by one of many concurrent welfare schemes (see Box 3.1). Many of these benefits follow a social insurance rationale, as allowances are based on previous earnings. A wide range of risks is covered, although workers considered as employable, as well as pensioners affected by work incapacity, have been affected by reforms reducing the generosity of extant programmes (Welti 2019, pp. 174–175).

Second, relevant professional and legal norms refer to the WHO/ICF-based 'bio-psycho-social logic' of tackling a given functional incapacity in its relation to physical and mental health, as well as the (social and

Box 3.1 Monetary Benefits for Citizens Covered by the German Rehabilitation System

Sickness allowance	For workers (up to 90% of net salary, up to 78 weeks within three years, renewable)
Transition allowance	For workers in medical rehabilitation (75% of net salary, paid during a measure, i.e. a treatment, a counselling, a job preparation, etc.)
Incapacity pension	For workers (depending on contribution records and degree of incapacity)
State benefits	For civil servants or victims of war (several varieties, generally quite generous)
Social assistance	* Basic rate of €424/month *plus* housing *plus* support in case of special needs; * Payment only if no further income and no further entitlements; * In case of *partial* employability, beneficiaries must show efforts to find a job or improve their employability; * Members of sheltered workshops receive a salary related to their relative productivity *plus* a minimum benefit

technical) environments of affected citizens (see Chaps. 1 and 13). Under the current legal framework, the overarching rationale must be participation in ordinary life (see, e.g. Xyländer and Meyer 2018, pp. 120–121), with all involved agencies expected to contribute to this purpose (§ 4 'Social Code' part IX). Citizens with impairments are entitled to support combining medical intervention and measures impacting on their professional and personal projects, enabling them to live in a self-determined way. Consequently, users are the fulcrum of the entire system and can always initiate a rehabilitation plan through a doctor's referral. Funding agencies only occasionally solicit potential users to file an application. However, it is these agencies that examine the aforementioned referrals (without conducting assessments themselves) and eventually decide on applications. As users enjoy a free choice of provider (*Wunsch- und Wahlrecht*, i.e. 'the right to wish and choose'), the result is often a multi-party dialogue involving the funding agency, a provider, and the user (see Sachverständigenrat zur Begutachtung der Entwicklung im Gesundheitswesen (SVR) 2014, pp. 294–295).

Third, support to those in need often takes place in specialized settings under a distinctive regulation. In these settings, available service packages are comprehensive if compared to acute healthcare or classical social work. Within the German welfare state, those settings are among the few institutions that explicitly follow a *socio-medical* orientation. The pivotal place for this is 'rehabilitation centres' (*Reha-Kliniken*), including clinics providing treatment to individuals with psychosomatic disorder. Although these centres only host users for a limited period (25 days on average), they offer a bundle of measures including medical care, social or psychological counselling, and employment-related actions (workplace adjustments, etc.). Multi-disciplinary and multi-modal intervention is a matter of fact here; team-based activities are the rule rather than an exception, even though their actual scope may vary in breadth (Xyländer and Meyer 2018, pp. 131–136).

This is particularly obvious in the field of medical rehabilitation, which co-exists with other subsectors (as detailed below). Here, the institutionalization of 'bio-psycho-social logic' is particularly pronounced, differing markedly from countries such as France—where much is left to the rehabilitation departments of ordinary hospitals—and from systems where nursing-based support predominates, as in the UK. The German welfare state has created a clear institutional separation between inpatient care in hospitals and rehabilitative endeavour, which is distinct from prominent arrangements in Nordic countries (e.g. Norway). Also, rehabilitation in Germany is relatively insulated from employers' interference, again contrasting with other European welfare states (e.g. in the Netherlands and Finland: see Mittag et al. 2018).

Interventions controlled by the pension fund (*Soziale Rentenversicherung*) are emblematic of the German rehabilitation system and its holistic orientation. Though there is evidently focus on employability, as only 15% of users do not return to gainful employment after a measure in this (sub) sector, service packages are particularly comprehensive. They can embrace treatment by medical doctors, psychological or social therapy, stress tests, and occupation-focused interventions. The latter, including expert advice and contact with employers, have recently been strengthened (Buschmann-Steinhage 2017, pp. 372–373). A further current focus is on the concept of 'medical-vocational orientation' (Bethge 2017); target groups are the long-term jobless and citizens with reduced employability, including users with little faith in their own (future) work capacity. Typical tools include diagnostic assessments addressing workplace challenges and psycho-social focus groups. Moreover, the pension fund supports preventive activities, paediatric rehabilitation, and post-hospital care. Current policies seem to be geared towards further enhancing the range of offered activities.

In all parts of the rehabilitation system, funding agencies endorse this holistic orientation by paying lump-sum day rates to the aforementioned centres. This differs markedly from acute hospital care which is funded by *activity*-based subsidies related to the so-called diagnosis-related groups (see below). In contrast to Nordic welfare states, most providers are outside the public sector and operate as private (for- or non-profit) organizations. Major purchasing agencies (i.e. Social Security units) are equally independent from state bureaucracy. From a Nordic perspective, this may be viewed as prone to disruptions. Yet the German purchaser-provider split is based on stable contractual relationships and commitments to find inter-party compromises (see below), and funding agencies can be owners of affiliated service centres, which is quite rare in Europe. Thus, one in four beds available for (residential) medical rehabilitation is run by the German pension fund, as the biggest funding agency in this (sub) sector. In this configuration, economic and operational issues can be 'reconciled' within one and the same institutional universe. Such reconciliation is equally possible in other sections of the rehabilitation system where special instances have a remit to coordinate funding and service delivery, which includes running 'unified service centres' (see below). All administrative agencies are mandatory members of a collaborative working party named B.A.R. (*Bundesarbeitsgemeinschaft Rehabilitation*), which also involves the Trade Union Federation and National Employer Federation, as well as the Association of Outpatient Doctors (Seel 2015, pp. 869–871). This is another dimension in which the German rehabilitation system appears rather fine-tuned.

3.2.2   Complex Infrastructure

Notwithstanding the holistic orientation detailed above, the technical infrastructure for rehabilitation in Germany appears rather complex (see overviews provided by SVR 2014, pp. 255–279; Buschmann-Steinhage 2017; Welti 2019). This is why developments concerning its *governance* are of crucial importance. The system comprises three pillars, with nine different funding agencies running the sector's administration and also, in some cases, its practical dimensions (see Box 3.2). Four agencies are related to the social insurance pillar, with two—the pension insurance and sickness funds—contributing two-thirds of total outlays. In addition, there is a social assistance pillar containing three schemes (one for children, one for working-age disabled people, and one for citizens without social insurance coverage). The two remaining pillars cover civil servants and victims of war.

Each of these pillars exhibits a distinctive regulatory framework and specific operational conditions. This, first of all, holds for long-term assistance to disabled people, referred to as *social rehabilitation* in Germany. As a major subsector of the country's rehabilitation system, it ensures practical support to citizens with permanent impairments, such as assisted living, residential care, housing, and places in sheltered workshops

Box 3.2 The 'Service Pillars' of the German Rehabilitation System

Pillar	Responsible agency	Budget 2016
Social insurance	**Pension fund** Medical rehabilitation (workers with assumed employability)	20%
	Sickness funds Medical rehabilitation (all categories)	9%
	Unemployment insurance Vocational rehabilitation (workers)	7%
	Social insurance for workers' compensation All kinds of rehabilitation (occupational accidents)	13%

Social assistance	**Support for disabled citizens (*Eingliederungshilfe*)**
	Social rehabilitation
	  Individual support for adults (daily living / institutions)
	  Support for children (daily living / institutions)
		46%

	Support for citizens lacking social insurance coverage Funding for all sorts of rehabilitation	4%
Provisions for civil servants and victims of war	Funding for all sorts of rehabilitation	1%

Source: B.A.R. (2018); author's calculations

(300,000 in 2015). If included in the calculation of total expenditure on rehabilitation, it consumes half of Germany's total expenditure on rehabilitation. Resources are basically sourced from earmarked (local or regional) tax-funded budgets (B.A.R. 2018), which have increased significantly over the last 20 years. The healthcare-related component is rather weak here.

A further subsector is *vocational rehabilitation*. Activities under this label include measures meant to facilitate a physically or mentally disadvantaged person's participation in the labour market, e.g. re-education or special training schemes. In this field, two-thirds of all submitted applications are accepted. Funding and administration are incumbent on either the (social) unemployment insurance scheme (*Bundesagentur für Arbeit*, 175,000 admissions in 2015) or on the German pension fund (150,000 cases). Vocational rehabilitation has grown markedly since 2000. Users are relatively young, with two of every three beneficiaries moving back into gainful employment following a measure under this programme.

The *medical rehabilitation* subsector is outstanding in that it orchestrates health-related interventions in combination with other types of support. Most services are organized (and funded) by two social insurance institutions: the *sickness funds* (*Krankenkassen*) pay for measures to help the chronically ill and, to a lesser extent, mental health patients. Post-hospital treatments consume by far the largest proportion of total outlays. Funding for cures was once considered important, but decreased in volume following budget cuts at the end of the 1970s. The sickness funds reject applications less often than administrators elsewhere in the German rehabilitation system; outlays follow assessed needs, with no caps applied to this part of the system. Day rehabilitation services have been strongly promoted in this sector in recent years, with 50% growth since 2006.

A much bigger part of medical rehabilitation is orchestrated by the *pension fund* and targeted to enrolees of this social insurance scheme (ordinary workers and employees), notwithstanding stagnating volumes since the 1970s and reduced budgets relative to total healthcare spending (see SVR 2014, p. 256), since the spending cap coevolves with gross salaries, rather than public health indicators. Nowadays, two-thirds of submitted applications are accepted, with a quite comprehensive range of offered services. This subsector still forms the core of the German rehabilitation system, featuring 1150 rehabilitation centres and 1.4 million cases under treatment (in 2015/2016, see Deutsche Rentenversicherung Bund 2018, pp. 47–48; Welti 2019, pp. 177–178).

Finally, the rehabilitative infrastructure contains some *peripheral segments*. For those with a *private healthcare insurance plan* (roughly 10% of the population), the respective insurance provider operates as a funding agency. For those not covered by any of the aforementioned payers (general) *social assistance* steps in; it provides long-term support to disabled people with no other income. Furthermore, the service package covered by *long-term care insurance* includes rehabilitative services, at least in theory (Klie 2017).

Overall, German citizens have *various opportunities* to receive rehabilitation services, but must often grapple with a *jungle of institutions* before accessing them. Besides the multitude of funding agencies, the supply side is fairly heterogeneous: for instance, among the 1150 rehabilitation centres contracted by the pension fund, more than half are owned by private companies. The highly pluralistic set-up of administrative and provider roles can make intervention trajectories rather multifarious. What becomes salient here is an 'institutional paradox', as the formal promise of holistic ('all-inclusive') rehabilitation services encounters a disintegrated infrastructure of administrative and service-providing entities.

3.2.3   Fragmentation in Various Respects

Institutional complexity chimes with *fragmentation* in numerous respects. First, the legal framework makes categorical distinctions between social, medical, and occupational or vocational rehabilitation. Accordingly, interventions are incumbent on a wide range of separate administrative entities and service providers, implying 'fragmented structures with many and often poorly connected actors' (Mittag et al. 2018, p. 7). Legal responsibilities depend upon causal factors and enrolment rules (related to the various social insurance schemes). As they nevertheless overlap in many instances, a complex clearing process is often required for a given user or patient (see SVR 2014, pp. 272–274). Since many of the existing programmes are underfunded (SVR 2014, pp. 281–282), agencies seek to devolve tasks onto others, which can be quite burdensome for users.

Second, there is (at least implicit) fragmentation in the role-set of the involved professions. While the latter do, by necessity, work together in many settings, *inter*professional divisions are obvious, given a striking 'dominance of the doctor's role' (Xyländer and Meyer 2018, p. 135) within various service settings. Due to this medical bias, rehabilitative endeavour may become fraught with over-specialization. At the same time, physicians employed by rehabilitation centres suffer inferior social status in their peer community, as doctors *outside* their industry, which can perturb *intra*professional communication.

Third, *practical* coordination is often poor. The formal independence of most service providers greatly limits the ability of (quasi-)public authorities to interfere in an intervention trajectory. This especially holds for the provision of 'post-residential' services. Collaboration within a given territory is patchy, for example, in the communication between GPs and rehabilitation centres. Following a rehabilitation measure or therapy, GPs receive a rehabilitation report or a physician's letter of discharge, yet direct inter-sectoral collaboration is rare. Furthermore, occupational health physicians (at company level) are seldom involved in the rehabilitative process (see Stratil et al. 2017; Bethge 2017, p. 433), attributable to data privacy regulation and intra-professional rivalry.

This fragmentation is accompanied by biases in terms of coverage. The German rehabilitation system has a strong residential orientation, whereas day-care services are still in their infancy; this pertains to both long-term support schemes for disabled citizens (e.g. assisted work or housing) and medical rehabilitation. Moreover, large sections of the German rehabilitative system focus on re-establishing or preserving users' or patients' employability, implying that geriatric intervention is neglected within this system (Klie 2017). In addition, social care insurance—the dominant funding source for elderly care services in Germany (see Bode 2008)—is often (mis)understood as a non-rehabilitative institution. Although the regulatory framework is quite flexible on the services covered by this scheme, activating nursing and personal care—theoretically fulfilling rehabilitative functions—remain small-scale in many places. This holds irrespective of recent reforms, through which benefits from the social care insurance scheme can be used for *social* rehabilitation, such as day-to-day company for frail persons.

3.3   Changes in the Governance of Rehabilitation in Germany

3.3.1   The Corporatist Legacy

From an international perspective, the institutional pluralism instilled in the German rehabilitation system may appear awkward, yet it arguably accords well with the complexity of any advanced human service sector. The regulatory framework gives voices and veto points to various stakeholders, which enhances the system's capacity to develop in line with manifold and evolving concerns. There is ample space for network-based deliberation and multi-party arrangements, both deemed a timely approach to regulating public affairs by scholarship on the organization of contemporary welfare states. This steering mode, labelled *governance*, has come to be viewed as a superior alternative to more classical techniques of govern*ment* (Verschraegen 2015; Treib et al. 2007), since it involves multiple stakeholders, can handle complex needs, and responds to 'wicked problems'. Concerning rehabilitation, such problems can include the multiplication of involved specialties or increased multimorbidity. Governance theory submits that such problems cannot be tackled via a unitary, command-and-control bureaucracy; rather, it is assumed that classical forms of govern*ment* tend to let essential operations proceed below the (public) radar, and leave their coordination to fortuitous (local) forces.

The German tradition of multi-party steering in social welfare and healthcare provision (Bode 2011) is of particular interest for this debate within contemporary political sociology. Interest intermediation in the German welfare state is based on the systematic involvement of well-organized membership organizations, and underpins a configuration known as *corporatism*, which is an early variety of what is termed 'governance' today (Kjaer 2016). In essence, corporatism has evolved as a mode of steering by which major interest groups negotiate regulatory norms, whether in politics, through industrial relations, or within human service sectors. It was a typical feature of West Germany's socio-political fabric in the twentieth century, extending to an ever-broader area of sectors, including rehabilitation. Although the former German Democratic Republic established a distinctive (state-dominated) rehabilitation system (see Ramm 2017), institutions originally constructed in the East were generally rendered compatible with the Western legacy following reunification in 1990.

In this legacy, corporatist governance implies the wide-reaching involvement of professional groups, including non-medical entities. This is most salient in medical rehabilitation, which received a strong boost during the post-war decades and assumed the 'mission' of providing vulnerable citizens with opportunities for convalescence, even when several professions must participate. This mission became somewhat medicalized as physicians' expertise was given ever greater value over time. In the later 1970s, the rehabilitation system was curtailed in quantitative terms, when reform reduced its earmarked expenditure by one-third, with non-medical intervention becoming particularly devalued within the system. However, the mission itself survived.

Nowadays, rehabilitative endeavour in Germany is still based on a steering arrangement through which the many funding agencies, service providers, and professional groups, while operating as independent entities, remain firmly involved in running the industry. Moreover, typical organizational settlements make different professional communities work side by side in many places. In some ways, then, the entire system has developed as a 'negotiated order', to cite a concept developed to portray the inner life of modern healthcare organizations (Strauss et al. 1963).

The cornerstones of this order have been long-term *contractual relations* and *expert deliberation* on regulatory and procedural issues. Concerning *contracts*, the German rehabilitation system is operated by individual agreements between funders and providers (SVR 2014, p. 291). Notwithstanding the formal purchaser-provider split in most parts of the industry, these agreements always used to be quite stable (though updated periodically). This avoids disruptions in the 'terms of trade' for service delivery. At present, typical agreements contain structural and (some) process quality standards, as well as fixed lump-sum day rates for various categories of users suffering from a similar impairment or disorder. Importantly, this input-oriented funding differs from the fee-per-service schemes established in the acute inpatient care sector.

As capacity development is sluggish, providers can expect a steady influx of users, although the power of the various (quasi-)public funding agencies is considerable in allocating patients to clinics.

As for *deliberative processes*, policies affecting the social welfare and healthcare sector still are negotiated with the industry's major stakeholders. The corporatist steering mode extends to fora in which relevant stakeholders can discuss regulatory issues on a regular basis; one of these fora is the aforementioned permanent working party (B.A.R.) focused on the current problems and future prospects of rehabilitation. Moreover, as the most important funding agency for medical rehabilitation, the German pension fund operates a scheme through which permanent 'advisers' discuss issues with providers individually. Hence, large sections of the system are based on 'strong ties' between the funding (administrative) side and those who run the industry in practical terms.

3.3.2   Towards a Post-corporatist Configuration Putting the Onus on Users

Recent decades have seen a destabilization of long-established governance arrangements, which sits uneasily with concurrent attempts to make services more seamless and to improve inter-party coordination. The institutional paradox—instilled early in the set-up of the German rehabilitation system—now manifests in a new version, featuring both a stronger emphasis on integrated service provision *and* enhanced fragmentation. These contradictory dynamics can be illustrated in greater detail for two subsectors of the rehabilitation system.

A first case in point is the area of *social rehabilitation* (addressing long-term disabled citizens). A new legal framework has recently been introduced, titled the Federal Law on Participation (*Bundesteilhabegesetz*), to be fully implemented by 2023. This framework focuses on services outside healthcare and shifts the most relevant legal provisions from social assistance to section 9 of the Social Code, which applies to all other rehabilitation services (Welti 2019, pp. 181–182). The approach aims to make welfare state support to citizens with impairments more 'inclusive', 'personalized', and 'participatory'. Besides extended rights for employees in sheltered workshops and higher income limits for means-tested benefits eligibility, the reform brings new entitlements to integrated service packages; a standard application scheme covering all potential benefits; a merger of need assessment tools across administrative boundaries; and the first steps towards cross-agency case management that may comprise 'grand rounds' involving relevant specialists. It also guarantees free choice of housing and fosters disabled citizens' access to peer counselling services, via seed funding to independent agencies that provide this counselling.

At the same time, however, the new framework is embedded in activation policies related to labour market participation. These were enacted in the early 2000s, weakening the traditional status-protection logic of the German welfare regime and shifting many benefit claimants to social *assistance* schemes (Bothfeld and Rosenthal 2018). As in other countries (see Chap. 2 of this volume), this particularly affects workers with limited employability, who become obliged to accept 'bad jobs' offering salaries far below previous earnings; these persons may also receive wage-related unemployment benefits for much shorter periods than in the pre-reform era. Moreover, incapacity benefits were considerably curtailed by pension policies in the 2000s (Bode 2008), and it remains to be seen whether revisions taking effect in 2019 will compensate their impact. Thus, for many people needing rehabilitation, material living conditions have markedly deteriorated.

Concerning access to rehabilitative support, new regulations aim to incentivize major target groups to operate as 'consumers', purchasing individualized assistance and bargaining with provider organizations as if market-oriented service suppliers. A key innovation is personalized budgets, through which entitlements to allowances from various benefit-granting agencies are merged in a single payment. There are enhanced opportunities to use benefits in flexible ways, for example, for preferred types of personal assistance. Moreover, firms outside the traditional work rehabilitation sector have been invited to offer beneficiaries opportunities for assisted employment, thereby becoming rivals of long-established sheltered workshops. All this may certainly serve the personal interests of numerous users, but it also opens the door to erratic decisions and new social divisions. Disadvantaged groups may become lost in the aforementioned jungle of institutions, even when sporadically advised by an agency. Those from a lower social class background may be incapable of operating as consumers or do so only inconsistently and in a piecemeal manner. Other beneficiaries may abuse their new 'power' vis-à-vis personal assistants, hired from a deregulated labour market in which such assistants struggle to find decent jobs. Finally, personalization may also 'unburden' those institutions that must otherwise ensure seamless service provision for anyone (Mladenov et al. 2015).

These overall developments resemble international movements towards making disadvantaged citizens 'market subjects', focusing on individualized responsibility and understanding social support as an investment in human capital (see Murphy 2014, p. 158), rather than a state-guaranteed right. This policy targets *user-driven integration at 'micro level'*, attempting to push individuals to build their own *personal* interface with the different layers of the rehabilitation system, although this interface may remain fractured in many instances. It meshes with further developments concerning social support to long-term disabled citizens. In recent years, the mantra of New Public Management (NPM), though less influential in Germany than in the Anglo-Saxon world, has nonetheless influenced the regulatory framework through which interventions for these users are orchestrated. Although this framework still does not contain public tenders through which service packages are commissioned to non-statutory providers in a competitive process, new 'performance contracts' have been introduced by local and regional welfare departments. Frequently, these contracts pressurize service providers to become market-oriented and entrepreneurial (Weber 2014), incentivizing them to 'cherry pick' users by looking at the gravity or complexity of their impairment and keeping actual costs per case as low as possible. Thus, users encounter a more marketized supply side that may disregard actual needs if these deviate from what is defined as 'normal' by the contracts.

A similar paradox is apparent in the evolving regulation of *medical rehabilitation,* providing a second example of contradictory movements concerning the governance of Germany's rehabilitation system. Recent reforms were aimed at overcoming demand-side fragmentation (i.e. among the responsible funding agencies). One strategy was the creation of 'unitary service centres' (*Gemeinsame Servicestellen*; see Seel 2015) with a remit to establish operational links between the many components of the rehabilitation system throughout Germany. Today, 450 such centres offer support to users wanting to claim benefits and apply to a given service but unsure how to find the responsible funding agency and appropriate provider. Located within established institutions (e.g. a sickness fund branch office or a local Jobcentre) or in one-stop agencies co-managed by several of the aforementioned funding agencies, these entities operate standard procedures to provide early case management. However, they lack the power to compel action by other stakeholders, and so are viewed as failing bureaucracies by many experts. Again, this is indicative of a propensity to encourage '*integration at micro level*', as beneficiaries are incentivized to take action individually but are not guaranteed appropriate solutions; consequently, personal initiative may have a piecemeal character and is susceptible to (new) social inequalities.

On the supply side, inconsistencies are also blatant. On the one hand, there have been efforts to bolster the comprehensive approach to rehabilitation regarding the service packages on offer. The pension fund has invested in prevention programmes that today cover 1200 different measures, including new operational links to occupational health, paediatric rehabilitation, pilot schemes geared towards avoiding disability after severe illness, and intensified treatments for drug addicts. There are also initiatives to improve information transparency within the rehabilitation system, such as an internet-based service point for patients seeking an appropriate provider of post-hospital treatment. In addition, a growing proportion of users are offered non-residential services in their local environment. Nowadays, these services consume 20% of the pension fund's total outlays.

On the other hand, however, the comprehensiveness of the rehabilitative endeavour suffers from changes in this subsector's governance. First, the aforementioned budget cap has caused the pension fund to become more restrictive on the duration and range of rehabilitative services. Experts also observe that contracts with providers have become leaner. Although few data are available on providers' financial situation, their incurred costs have grown more than the increase in lump-sum rates, implying marked economic constraints on the supply side (SVR 2014, p. 292). Indeed, recent estimations suggest that one in four providers has high bankruptcy risk.

Second, the behaviour of neighbouring welfare and healthcare providers aggravates the situation in the industry. Reforms affecting both acute inpatient and elderly care have made the task structure devolved on the rehabilitation system even more demanding. Following the aforementioned 'haircut' for medical rehabilitation at the end of the 1970s, providers had to invest in more sophisticated medical care facilities as users' needs became more challenging (due partly to population ageing). This pressure has subsequently been exacerbated by acute care hospitals referring patients to specialized rehabilitation centres at a much earlier stage than previously (von Eiff et al. 2011). A major reason is the exposure of acute care hospitals to individual 'market accountability' (Bode 2019a), imposing pressure to become a profitable enterprise within a competition-driven inpatient care industry. Early discharge has, consequently, become a priority prompted by a funding regime through which hospitals receive standardized 'per-case' payments for disorders listed in one 'diagnosis-related group', leaving the full economic risks related to unforeseeable complications entirely with the supply side.

A similar movement is affecting older users. Due to market pressures, elderly care homes are pressured to minimize staff expenditure, which entails a 'task enrichment' of rehabilitation centres insofar as the latter face a growing need for geriatric care (whereas the number of staff does not keep pace with this rise of their workload). As for domiciliary elderly care, which has expanded markedly since the 1990s, day-to-day support is often confined to mere nursing, with only rudimentary interventions for activating the cared-for. This sector has equally been exposed to strong market forces (Bode et al. 2013), with home care providers competing for 'good risks' and incurring the full economic risk when dealing (spontaneously) with needs not fully covered by long-term care insurance.

Such (quasi-)marketization undermines the inherited corporatist logic, with a growing proportion of coordination activities permeated by competitive orientations, at the expense of arrangements through which stakeholders (including funding agencies) discursively engage with both economic concerns and evidenced needs. Hence the German rehabilitation system is affected by the erosion of corporatist governance *in its environments*. Simultaneously, with poor coordination between rehabilitative institutions and mainstream medical or elderly care providers, the onus for organizing a sound rehabilitative trajectory shifts to the cared-for (and their relatives), again reflecting the agenda of *user-driven integration* regarding the access to relevant services.

Moreover, *within* the medical rehabilitation subsector, new policies tend to put providers under organizational strain. Thus, the operations of the sickness funds—a major funding source for rehabilitation—have become infused with 'NPM thinking' (Bode 2010). In medical rehabilitation, the funds tend to use benchmark indicators based on (often over-simplified) comparative performance data when negotiating standards and prices (with providers). Although this part of the German rehabilitation system has not yet shifted to radical market governance, the sickness funds may become motivated to move further in this direction by supply-side changes. As noted earlier, most providers are for-profit, and some have developed into fully-fledged capitalistic businesses, striving for a high return on investment to serve stockholders' interests, with strategies including union busting and low pay. A prominent recent example is the French company Orphea, which owns 160 facilities in Germany. Such experiences strongly incentivize funding agencies to establish new schemes for 'performance control'.

The 'zeitgeist' corroborates such ambitions. In the area of medical rehabilitation, the example of *quality assurance policies* is telling (Xyländer and Meyer 2018, pp. 122–131; Deutsche Rentenversicherung Bund 2018, pp. 35–46). These policies have come to emphasize *output* evaluation, for which purpose the pension fund runs its own monitoring scheme (covering 950 providers). Since 1994, it has invested in developing tools for quality inspection, based on: user satisfaction data; peer reviews (using discharge reports and evaluation guidelines); and information on minimum standards for input and process quality. The results feed into an internal benchmarking system. Meanwhile, there are legal provisions obliging all parties involved in medical rehabilitation to employ such tools. The sickness funds apply a distinctive scheme ('QS-Reha') which includes on-site inspections and currently covers 600 providers (on this particular scheme, see Farin et al. 2004).

The crucial question is how data on the relative performance of rehabilitative services are used to steer providers in economic terms. Internationally, the movement towards 'government by numbers' is proliferating across various areas of social welfare and healthcare provision

(Bode 2019b; Kersten et al. 2015). To date, the quality inspection policy of the pension fund remains largely corporatist. Available information is used to inspire a 'dialogue' with providers showing modest results (for instance, in terms of improved work capacities). While, in theory, the current regulatory framework allows a poor performer's contract to be cancelled, the pension fund's official policy is to share collected information with the underperforming provider and discuss possible causes and remedies. This corresponds to the de facto limits to both numeric performance control and ensuing 'process reengineering' (i.e. attempts to influence outputs by mechanical management tools), given the complex (bio-psycho-social) nature of rehabilitative endeavour. The traditional inspection policy contributes to preserving the comprehensive character of rehabilitation programmes, showing reluctance to devalue activities whose impact is particularly hard to measure (e.g. psychological or social support).

Again, however, one can discern a tendency to deviate from long-established habits. Under the pressure of experts deploring a lack of 'evidence-based regulation' (SVR 2014, p. 212) and advocating 'market transparency' (see, e.g. Klie 2017, p. 279), the pension fund has developed a discourse promoting inter-provider competition for evidence-based quality. The fund already experiments with comparative benchmarking, using data on social insurance contribution records (e.g. on the number of patients returning to full-time employment after rehabilitation). Over the coming years, such data are supposed to be used as *one* criterion for contracting providers and allocating users to them. All of these developments endorse the incremental shift towards post-corporatist governance in the German rehabilitation system.

3.4   Conclusion

This chapter opened by highlighting the *paradox* inherent in rehabilitative endeavour in Germany (as in other parts of the Western world). On the one hand, we find a holistic approach to rehabilitation, applied in specialized clinical settings (outside the acute care sector) and by multi-professional interventions *within* these settings. On the other hand, the funding and supply-side infrastructure for rehabilitation is disintegrated, and the orchestration of service provision proves fragmented in many instances. Recent regulatory changes have amplified this paradox. There are even signs that the German rehabilitation system is currently at a crossroads.

As illustrated by the example of quality assurance, final decisions are yet to come. In general, the system still exhibits *high potential* in providing decent financial support to many (albeit not all) citizens in need, as well as diversified service packages combining medical, social, and work-related aspects. The infrastructure for service provision is well-developed; the relevant funding agencies, professional communities, and wider social forces appear strongly committed; and recent steps towards programme innovation look promising. Both the pluralistic landscape of the industry and its long-standing embeddedness in institutionalized partnerships provide interesting opportunities. Rehabilitation in Germany has long developed in the shadow of the NPM mantra, which has proved much more influential in acute healthcare and elderly care settings. Moreover, action has been taken to make service provision more comprehensive, with new programmes, enhanced entitlements, and attempts to improve collaboration. All these factors seem to endorse the traditional holistic approach.

However, there are *critical moments* regarding the near future. Both fundamental change in the system's key *environments* and the very *instruments* by which the system is to be modernized conflict with the traditional holistic orientation. Activation policies and their work-first rationale, though of limited importance regarding long-term disabled citizens, have often placed extra strain on citizens with limited employability and those receiving incapacity pension benefits. Moreover, current attempts to bridge inter-sectoral boundaries at micro level (e.g. by personal budgets) impose a boundary-spanning role on users who will often fulfil this role in only a piecemeal manner. Meanwhile, providers are pushed towards behaving as 'egocentric' organizations, complying with both formalized 'performance control' and the preferences of a market-minded clientele. The movement towards 'government by numbers' (or 'evidence'-based funding) is equally prone to strain the system, since managed (cure and) care and economic competition reduce space for dialogue, information sharing, and collaborative endeavour in many instances.

In the past, the integration of the German rehabilitation system was already patchy in several respects. Thus, the strong role of profit-seeking providers was always a potential stumbling block for ensuring a smooth interaction between the funding and supply side; meanwhile, the rising influence of capitalistic companies on the supply side seems to have stiffened this barrier. Furthermore, despite high symbolic value attached to the very concept of rehabilitation, legal divisions within the multi-pillar system have proved considerable during the post-war decades, and they still appear rather solid. In addition, while interprofessional collaboration within one and the same setting is remarkable when considered against common practice in major social welfare and healthcare industries, the dominance of the medical profession within the rehabilitation industry does pose problems.

That said, recent regulatory trends are tending to destabilize achievements in collaborative endeavour and impede possible improvements. Despite growing awareness of detrimental divisions, opportunities for transcending institutional boundaries are being missed. Indeed, recent policies are inducing greater fragmentation. For instance, pressures to use (rough) output assessments as a tool for selecting providers not only risks reducing the role of 'soft' (and often intangible) rehabilitative activities that are crucial to person-centred services; they also entail a loss of faith in both inter-party dialogue and open deliberation between funding agencies and providers to improve quality. On the horizon is a post-corporatist settlement in which attempts to strengthen the system's integration coincide with regulatory trends susceptible to creating new disruption.

A general insight from this chapter may be that similar trends, though taking shape in country-specific ways, penetrate dissimilar rehabilitation systems. This applies to both sides of the paradox: the one concerning commitments to integrated service provision (across various social welfare and healthcare services) or even the human right to social inclusion; the other epitomized by movements towards personalization, quasi-market pressure, and 'mechanic' performance control. More generally, the case of Germany suggests that rehabilitative endeavour can be institutionalized in *specific* ways that may *all* entail promising outcomes. Yet it also bears witness to such endeavour being unsettled by regulatory approaches fostering competitive thinking and distrust. Thus, countries that seek to establish (more) pluralistic governance within their rehabilitation system should pay attention to the wider circumstances under which such governance is operated.

References

B.A.R. (Bundesarbeitsgemeinschaft Rehabilitation). (2018). Trägerübergreifende Ausgaben für Rehabilitation und Teilhabe [Expenditure for rehabilitation and participation across providers] Rehab-Info 1-2018. www.bar-frankfurt. de/publikationen/reha-info/reha-info-012018/traegeruebergreifende-ausgaben-fuer-rehabilitation-und-teilhabe/. Accessed 15 Dec 2018.

Bethge, M. (2017). Rehabilitation und Teilhabe am Arbeitsleben [Rehabilitation and participation in working life]. *Bundesgesundheitsblatt, 60,* 427–435.

Bode, I. (2008). Aging and the welfare state in Germany. In C. Aspalter & A. Walker (Eds.), *Securing the future for old age in Europe* (pp. 223–250). Taipei: Casa Verde.

Bode, I. (2010). Towards disorganised governance in public service provision? The case of German sickness funds. *International Journal of Public Administration, 33*(2), 61–72.

Bode, I. (2011). Creeping marketization and post-corporatist governance: The transformation of state–nonprofit relations in continental Europe. In S. D. Phillips & S. Rathgeb Smith (Eds.), *Governance and regulation in the third sector* (pp. 115–141). London: Routledge.

Bode, I. (2019a). Publicness in times of market accountability: Lessons from a changing hospital industry in Germany. *Public Policy and Administration, 34*(1), 3–21.

Bode, I. (2019b). Let's count and manage – And forget the rest. Understanding numeric rationalization in human service provision. *Historical Social Research, 43*(2), 131–154.

Bode, I., Champetier, B., & Chartrand, S. (2013). Embedded marketization as transnational path departure. Assessing recent change in home care systems comparatively. *Comparative Sociology, 12*(6), 821–850.

Bothfeld, S., & Rosenthal, P. (2018). The end of social security as we know it – The Erosion of status protection in German labour market policy. *Journal of Social Policy, 47*(2), 275–294.

Buschmann-Steinhage, R. (2017). Trends in der medizinischen rehabilitation. Angebotsstruktur und Zielgruppen [Trends in medical rehabilitation. The supply-side structure and target groups]. *Bundesgesundheitsblatt, 60*(4), 368–377.

Deutsche Rentenversicherung Bund. (2018). *Reha-Bericht 2018.* Berlin.

Farin, E., Follert, P., Gerdes, N., Jaeckel, W. H., & Thalau, J. (2004). Quality assessment in rehabilitation centers: The indicator system 'quality profile'. *Disability and Rehabilitation, 26*(18), 1096–1104.

Kersten, P., Lundgren-Nilsson, A., & Batcho, C. S. (2015). Rethinking measurement in rehabilitation. In K. McPherson, B. Gibson, & A. Leplège (Eds.), *Rethinking rehabilitation. Theory and practice* (pp. 209–226). Boca Raton: CRC Press.

Kjaer, P. F. (2016). From corporatism to governance: Dimensions of a theory of intermediary institutions. In E. Hartmann (Ed.), *The evolution of intermediary institutions in Europe. From corporatism to governance* (pp. 11–28). Berlin: Springer.

Klenk, T., & Pavolini, E. (Eds.). (2015). *Restructuring welfare governance. Marketization, managerialism and welfare state professionalism.* Cheltenham: Edward Elgar.

Klie, T. (2017). Kooperation und Integration: die Herausforderung Rehabilitation vor Pflege [Cooperation and integration: The challenge of prioritizing rehabilitation over elderly care]. In K. Brandhorst (Ed.), *Kooperation und Integration – das unvollendete Projekt des Gesundheitssystems* [Cooperation and integration: The unfinished mission of the healthcare system] (pp. 263–283). Wiesbaden: Springer VS.

Meinert, R. G., & Yuen, F. (Eds.). (2014). Introduction. In *Controversies and disputes in disability and rehabilitation* (pp. 1–4). New York/London: Routledge.

Mittag, O., Kotkas, T., Reese, C., Kampling, H., Groskreutz, H., de Boer, H., & Welti, F. (2018). Intervention policies and social security in case of reduced working capacity in the Netherlands, Finland and Germany. A comparative analysis. *International Journal of Public Health, 63*(9), 1081–1088.

Mladenov, T., Owens, J., & Cribb, A. (2015). Personalisation in disability services and healthcare: A critical comparative analysis. *Critical Social Policy, 35*(3), 307–326.

Murphy, J. W. (2014). Service delivery, community development, and disability. In R. Meinert & F. Yuen (Eds.), *Controversies and disputes in disability and rehabilitation* (pp. 155–164). New York/London: Routledge.

Ramm, D. (2017). *Die Rehabilitation und das Schwerbeschädigtenrecht der DDR im Übergang zur Bundesrepublik Deutschland. Strukturen und Akteure* [Rehabilitation and disability law in the GDR during the transition to the Federal Republic of Germany. Structure and actors]. Kassel: Kassel University Press.

Safilios-Rothschild, C. (1970). *The sociology and social psychology of disability and rehabilitation*. New York: Random House.

Seel, H. (2015). Zentrale, trägerübergreifende Anlaufstellen – Ansätze, Hindernisse, Perspektiven [One-stop service units – approaches, barriers, prospects]. In L. Mülheims, K. Hummel, S. Peters-Lange, E. Toepler, & I. Schuhmann (Eds.), *Sozialversicherungswissenschaft* [The science of social security] (pp. 867–881). Wiesbaden: Springer VS.

Stratil, J. M., Rieger, M. A., & Völter-Mahlknecht, S. (2017). Cooperation between general practitioners, occupational health physicians, and rehabilitation physicians in Germany: What are problems and barriers to cooperation? A qualitative study. *International Archive for Occupational and Environmental Health, 90*(6), 481–490.

Strauss, A. L., Schatzman, L., Ehrlich, D., Bucher, R., & Sabshin, M. (1963). The hospital and its negotiated order. In E. Freidson (Ed.), *The hospital in modern society* (pp. 147–169). London: Collier-Macmillan.

SVR (Sachverständigenrat zur Begutachtung der Entwicklung im Gesundheitswesen) [Expert Group for Reviewing the Development of the Healthcare System]. (2014). *Bedarfsgerechte Versorgung – Perspektiven für ländliche Regionen und ausgewählte Leistungsbereiche* [Need-based services – Perspectives for rural regions and selected service areas]. Bern: Verlag Hans Huber.

Treib, O., Bähr, H., & Falkner, G. (2007). Modes of governance: Towards a conceptual clarification. *European Journal of Public Policy, 14*(1), 1–20.

Verschraegen, G. (2015). The evolution of welfare state governance. In K. Van Assche, R. Beunen, & M. Duineveld (Eds.), *Evolutionary governance theory* (pp. 57–71). Berlin: Springer.

von Eiff, W., Schüring, S., & Niehues, C. (2011). *REDIA: Auswirkungen der DRG-Einführung auf die medizinische Rehabilitation. Ergebnisse einer prospektiven und medizin-ökonomischen Langzeitstudie 2003 bis 2011* [The impact of the introduction of DRGs on medical rehabilitation. Findings of a prospective and medical-economic long-term study]. Münster: LIT.

Weber, S. (2014). *Leistungsverträge in der Behindertenhilfe. Wohlfahrtspflege zwischen Tradition und Ökonomisierungserwartung* [Performance contracts in support for disabled people. Welfare provision between tradition and expectations to make it more economic]. Marburg: Tectum.

Welti, F. (2019). Work disability policy in Germany: Experiences of collective and individual participation and cooperation. In E. MacEachen (Ed.), *The science and politics of work disability prevention* (pp. 171–188). New York/ London: Routledge.

Xyländer, M., & Meyer, T. (2018). Qualitätsentwicklung in Gesundheitsorganisationen am Beispiel der medizinischen Rehabilitation mit einem besonderen Blick auf Ergebnisqualität und die Rolle der Professionen [Quality management in healthcare organizations. The example of medical rehabilitation, focusing quality performance and the role of professions]. In P. Hensen, & M. Stamer (Eds.), *Professionsbezogene Qualitätsentwicklung im interdisziplinären Gesundheitswesen. Gestaltungsansätze, Handlungsfelder und Querschnittsbereiche* [Professional quality management in an interdisciplinary healthcare system. Management models, action fields, and cross-sectional areas] (pp. 119–140). Wiesbaden: Springer VS.

4

From Quotas to Sanctions: The Political Economy of Rehabilitation in the UK

Clare Bambra

4.1 Introduction

This chapter examines UK social policy towards people who are out of work on a long-term basis due to a chronic illness or disability (Gabbay et al. 2011). A 'disability', in this context, is defined as an illness or impairment that limits the usual activities of daily living, including work ability (Organisation for Economic Co-operation and Development (OECD) 2009, p. 11). Across advanced market democracies, poor health is a significant risk factor for unemployment, as well as remaining unemployed. In 2018, the UK employment rate for people with a disability was 51%, compared to 81% for those without an illness or disability (House of Commons Library 2018). There was also a small gender gap, with women with a disability having a slightly lower employment rate than men with a disability (51% vs. 52%) (House of Commons Library 2018). People with a disability in the UK are also 50% more likely to work part-time: 24% of people

C. Bambra (✉)
Institute of Health & Society, Faculty of Medical Sciences,
Newcastle University, Newcastle, UK
e-mail: Clare.Bambra@newcastle.ac.uk

© The Author(s) 2019
I. Harsløf et al. (eds.), *New Dynamics of Disability and Rehabilitation*,
https://doi.org/10.1007/978-981-13-7346-6_4

69

with disabilities were working part-time compared to 36% of people without disabilities (House of Commons Library 2018). However, disability-related unemployment is also unequally distributed both socioeconomically and geographically. Men and women from lower educational or occupational backgrounds are significantly more likely to experience disability-related unemployment in the UK, as well as in other European countries (Pope and Bambra 2005; Bambra and Pope 2007). The employment of people with a disability in the UK is also geographically skewed, with the lowest rates in de-industrialized areas reflecting wider patterns of ill health and unemployment (Norman and Bambra 2007). In 2018, for example, the employment rate for people with a disability was highest in South East England (58%) and lowest in Scotland (45%), Wales (43%), North East England (41%), and Northern Ireland (35%) (House of Commons Library 2018). Poverty, social exclusion, and downward social mobility are also important issues for people with a disability in the UK (Bambra 2011a).

As in most other advanced market economies, the UK state provides financial support to individuals whose unemployment is disability-related, in the form of sickness and disability pensions (see Box 4.1) (Bambra 2011b). Rates of receipt of these disability-related benefits have increased rapidly since the 1970s: in the UK, they have increased from 0.5 million recipients in 1975 to 2 million in 2018, meaning that around 7% of the UK working-age population currently receives disability-related benefits (Office for National Statistics 2018). This accounts for over 10% of UK social security expenditure and almost 2% of gross domestic product (GDP) (Gabbay et al. 2011). The probability of returning to work after receiving long-term health-related benefits is just 2% annually (OECD 2003, 2009), with most recipients who have been without work for six months or more having only a 20% chance of returning to work within five years (Waddell and Burton 2006). The most common causes of long-term sickness absence in the UK are musculoskeletal conditions (including obesity-related) and mental health problems (including drug and alcohol addictions) (Black 2016).

Concern over the rising numbers of disability-related benefit recipients has meant that in the UK, as in most other European countries, disability-related benefits have had a high political profile over the last three decades. This has led to substantial changes to rehabilitation medicine, vocational services, and the social security support provided to disabled people.

Box 4.1 Main Disability-Related Social Security Benefits in the UK (1994–Date)

Incapacity Benefit (1994–2008) replaced Invalidity Benefit in 1994. It was a non-means-tested social security cash benefit, paid to people in the UK who were medically certified as incapable of work due to illness or disability and who had contributed sufficient National Insurance payments. Incapacity Benefit was paid at a higher rate than usual unemployment benefit (c.33% higher). It was similar in remit to the long-term sickness and disability insurance schemes of other Western countries, such as the USA's Social Security Disability Insurance and the disability pensions of Germany and Sweden. There were three rates of Incapacity Benefit. In the short-term, a lower rate was paid for the first 28 weeks of sickness, and a higher rate for weeks 29–52. The third (long-term) rate applied to people who had been sick for more than a year; this group comprised the largest number of claimants. Incapacity Benefit could be received up to pensionable age. It was discontinued in 2008 and gradually replaced for new and existing recipients with the Employment and Support Allowance.

Employment and Support Allowance (2008–date) was introduced in 2008 to replace Incapacity Benefit. It has a two-tier system of benefits, based on a medically administered Work Capability Assessment. Those judged unable to work or with limited work capacity due to the severity of their physical or mental condition receive a higher level of benefit with no conditionality. By contrast, those deemed 'sick but able to work'—the work-related activity group—only receive an additional Employment Support premium if they participate in employability initiatives. Those who fail to do so are only entitled to the basic Employment and Support Allowance (paid at the same rate as unemployment benefit—Jobseeker's Allowance). Since 2010, receipt of Employment and Support Allowance for the 'work-related activity' group is limited to a maximum of one year.

Universal Credit (since 2017) is a single working-age benefit which replaced Jobseeker's Allowance (unemployment benefit), Income Support (means-tested social assistance), and Employment and Support Allowance (disability-related benefit) from 2015 (Department for Work and Pensions 2010b). Compulsory work-for-benefit, as well as a 'claimant contract' with benefit sanctions (of three months', six months', or up to three years' benefit removal for recipients who refuse to accept a job offer), are key components of Universal Credit, and they apply to recipients of all, including disability-related, benefits.

Rehabilitation medicine in the UK is both clinical (provided by the National Health Service [NHS]) and vocational (provided by the Department for Work and Pensions [DWP]). It can be broadly divided into: neurological rehabilitation (including brain, spinal cord, and peripheral nerve conditions and injuries), musculoskeletal rehabilitation, and mental health conditions (Royal College of Physicians 2010). The latter two conditions account for over 60% of unemployment amongst people with a disability. All areas of clinical rehabilitation medicine practice include the management of pain, health and employment behaviours, emotional disturbances, and cognitive issues (Royal College of Physicians 2010). In the provision of rehabilitation services, the UK lags behind other European countries: for example, it has only 0.26 rehabilitation specialist doctors per 100,000 population compared to 1.88 in Sweden and 2.87 in France (Ward 2005). Rehabilitation medicine also works closely with vocational rehabilitation services to promote employment opportunities for disabled adults of working age, working in liaison with occupational medicine, occupational therapists, vocational services, and employers (Royal College of Physicians 2010).

This chapter focuses on the vocational aspects of rehabilitation medicine in the UK, examining key policy regime shifts in the UK context. It outlines the moves away from the *passive welfare* of the 1970s and 1980s (typified by compulsory employment quotas and passive welfare benefits); through the *active welfare* of the 1990s and 2000s (including anti-discrimination legislation, welfare to work, and active welfare benefits); to the *workfare* approach entrenched in the present system and accelerated under austerity (typified by benefit sanctions, benefit cuts, and compulsory work-for-benefit). These significant social policy shifts are then analysed from a political economy perspective, exploring the broad context of neoliberal restructuring of the state and the specific issues of reasserting labour discipline and reclassifying people with a disability from 'deserving' to 'undeserving' subjects (Bambra and Smith 2010; Bambra 2011a; Schrecker and Bambra 2015).

4.2   The Evolution of UK Disability Policy

This section summarizes the historical evolution of UK social policy for people with a disability from 1944 to today. It identifies and outlines four key and distinct phases: (1) 'passive welfare'; (2) 'active welfare'; (3) 'towards workfare'; and (4) 'austerity'. The effects of these policy changes on the employment of people with a disability are also examined, noting their limited impacts.

4.2.1 Passive Welfare (1970s–1990s)

The first phase of UK public policy towards the employment of people with a disability was framed by the Disabled Persons (Employment) Act 1944, under which employment programmes (such as Remploy), medical rehabilitation services, and the post-war employment quota were established (Table. 4.1). In the 1970s, these measures were supplemented by several health-related cash benefits for out-of-work individuals, such as

Table 4.1 'Passive Welfare' phase of UK disability policy (1944–1994)

1944	**Disabled Persons (Employment) Act** Launched the post-war disability employment quota of 3% for employers with over 20 staff. Some vocational services initiated and special, initially sheltered, employment started ('Remploy')
1970	**Chronically Sick and Disabled Persons Act** Improved access to local authority public buildings and services
1971	**National Insurance Act** Invalidity Benefit established
1973	**Employment and Training Act** Introduced employment rehabilitation centres and resettlement officers **Social Security Act** Attendance Allowance introduced: subsidies for costs of home care/assistance
1975	**Social Security Benefits Act** Introduced the Mobility Allowance: cash benefit paid for transport costs **Social Security Pensions Act** Non-Contributory Invalidity Pension (later known as Severe Disablement Allowance)
1980	**Social Security Act** Reduced benefit levels
1991	**Disability Living Allowance and Disability Working Allowance Act** Disability Living Allowance combined the Attendance and Mobility Allowances Disability Working Allowance: wage top-up for low-paid workers (replaced with tax credit in 1999) **Placement, Assessment, and Counselling Teams (PACTs)** Vocational preparation and placement services (renamed Disability Service Teams in 1999)

Adapted from Bambra et al. (2005)

Invalidity Benefit in 1971 (renamed Incapacity Benefit in 1994). Ill-health-based cash benefits were higher than unemployment benefits, which recognized the long-term nature of ill health and the additional associated costs (Bambra 2011a). The social security reforms of the 1980s and early 1990s placed additional restrictions on these cash benefits (e.g. the introduction of the 'all work' test in 1994). However, fuelled by growing government concerns about the costs of disability-related benefits, alongside pressure from disability campaign groups regarding social exclusion (Barnes 1991), a more radical policy shift occurred in the mid-1990s.

The Disability Discrimination Act 1995 (and subsequent amendments) abolished the post-war disability employment quota and instigated a more rights-based approach to the employment of disabled people (Oliver and Barnes 1998). This Act introduced a distinction in social policy between people with a legally recognized disability (including *limiting* long-term illnesses) and those with other forms of chronic illness. Key features of the Disability Discrimination Act 1995 (later subsumed into the wider Equalities Act 2010) are presented in Box 4.2.

Box 4.2 Disability Discrimination Act 1995 (Now Subsumed into Equalities Act 2010)

The 1995 Act made it illegal to discriminate on the grounds of physical or mental disability or limiting long-term illness: since its implementation in 1996, it has been unlawful to '*discriminate against disabled persons in connection with employment, the provision of goods, facilities and services, or the disposal or management of premises*'.

Employers are required to make '*reasonable adjustments*' to work and premises to cater for people with a disability.

The Act defines disability as '*a physical or mental impairment that has a substantial and long-term adverse effect on [the individual's] ability to carry out normal day-to-day activities*':

- *Physical impairment*—includes weakening or adverse change of a part of the body caused through illness, by accident or from birth such as blindness, deafness, heart disease, the paralysis of a limb or severe disfigurement.
- *Mental impairment*—can include learning disabilities and all recognized mental illnesses.
- *Substantial*—does not have to be severe, but is more than minor or trivial.

- *Long-term adverse effect*—has lasted or is likely to last more than 12 months.
- *A normal day-to-day activity*—mobility; manual dexterity; physical co-ordination; continence; ability to lift, carry, or otherwise move everyday objects; speech, hearing, or eyesight; memory or ability to concentrate, learn, or understand; or perception of the risk of physical danger.

4.2.2 Active Welfare (1990s–2000s)

The UK welfare state has always contained an element of active welfare: for example, many of the initial post-war cash benefits, such as pensions, were only available to those who had previously paid National Insurance contributions (Fulcher and Scott 2003). However, this feature has become more prominent and far reaching in recent decades. In the second phase of government action, people with a disability or long-term condition were re-conceptualized as a key group of working-age benefit recipients and, as such, became the targets of *activation* policies and subject to diverse active labour market policies (ALMPs). 'Activation' has also emerged as a dominant reform theme across other European welfare states, with benefits and services for working-age people becoming more focused on re-connecting recipients with the labour market, requiring them to actively seek employment (Houston and Lindsay 2010). In the UK, for example, the early ALMPs of the Disability Working Allowance, the New Deal for Disabled People, and the Access to Work programme all targeted people with a disability in the 1990s (Table 4.2). These interventions generally tried to overcome the different barriers faced by people with a disability or chronic illness when trying to enter employment, including: lack of experience or skills; employers' uncertainty; problems with physical access to work; and concerns over pay, hours, and conditions (Goldstone and Meager 2002). However, the majority of interventions focused on the supply side, with little consideration of actual labour market demand (Bambra 2006). In this period, participation by benefit recipients was largely on a voluntary basis (Bambra et al. 2005).

Table 4.2 'Active Welfare' phase of UK disability policy (1994–2003)

1994	**Social Security (Incapacity for Work) Act** Introduced the All Works Test and Incapacity Benefit **Access to Work Programme** Provided financial assistance towards practical aids, workplace adaptation, fares to work, and personal support
1995	**Disability Discrimination Act** Since 1996, it has been unlawful to discriminate in recruitment, promotion, training, working conditions, and dismissal on the grounds of disability or ill health (restricted to employers with over 20 employees, reduced to 15 in 1998). Abolished the 3% employment quota of 1944
1998	**New Deal for Disabled People Pilots** A package of different interventions including the Personal Adviser service, the Innovative Schemes, and smaller projects such as the Job Finders Grant
1999	**Tax Credit Act** Introduced the Disabled Person's Tax Credit—a wage top-up for people with disabilities in low-paid employment (merged into the Working Tax Credit in 2002) **Disability Rights Commission** Monitored implementation of the Disability Discrimination Act from 2000 onwards **Welfare Reform and Pensions Act** Incapacity Benefit became means-tested, Severe Disablement Allowance was age-restricted, and the Personal Capacity Test replaced the All Works Test **ONE Pilot** People applying for benefits were given an adviser to discuss work options. Compulsory after 2000
2000	**WORKSTEP programme** Assists with transition from segregated supported work into mainstream employment
2001	**Special Educational Needs and Disability Act** Extended the provisions of the Disability Discrimination Act to education providers (provisions in force from 2002) **New Deal for Disabled People National Extension** Introduced Job Brokers (public, vocational advisers) **Job Centre Plus** Services of the Employment Service and the Benefits Agency were combined

(continued)

Table 4.2 (continued)

2002	Tax Credits Act
	Disabled Persons Tax Credit merged into the Working Tax Credit for all low-paid workers
	Permitted Work Rules
	Allows benefit claimants to undertake paid work for up to 16 hours per week

Source: Adapted from Bambra et al. (2005)

4.2.3   Towards 'Workfare' (2003–2010)

Despite a rapid increase in the use of ALMPs in the UK since the 1990s, the employment rate for people with a disability remained very low. In the 2000s, there were still over 2.5 million people receiving disability-related benefits in the UK. They remained, therefore, at the centre of the welfare reform agenda, with the benefits of (re)employment for health and well-being increasingly emphasized in policy circles (Black 2008). Voluntary engagement with ALMPs was replaced by compulsory engagement and conditionality in the new policy approach. In 2003, for example, pilots for the Pathways to Work programme introduced compulsory Work Focused Interviews for all new benefit recipients (Table 4.3). Most significantly, in 2008, Incapacity Benefit was phased out for new recipients and replaced with the two-tiered Employment and Support Allowance (ESA) (see Box 4.1).

Using a new test administered by the private sector (first Atos, then Maximus), called the Work Capability Assessment (WCA), the ESA required all but the most severely sick or disabled recipients to be work-ready by, for example, undergoing rehabilitation or retraining (Warren et al. 2014). All existing Incapacity Benefit recipients were gradually re-evaluated and moved onto ESA or the lower-value Jobseeker's Allowance (JSA; unemployment benefit). Contracting private sector providers to deliver the WCA has been criticized for incentivizing claim rejection, as well as being expensive, impersonal, mechanistic, and insufficiently transparent, with a high rate of appeals (Warren et al. 2014). The ESA introduced new distinctions between disability-related recipients: (1) those deemed 'fit for work' were immediately transferred onto the lower-paying

78   C. Bambra

Table 4.3 Towards 'Workfare' phase of UK disability policy (2003–2010)

2003	**Disability Discrimination Act 1995 (Amendment) Regulations 2003** Incorporates the disability provisions of recent EU Employment Directives, removed small employer exemption. Came into force in October 2004 **Pathways to Work Pilots** 'Return to work' credit for new claimants leaving Incapacity Benefit, Condition Management Programmes, and mandatory Work Focused Interviews
2004	**Pathways to Work Extension 1** Job Preparation Premium paid to those on Incapacity Benefit undertaking return to work activity, extended to Incapacity Benefit claims started in last two years
2005	**Disability Discrimination Act 2005** Extends service provisions to transportation. Definition of disability broadened to cover more people with HIV, cancer, and multiple sclerosis. New duty placed on public authorities to promote equality of opportunity for disabled people **Pathways to Work Extension 2** Pilot measures extended to cover around one-third of the UK **Job Retention and Rehabilitation pilot** Examines retention in work comparing employment-focussed support and health-based support
2007	**Welfare Reform Act** Announced the phase-out of Incapacity Benefit and introduced the Employment and Support Allowance from 2008 (see Box 4.1). Established Work Capability Assessment to assess entitlement to Employment and Support Allowance
2010	**Fit Note** Assesses fitness for work, as opposed to sickness and incapacity—active from 2010 **Equality Act** Merged previous antidiscrimination legislation relating to age, disability, gender, race, religion and belief, sexual orientation and gender reassignment into one piece of legislation. Set up the Equality and Human Rights Commission (which incorporated the Disability Rights Commission amongst others)

Source: Adapted from Bambra et al. (2005) and Bambra (2006)

Jobseeker's Allowance (a very conditional benefit worth around a third less in cash per week); (2) those deemed too 'incapacitated' for work were placed on the ESA with a 'support' premium and no conditionality (few recipients met the threshold for this classification); and (3) those considered 'sick but able to work' were placed on ESA with a 'work-related activity' premium (see Box 4.1). Those in the third group who failed to engage in compulsory 'work-related activity' lost the premium and received only the ESA basic rate (worth a third less than the 'work-related activity' benefit).

Also during this period, a new 'fit note' replaced the old general practitioner-administered 'sick note' (DWP 2009). The 'sick note' traditionally used by general practitioners (primary care physicians) to certify sickness absence operated on a zero-sum basis: an individual was either too sick to work or well enough to work. The aim of the 'fit note' was to assess fitness for work, as opposed to sickness, adding the option of being partially fit for work if certain issues are taken into account, including a phased return to work, altered hours, amended duties, and workplace adaptations. The fit note was intended to reduce the number of people on short-term sickness absence who then lose their employment and become long-term benefit recipients. It was also intended to address concerns that general practitioners were too close to their patients and too keen to sign people off—'on the sick'—particularly in areas or times of high unemployment (OECD 2009).

Although these reforms clearly built on the previous period of active welfare reform, the addition of such overt conditionality for people receiving disability-related benefits marked a new turn in UK social policy, signalling a clear break from the voluntary nature of previous participation in ALMPs (Bambra and Smith 2010). Therefore, it arguably marked the beginning of a third phase of policy towards the employment of people with a disability, distinguished by a move towards subjecting these recipients to a form of 'workfare' (Bambra 2011a). Indeed, in a report titled *Building Bridges to Work,* the government explicitly stated that *'the old-style, passive, incapacity benefits have been replaced by the new, active Employment and Support Allowance'* (DWP 2010, p. 7). The aim was to create a *'something for something'* approach that widens *'the right to support and deepens the responsibility to take up this support: individuals have the responsibility to move towards and into work, in return they should get the help they need to do so'* (DWP 2010, p. 21).

4.2.4   Austerity (Since 2011)

The term 'workfare' refers to those welfare reforms that link participation in employment programmes to ongoing receipt of benefits. Workfare is, thus, the obligation on welfare recipients to 'earn' their benefit payments via compulsory participation in training or compulsory 'work-for-benefit' style employment, including compulsory work for charities (Burghes 1987; Gibson et al. 2018). Workfare originated in the USA with the Clinton-era reforms of 1996, when the Personal Responsibility and Work Opportunity Reconciliation Act (PRWORA) introduced sanctions and benefit limits for millions of poor Americans, particularly lone mothers and their children: the so-called '99ers' (as benefit receipt is limited to 99 weeks). The PRWORA was considered a success, as welfare rolls more than halved in the first five years, from 12.2 million in 1996 to 5.3 million in 2001. However, the social and economic costs for individuals have been far more problematic, with only around 10–20% of those leaving welfare rolls actually finding employment that pays above the federal poverty line (Bambra 2011a).

Similar workfare-style reforms for disability-related benefits were enacted in the UK from 2010 onwards as part of the national austerity programme (Table 4.4). In economics, 'austerity' refers to reducing budget deficits in economic downturns by decreasing public expenditure, particularly on welfare, and/or increasing taxes (Bambra et al. 2016). Since 2010, the UK government has responded to the economic recession that followed the 2007–2008 global financial crisis by implementing a programme of austerity. This has been characterized by large-scale cuts to central and local government budgets, healthcare (NHS) privatization, and associated cuts to welfare services and benefits. Reductions in local government budgets and welfare cuts have hit the poorest parts of the country hardest (Beatty and Fothergill 2016), and the effects of tax and benefit reforms have largely been regressive, with low-income households of working age losing the most (Browne and Levell 2010). Working-age benefits have been particularly targeted, including disability-related benefits, with reductions, restrictions, and the introduction of sanctions (Bambra 2016; Bambra et al. 2016).

Table 4.4 'Austerity' phase of UK disability policy (since 2011)

2011	**Welfare Reform White Paper**
	Outlined plans for a new Universal Working Age benefit to replace Jobseeker's Allowance, Employment and Support Allowance, Income Support and so on. A new 'claimant contract' announced
2012	**Employment and Support Allowance 1-year limit**
	A one-year time limit to the receipt of contributory ESA for people in the Work Related Activity Group
	Claimant Contract
	Applies sanctions of three months', six months', and up to three years' benefit removal for those benefit recipients who refuse to take up a job offer
2013	**Personal Independence Payment (PIP)**
	Replacement of Disability Living Allowance (DLA) by Personal Independence Payment (PIP) for all new claims. Migration of all existing working-age DLA claimants onto PIP
	Universal Credit Roll out commences
	A single working-age benefit replacing ESA, JSA, and Income Support is implemented for all new claimants, gradually across the country
2015	**Working-age benefits value frozen**
	Value frozen for four years from 2016 (not uprated with inflation)
	ESA Payments Reduced
	Work-related activity element of Employment and Support Allowance (ESA) payments reduced to Jobseeker's Allowance (JSA) levels
2017	**Universal Credit Roll Full Implementation**
	A single working-age benefit replacing ESA, JSA, and Income Support is rolled out across the country for all existing claimants

Source: Adapted from Bambra (2016)

ESA was reformed in 2011, limiting entitlement to ESA to one year for recipients in the 'work-related activity' group. After one year, they had no right to insurance-based benefits (not even Jobseeker's Allowance), and so became reliant on support from their family, charities, or means-tested public assistance (Income Support). For the great majority of recipients, ESA thus became a temporary benefit, designed to 'activate the aspirations' of recipients and encourage them to look for and take up paid work, marking a shift in the 'culture' of 'incapacity benefits' from 'invalidity to employability' (Bambra 2011a). In 2012, a 'claimant contract' with benefit sanctions (of three months', six months', or up to three years' benefit removal) was introduced for all 'active' benefits: the sanctions applied to recipients who refused to accept a job offer or missed their appointments with vocational services. In 2015, the value of the 'work-related activity' element of ESA was reduced to the level of Jobseeker's Allowance, thus removing the premium of a 33% higher rate in weekly income.

With the phased rollout of the new Universal Credit benefit, which began in 2013 and continues today (see Box 4.1), ESA is being gradually abolished. Universal Credit is a single working-age benefit intended to replace Jobseeker's Allowance (unemployment benefit), Income Support (means-tested social assistance), and ESA (disability-related benefit). Compulsory work-for-benefit and the claimant contract are key components of Universal Credit, and they apply to recipients of all benefits, including disability-related payments. Other significant welfare reforms applied to all working-age benefits (such as the under-occupancy charge [more commonly referred to as the 'Bedroom Tax']) have also impacted on disability-related benefit claimants (for a full overview of austerity and welfare reform, see Schrecker and Bambra 2015).

4.2.5   Employment Effects of Policy Changes

The shifts from passive to active/workfare approaches to disability support were justified by politicians and policymakers as means to increase the employment and labour market participation of people with a disability. However, various reviews of the effectiveness of such ALMPs and benefit entitlement restrictions have found very little evidence of positive contribution to the employment of disabled people (Bambra et al. 2005; Bambra 2006; Barr et al. 2010; Clayton et al. 2011, 2012). For example, one review concluded that *'no large-scale programme has demonstrated through a scientifically rigorous study that it improves employment rates by more than a few percentage points'* (Bambra 2006); another found that benefit restrictions have had no positive impacts on employment (Barr et al. 2010). UK policy has largely focused on supply-side measures, rather than trying to increase employer demand (Bambra 2006, 2011a).

Supply-side ALMP interventions (such as training, work placements, advice and support services, or in-work benefits) are concerned with increasing the availability and work readiness of individuals with a disability. Accordingly, they are designed to overcome some of the employment barriers faced by people with a disability, particularly their lack of skills or work experience, and financial uncertainty about the transition into paid employment. UK evidence suggests that some training and advice interventions can have small positive impacts on employment rates, depending on the characteristics of participants, such as 'job-readiness' or type of illness, as well as the local labour market context (Bambra et al. 2005). However, given the small-scale and poor-quality nature of the evaluations, it is impossible to determine if improved employment chances were due to the effectiveness of the interventions themselves or to external factors, such as a general upturn in employment rates in the early 2000s. There is little evidence that in-work benefits were effective in increasing employment (Bambra 2006).

Further workfare-style interventions (including benefit restrictions, sanctions, and conditionality) can be considered as another type of supply-side ALMP intervention, albeit a very radical one, which aims to increase the employment of disabled people by making it harder for them to survive outside the labour market. Barr et al. (2010) performed an international systematic review of the employment effects of restricting entitlements to welfare benefits for people with a disability, considering the UK, Canada, Denmark, Sweden, and Norway. They concluded that 'there is insufficient evidence, and what there is [is] equivocal, to indicate whether [restrictive] changes in benefit eligibility requirements ... will have an impact on the employment of people with disabilities and chronic illness in well-developed welfare states' (Barr et al. 2010, p. 1106). Another international study suggests that conditionality interventions raise employment rates in non-disabled people but lower them among disabled people (Baumberg Geiger 2017). Research in the UK links the WCA to deterioration in mental health among those assessed (Barr et al. 2016), and benefit sanctions have been associated with decreased return to work among disabled people (National Audit Office 2016). Although the evidence is inconclusive, a suggested explanation for this latter finding is that people completely drop out of the system, preferring to suffer economic hardship or rely on unreported income or support from local authorities, charities, or friends and family (National Audit Office 2016).

Demand-side ALMP interventions (such as financial incentives for employers, disability discrimination legislation, and accessibility interventions) focus on increasing the demand for disabled workers among employers (Bambra 2006). They attempt to combat the other type of employment barriers faced by people with a disability: employer uncertainty and the physical difficulties of workplaces. Demand-side interventions have been less well used in the UK (Bambra 2006, 2011a), with evidence suggesting that their impact on employment has been very limited. For example, financial interventions designed to incentivize employers were ineffective because they did not adequately off-set the perceived risks and costs of employing a disabled person (Bambra 2006). Likewise, disability legislation had no effect on employers' recruitment decisions, with the majority of employers unaware of its employment provisions (Roberts et al. 2004); the employment gap between those with and without a health condition or disability actually increased after the Disability Discrimination Act was introduced (Pope and Bambra 2005). Only accessibility interventions (workplace adjustments) appear to have a more positive employment impact, but uptake by employers has been very low (Clayton et al. 2012).

4.3   The Political Economy of UK Disability Policy

Through compulsory involvement in ALMPs, sanctions, and time-limits on benefit receipt, UK policy on disability-related benefits has clearly abandoned the 'passive' approach that characterized most of the post-war period. However, embracing conditionality is consistent with the reform of other UK out-of-work benefits (such as the reforms to unemployment benefit of the 1980s and 1990s) and changes to disability-related benefits elsewhere, such as in Australia, the USA, and other EU countries (OECD 2009). In the UK, these welfare reforms are usually presented (by politicians from both the centre-left and centre-right) as attempts to reintroduce recipients to the labour market or incentivize unemployed people to seek and return to work. However, a political economy perspective provides an alternative explanation for these disability reforms, framing them as a key part of wider neoliberal restructuring of the welfare state; specifically, they contribute to reasserting labour discipline and reclassifying people with a disability as the 'undeserving' poor (Bambra and Smith 2010; Bambra 2011a; Schrecker and Bambra 2015).

4.3.1 The Neoliberalization of the Welfare State

The different phases of disability policy in the UK reflect wider trends in the general development of the welfare state. Indeed, the most recent shift towards workfare is the culmination of the neoliberalization project to 'hollow out' the welfare state (Rhodes 1994).

For most of the nineteenth century, there was minimal state provision of welfare beyond very basic 'poor relief', comprising basic food rations and shelter (often provided via institutions, such as the English workhouse system). Beyond these provisions, welfare came via family members or charity (particularly the Church). This began to change in the early twentieth century with the introduction of rudimentary state-organized welfare systems, which provided basic pensions, unemployment, and sickness benefits funded via social insurance payments (e.g. the 1911 National Insurance Act in the UK or the Bismarckian welfare reforms of 1880s Germany). Such schemes were highly selective in terms of population coverage, typically excluding non-workers, and therefore most women.

It was not until after the Second World War (1945) that a more comprehensive welfare state—often termed the 'Keynesian welfare state'—was established in most market democracies. To a greater or lesser extent, this 'golden age' of welfare state capitalism was characterized by centralism, universalism, and Keynesian economics. Keynesian economic models entailed active macroeconomic management by the state (such as interventionist fiscal policy, a large public sector, and a mixed economy), full (male, able-bodied) employment, high public expenditure, and the promotion of mass consumption via a more redistributive tax and welfare system. There was also mainstream political consensus in favour of the welfare state and the redistribution it encompassed. In the golden age of welfare state expansion (1940s–1960s), Western countries experienced significant improvements to public housing and healthcare, and workers enjoyed their highest ever share of national income (Schrecker and Bambra 2015).

However, golden-age welfare states varied considerably in the services they provided and the generosity and coverage of social insurance and welfare benefits (Esping-Andersen 1990). The UK welfare state was a broadly liberal regime (like the other Anglo-American countries of Australia, Canada, Ireland, New Zealand, and the USA). State provision of welfare was fairly minimal; social insurance benefits were modest and often had strict entitlement criteria; and recipients were often subject to means-testing, with receipt stigmatized. In this model, even in the post-war period, the dominance of the market was encouraged by guaranteeing only a minimum level of state support, alongside the subsidizing of private welfare schemes. A stark division existed between those who relied on state aid (largely the poor) and those able to afford private provision.

This golden age of the welfare state effectively ended with the economic crisis of the 1970s (when rising oil prices combined with high inflation and high unemployment), combined with the simultaneous rise of neoliberalism—or 'market fundamentalism'—as the dominant political and economic ideology (Schrecker and Bambra 2015). The fundamental presuppositions of neoliberalism are as follows: (1) markets are the normal, natural, and preferable way of organizing human interaction; (2) the primary function of the state is to ensure the efficient functioning of markets; and (3) institutions or policies whose outcomes differ from what would be expected in a functioning market require justification (Ward and England 2007). The core tenets of neoliberalism remained on the margins of mainstream politics in the wealthy world until the 1970s (Harvey 2005). At that point, the economic uncertainties of 'stagflation'—the simultaneous occurrence of high inflation and high unemployment—'created a newly receptive climate among both elites and, in many countries, electorates' (Schrecker and Bambra 2015, p. 13).

The literature offers various narratives of the advance of neoliberalism. One regards neoliberal policies as pragmatic responses to a changing global economic environment, largely outside the control of individual national governments. Under these new conditions, neoliberal policies were the only ones that 'worked' (Fourcade-Gourinchas and Babb 2002). Another views neoliberalism as a political project aimed at restoring the class power of business (capital), which had been eroded by the rise of the welfare state and associated redistributive policies (Harvey 2005). It is clear, however, that neoliberalism is best understood as having multiple dimensions, including: concrete policy programmes and innovations (e.g. scaling back the welfare state); more general reorganization of state institutions (e.g. privatization and contracting-out); and an implicit ideology that gives primacy to the individual, as opposed to the collective. The latter is exemplified by Margaret Thatcher's (in)famous comment: 'there is no such thing as society, only individuals and their families' (Ward and England 2007).

The elections of Thatcher's Conservatives in the UK (1979), Republican Ronald Reagan as US president (1980), and Helmut Kohl as West German Chancellor (1982) represented key turning points. The political consensus of the golden age began to break down as governments started to dismantle and restructure the welfare state. The 'reforms' were characterized by the privatization and marketization of welfare services; entitlement restrictions and stricter qualifying conditions for welfare benefits; a shift towards targeting and means-testing; cuts or limited increases to the actual cash values of benefits; modified funding arrangements (with a shift from business taxation towards consumption taxes); increased emphasis on active, rather than passive, welfare policies; deregulation of the economy, with the promotion of labour market flexibility, supply-side economics, and a desire to minimize public social expenditure; and the subordination of social policy to market demands (Bambra et al. 2010). This significantly reduced the support provided to people out of work. Analysis of the unemployment replacement rate—the percentage of an average worker's wage replaced by unemployment benefits—provides a telling illustration. In the UK, the rate for one earner supporting a partner and two children declined from 69% in 1971 to 36% in 1990. For a single worker with no dependents, the decline was even more dramatic, falling from 54% in 1971 to 20% or less from 1990 onwards (Scruggs et al. 2014).

This neoliberal restructuring of the welfare state has been analysed by some commentators as a shift from Keynesian welfare state capitalism, which could afford and required a high level of public welfare expenditure, to a system of 'workfare state capitalism', in which high welfare expenditure is considered incompatible with a profitable economy (Jessop 1991). Like welfare states, there are variants on the workfare model, reflecting the ongoing influence of historical welfare structures and politics, alongside inter-state variations in public opinion and regime differences in policy responses to common challenges (Jessop 1991). The neoliberal workfare state emphasizes privatizing state enterprise and welfare services and deregulating the private sector (Jessop 1991).

Since the 2007–2008 financial crisis, the austerity policies pursued by the UK government have led to further welfare state reforms advancing the neoliberal model, termed neoliberalism 2.0 (Schrecker and Bambra 2015). The financial crisis was triggered by a downturn in the US housing market, inducing a massive collapse in financial markets across the world. Banks increasingly required state bailouts: for example, the retail bank Northern Rock was nationalized in the UK, whilst Lehmann Brothers investment bank filed for bankruptcy and the mortgage companies Freddie Mac and Fannie Mae were given major government bailouts in the USA. Stock markets fell precipitously as effects in the 'real' economy began to be felt, with unemployment rates exceeding 10% in the USA and the Eurozone. In 2009, the International Monetary Fund announced that the global economy was experiencing its worst period for 60 years (Gamble 2009). The global economic recession continued throughout 2009 and 2010. Although many wealthy governments injected liquidity into their economies (so-called quantitative easing), this was accompanied in many European countries (including the UK, but most notably Greece and Spain) by escalating public expenditure cuts.

Though less affected than the Eurozone by the financial crisis and subsequent recession, the UK still embarked on a programme of austerity. From 2010 to 2015, the coalition government of the Conservatives and Liberal Democrats enacted large-scale cuts to central and local government budgets, increased health service (NHS) privatization, and made steep cuts to welfare services and benefits (including those for people with disabilities). It has been estimated that the UK welfare reforms enacted up to 2015 will take nearly £19 billion a year out of the economy by 2020 (Beatty and Fothergill 2016). This is equivalent to around £470 a year for every working-age adult in the country. The biggest financial losses arise from reforms to disability-related benefits, estimated at £4.3 billion a year (Beatty and Fothergill 2016). In England, local government spending (which includes social care) also fell by nearly 30% in real terms between 2008 and 2015. With the austerity programme continuing since the Conservatives won an electoral majority in 2015, this is the wider neoliberal context within which UK disability and rehabilitation policy has developed.

4.3.2   Reasserting Labour Discipline and No Longer Deserving

Regarding UK disability policy, two trends in the wider neoliberalization of the welfare state require particular attention: the reassertion of labour discipline and the shift from 'deserving' to 'undeserving' poor (Bambra and Smith 2010). The reforms to disability-related welfare benefits can be conceptualized as reasserting labour discipline and instilling the work ethic, accompanied by a notable shift in the language for classifying disability-related benefit recipients, who are no longer perceived as deserving of public/welfare state support. This discourse and the associated policy changes impact on all people with a disability, particularly those with poor mental health (and other 'hidden disabilities') or musculoskeletal problems. However, whilst those with very complicated or severe disabilities (e.g. resulting from an accident or terminal condition) receive more public sympathy and support, they are still subject to the same surveillance regime and poverty-level benefits (see, e.g. The Independent 2016, March 17).

There are four salient aspects of the labour discipline thesis for UK disability policy. First, commentators such as Ginsburg argue that the social security benefits system disciplines the labour force by attaching conditions to benefits, which 'ensure that the intransigent worker cannot so easily turn to the welfare state for support' (Ginsburg 1979). This reasoning is evident in the UK reforms, as recipients of the ESA must participate in employability schemes to receive full benefits. Second, following Piven and Cloward (1971), the reforms can be seen as part of a wider welfare state retrenchment, whereby welfare provisions serve to 'regulate the poor'. On this basis, the provision tends to be expanded at times of political unrest and subsequently reduced once social peace is restored. For example, in the USA, the civil unrest of the 1960s was associated with a subsequent expansion of the welfare state, followed up by a series of cut backs under the 1980s Reagan administration after social order had been restored. Since the UK has recently experienced a period of relative 'peace', it might be expected for welfare benefits to be cut back, with the financial crisis and austerity programme providing a narrative cloak. Third, Katz (1986) argues that the stigma associated with benefit receipt also serves to discipline the labour force, with dependency on state benefits considered not only a misfortune but also a moral failure. The tiered approach of the ESA system may heighten this aspect of labour discipline, with those deemed 'sick but able to work' feeling particularly stigmatized. Finally, as Byrne (2005) contends, the last two decades' reforms to welfare provision in the UK and elsewhere (particularly the USA) have aimed not to end benefit dependency but to link benefit receipt more closely to work. The welfare reforms can, thus, be seen as the somewhat logical extension of using the benefits system to assert the work ethic. The reforms similarly reinforce divisions of who is (*working poor*) and who is not (*non-working poor*) deserving of state support.

The separation of disability-related claims into two distinct categories of deserving and less- or non-deserving is, on the one hand, a logical consequence of the welfare reform philosophy of '*work for those who can, welfare for those who cannot*'. It also acknowledges that previous, more passive approaches have often exacerbated the labour market exclusion experienced by people with a disability or chronic illness (Barnes 1991). On the other hand, the division into two levels of benefits is inevitably tied to notions of the 'deserving' and 'undeserving' poor (Katz 1986; van Oorschot 2006). Disability-related benefits were the last in the UK to be extensively reformed and, until recently, did not attract as much popular stigma as other benefit types (most notably lone-parent benefits). This is also the case in other countries, where people receiving benefits due to ill health or disability have been viewed and treated as more 'deserving' or morally worthy than recipients of other types of benefit (van Oorschot 2006). Indeed, as Stone argues in *The Disabled State* (1986), disability was long considered a special administrative category in the welfare states of many Western countries, with distinctive entitlements in the form of social aid and exemptions from certain obligations of citizenship, such as the duty to work (Stone 1986, p. 4). Welfare reform in this area can, thus, be seen as a clear departure from the more accommodating perspective of the 'passive welfare' period, as a new political discourse dictates that certain types of disability are less deserving of public support than others.

People with a disability or chronic illness are variously categorized and re-categorized within the 'deserving' and 'undeserving' poor dichotomy. The relations of production which arose from capitalist industrialization established a discourse of 'able-bodiedness' which excluded the impaired and the chronically ill from the workplace and the general discourse of employability (Oliver 1990; Stone 1986). However, this has been renegotiated at various times and on different terms. For example, the context of the Second World War forced employers to recruit groups traditionally regarded as unemployable, such as women or people with disabilities. The Disabled Persons (Employment) Act 1944 established the long-term sick and disabled as the 'deserving' poor. In the welfare reforms implemented since the 1990s, this 'deserving' and 'undeserving' dichotomy has clearly been renegotiated. This redrawing was gradual, with those defined as sick but not disabled the first to be moved from the 'deserving' to the 'undeserving' poor category (the ESA Work Related Activity group). The workfare reforms implemented since the early 2000s then led to nearly *all* people with a disability being re-categorized (as the threshold for receiving unconditional support became much harder to meet). Further, the programme of austerity, with its associated sweeping benefit cuts, started a process whereby even those 'deserving' of unconditional support had their entitlements significantly curtailed. This has arguably diminished the status of people with a disability and subjected them to significant new levels of surveillance, previously reserved for the able-bodied 'undeserving' poor (Katz 1986).

4.4   Conclusion

This chapter has examined vocational rehabilitation services and support for people with disabilities in the UK, placing them within a wider welfare, labour market, and social policy context. It has overviewed the historical evolution of social policy in the UK regarding the employment of people with a disability, considering four key phases: passive welfare of the 1970s and 1980s (typified by compulsory employment quotas and passive welfare benefits); active welfare of the 1990s and early 2000s (including antidiscrimination legislation, welfare to work, and active welfare benefits); the workfare approach of the mid-2000s (typified by conditionality and compulsory work-for-benefit); and the austerity phase since 2011 (typified by sanctions, reductions, and restrictions). These policy changes have been analysed from a political economy perspective, exploring the broader context of the neoliberal restructuring of the welfare state and the specific issues of reasserting labour discipline and reclassifying people with a disability from 'deserving' to 'undeserving' subjects. Disability and rehabilitation policy in the UK has shifted radically, particularly since the 1990s. However, the effects of these reforms on employment rates and labour market inclusion has been very limited; instead, they have only served to further marginalize and stigmatize disabled people.

References

Bambra, C. (2006). The influence of government programmes and pilots on the employment of disabled workers. In K. Needels & B. Schmitz (Eds.), *Economic and social costs and benefits to employers for retaining, recruiting and employing disabled people and/or people with health conditions or an injury: A review of the evidence*. London: DWP Research Report no. 400.

Bambra, C. (2011a). *Work, worklessness and the political economy of health*. Oxford: Oxford University Press.

Bambra, C. (2011b). Work, worklessness and the political economy of health inequalities. *Journal of Epidemiology and Community Health, 65*, 746–750.

Bambra, C. (2016). *Health divides*. Bristol: Policy Press.

Bambra, C., & Pope, D. (2007). What are the effects of anti-discriminatory legislation on socioeconomic inequalities in the employment consequences of ill health and disability? *Journal of Epidemiology and Community Health, 61*, 421–426.

Bambra, C., & Smith, K. (2010). No longer deserving? Sickness benefit reform and the politics of (ill) health. *Critical Public Health, 20*, 71–84.

Bambra, C., Whitehead, M., & Hamilton, V. (2005). Does "welfare to work" work? A systematic review of the effectiveness of the UK's welfare to work programmes for people with a chronic illness or disability. *Social Science and Medicine, 60*, 1905–1918.

Bambra, C., Netuveli, G., & Eikemo, T. (2010). Welfare state regime life courses: The development of Western European welfare state regimes and age-related patterns of educational inequalities in self-reported health. *International Journal of Health Services, 40*(3), 399–420.

Bambra, C., Garthwaite, K., Copeland, A., & Barr, B. (2016). Chapter 12: All in it together? Health inequalities, welfare austerity and the 'great recession'. In K. E. Smith, S. Hill, & C. Bambra (Eds.), *Health inequalities: Critical perspectives* (pp. 164–176). Oxford: Oxford University Press.

Barnes, C. (1991). *Disabled people in Britain and discrimination: A case for anti-discrimination legislation*. London: Hurst Calgary.

Barr, B., Clayton, S., Whitehead, M., Thielen, K., Burstrom, B., Nylen, L., & Dahl, E. (2010). To what extent have relaxed eligibility requirements and increased generosity of disability benefits acted as disincentives for employment? A systematic review of evidence from countries with well-developed welfare systems. *Journal of Epidemiology and Community Health, 64*, 1106–1114.

Barr, B., Taylor-Robinson, D., Stuckler, D., Loopstra, R., Reeves, A., & Whitehead, M. (2016). 'First, do no harm': Are disability assessments associated with adverse trends in mental health? A longitudinal ecological study. *Journal of Epidemiology and Community Health, 70*(4), 339–345.

Baumberg Geiger, B. (2017). Benefits conditionality for disabled people: Stylised facts from a review of international evidence and practice. *Journal of Poverty and Social Justice, 25*(2), 107–128.

Beatty, C., & Fothergill, S. (2016). *The uneven impact of welfare reform. The financial losses to places and people*. Centre for Regional Economic and Social Research Sheffield Hallam University. http://www.shu.ac.uk/research/cresr/sites/shu.ac.uk/files/welfare-reform-2016_1.pdf. Accessed 21 Mar 2018.

Black, C. (2008). *Dame Carol Black's review of the health of the working age population – Working for a healthier tomorrow*. London: The Stationery Office (TSO).

Black, C. (2016). *An independent review into the impact on employment outcomes of drug or alcohol addiction, and obesity.* London: Her Majesty's Stationery Office (HMSO).

Browne, J., & Levell, P. (2010). *The distributional effect of tax and benefit reforms to be introduced between June 2010 and April 2014: A revised assessment.* London: Institute for Fiscal Studies.

Burghes, L. (1987). *Made in the USA: A review of workfare.* London: Unemployment Unit.

Byrne, D. (2005). *Social exclusion.* Milton Keynes: Open University.

Clayton, S., Bambra, C., Gosling, R., Povall, S., Misso, K., & Whitehead, M. (2011). Assembling the evidence jigsaw: Insights from a systematic review of UK studies of return to work initiatives for disabled and chronically ill people. *BMC Public Health, 11,* 170.

Clayton, S., Barr, B., Nylen, L., Burstrom, B., Thielen, K., Diderichsen, F., et al. (2012). Effectiveness of return-to-work interventions for disabled people: A systematic review of government initiatives focused on changing the behaviour of employers. *European Journal of Public Health, 22,* 434–439.

DWP. (2010). *Building bridges to work – Helping the long term unemployed back to work.* London: TSO.

DWP (Department for Work and Pensions). (2009). *Building Britain's recovery: Achieving full employment.* London: TSO.

Esping-Andersen, G. (1990). *The three worlds of welfare capitalism.* London: Polity.

Fourcade-Gourinchas, M., & Babb, S. L. (2002). The rebirth of the liberal creed: Paths to neoliberalism in four countries. *American Journal of Sociology, 108*(3), 533–579.

Fulcher, J., & Scott, J. (2003). The state, social policy and welfare. In *Sociology.* Oxford: Oxford University Press.

Gabbay, M., Taylor, L., Sheppard, L., Hillage, J., Bambra, C., Ford, F., et al. (2011). National Institute for Health and Clinical Excellence (NICE) Guidance on long term sickness and incapacity. *British Journal of General Practice, 61,* e118–e124.

Gamble, A. (2009). *The spectre at the feast: Capitalist crisis and the politics of recession.* Basingstoke: Palgrave.

Gibson, M., Thomson, H., Banas, K., Lutje, V., McKee, M., Martin, S., et al. (2018). Welfare to work interventions and their effects on the health and well-being of lone parents and their children (Review). *Cochrane Database of Systematic Reviews,* (2), CD009820.

Ginsburg, N. (1979). *Class, capital and social policy.* London: Macmillan.

Goldstone, C., & Meager, N. (2002). *Barriers to employment for disabled people.* London: Department for Work and Pensions.

Harvey, D. (2005). *A brief history of neoliberalism.* Oxford: Oxford University Press.

House of Commons Library. (2018). *People with disabilities in employment.* http://researchbriefings.files.parliament.uk/documents/CBP-7540/CBP-7540.pdf. Accessed 7 Dec 2018.

Houston, D., & Lindsay, C. (2010). Fit for work? Health, employability and challenges for the UK welfare reform agenda. *Policy Studies, 31,* 133–142.

Jessop, B. (1991). The welfare state in transition from Fordism to post-Fordism. In B. Jessop (Ed.), *The politics of flexibility: Restructuring state and industry in Britain, Germany and Scandinavia* (pp. 82–105). Aldershot: Edward Elgar.

Katz, M. B. (1986). *In the shadow of the poorhouse: A social history of welfare in America.* New York: Basic Books.

National Audit Office. (2016). *Benefit sanctions.* London: HMSO.

Norman, P., & Bambra, C. (2007). The utility of medically certified sickness absence as an updatable indicator of population health. *Population, Space and Place, 13,* 333–352.

OECD. (2009). *Sickness, disability and work: Background paper.* http://www.oecd.org/dataoecd/42/15/42699911.pdf. Accessed 5 Apr 2018.

OECD (Organisation for Economic Co-operation and Development). (2003). *Transforming disability into ability: Policies to promote work and income security for disabled people.* Paris: OECD.

Office for National Statistics. (2018). *Labour force statistics.* https://www.ons.gov.uk/employmentandlabourmarket/peopleinwork/employmentandemployeetypes/bulletins/uklabourmarket/november2018#economic-inactivity. Accessed 7 Dec 2018.

Oliver, M. (1990). *The politics of disablement.* London: Macmillan.

Oliver, M., & Barnes, C. (1998). *Disabled people and social policy.* London: Longman.

Piven, F., & Cloward, R. (1971). *Regulating the poor: The functions of public welfare.* New York: Vintage Books.

Pope, D., & Bambra, C. (2005). Has the Disability Discrimination Act closed the employment gap? *Disability and Rehabilitation, 27,* 1261–1266.

Rhodes, R. (1994). The hollowing out of the state: The changing nature of the public service in Britain. *The Political Quarterly, 65,* 138–151.

Roberts, S., Heaver, C., Hill, K., et al. (2004). *Disability in the workplace: Employers' and service providers responses to the Disability Discrimination Act in 2003 and preparations for the 2004 changes.* London: DWP.

Royal College of Physicians. (2010). *Medical rehabilitation in 2011 and beyond.* Report of a working party. London. https://www.bsrm.org.uk/downloads/medical-rehabilitation-2011-and-beyond.pdf. Accessed 6 Dec 2018.

Schrecker, T., & Bambra, C. (2015). *How politics makes us sick – Neoliberal epidemics.* London: Palgrave Macmillan.

Scruggs, L., Detlef, J., & Kuitto, K. (2014). *Comparative welfare entitlements dataset 2, version 2014-03 2014.* University of Connecticut & University of Greifswald. http://cwed2.org/. Accessed 15 Apr 2019.

Stone, D. A. (1986). *The disabled state.* New York: Templeton.

The Independent. (2016, March 17). *Terminally ill cancer patient 'told she is not disabled enough for benefits'.* https://www.independent.co.uk/news/uk/politics/terminally-ill-cancer-patient-told-she-is-not-disabled-enough-for-benefits-a6936831.html. Accessed 6 Dec 2018.

van Oorschot, W. (2006). Making the difference in social Europe: Deservingness perceptions among citizens of European welfare states. *Journal of European Social Policy, 16,* 23–42.

Waddell, G., & Burton, A. (2006). *Is work good for your health and wellbeing?* London: TSO.

Ward, A. B. (2005). Rehabilitation medicine: The European perspective. *American Journal of Physical Medicine & Rehabilitation, 84,* 233–237.

Ward, K., & England, K. (2007). Introduction: Reading neoliberalization. In *Neoliberalization: States, networks, peoples* (pp. 1–22). Oxford: Blackwell.

Warren, J., Garthwaite, K., & Bambra, C. (2014). After ATOS: Is ESA fit for work and does the WCA have a future? *Disability and Society, 29*(8), 1319–1323.

5

The Redesigning of Neurorehabilitation in Denmark and Norway

Marte Feiring and Inge Storgaard Bonfils

5.1 Introduction

A strong impulse towards evidence-based policies and practices increasingly characterizes the services for disability and rehabilitation. The British National Clinical Guideline for Stroke presents the following problem-solution model, linking the worldwide problem of disabling stroke to the need for more evidence-based guidelines:

> The Global Burden of Disease Study highlights how stroke represents one of the foremost burdens of lifelong disability around the world. The need for clear, evidence-based guidance for the everyday practice of many

M. Feiring (✉)
Department of Physiotherapy, Oslo Metropolitan University, Oslo, Norway
e-mail: mafei@oslomet.no

I. S. Bonfils
Department of Social Work, University College Copenhagen,
Copenhagen, Denmark
e-mail: inbo@kp.dk

© The Author(s) 2019
I. Harsløf et al. (eds.), *New Dynamics of Disability and Rehabilitation*,
https://doi.org/10.1007/978-981-13-7346-6_5

thousands of practitioners in stroke thus remains as great as ever. (Bowen et al. 2016, p. ii)

This chapter addresses the call for 'clear evidence-based guidance', analysing how political technologies, such as clinical guidelines and service guides, are made to redesign rehabilitation practices. Rehabilitation is an interprofessional and cross-sectoral practice involving the health, education, employment, and social welfare sectors. Acute medical rehabilitation is provided in hospitals and specialist rehabilitation centres, while longer-term rehabilitation takes place within local communities in primary health care centres, rehabilitation centres, schools, workplaces, prisons, or homes (WHO 2017). This confirms that rehabilitation is a multicomponent practice. For Hammell (2006), rehabilitation is client-centred practices aiming at enabling someone to live well with impairment. We will argue that such composite practices are characterized by uncertainty that challenges the possibilities for producing clear scientific evidence.

Recent decades have witnessed great political and social transformation in the Nordic countries. One major aspect is the change from relying on experiential knowledge to privileging evidence-based rehabilitation practices (Greenhalgh et al. 2015). Another is the reframing of conventional rehabilitation services into more composite, interprofessional approaches that aim to activate clients. A third shift is from traditional government to more complex, management-inspired ways of governing, known as new liberalism or advanced liberalism (Fairclough 2003; Rose 2006; Feiring 2016).

In this chapter, we will analyse the political technologies applied in rehabilitation services today. The term 'technology' is understood as 'the complex of mundane programmes, documents and procedures through which authorities seek to embody and give effect to governmental ambitions' (Rose and Miller 2010, p. 273). A study of political technologies can increase understanding of how governing authorities address and structure what they perceive as problems, solutions, and organizational conditions in rehabilitation practices.

Denmark and Norway are the national cases of this study. Both countries have undergone substantial welfare and health reforms, followed up by a redesigning and pluralization of political technologies, understood as the programmes, documents, and procedures regulating neurorehabilitation practices. Their respective healthcare sectors have performed rehabilitation under different administrative systems since the 1990s. The health ministry is the coordinating and overall authority of health-related rehabilitation in both countries. However, from 1945 until the mid-1990s, rehabilitation fell within the remit of the social authorities in Denmark and labour authorities in Norway.

In 1998, Denmark rolled out a major social reform involving the de-institutionalization of services for marginal groups, including chronically ill and disabled persons (Bonfils 2003). This was followed a decade later by the Structural Reform, which came into force in 2007. The Structural Reform reduced the number of municipalities from 271 to 98, the 13 counties to 5 regions, and altered the division of responsibility between the state, regions, and municipalities. It also further decentralized social and rehabilitation services from county to municipal level. The new municipalities have full authoritative and financial responsibility for longer-term rehabilitation matters, while the regions are mainly responsible for acute and specialist rehabilitation (Olsen 2008; Bonfils and Berger 2010).

In 2006, Norway merged its employment and national insurance administrations to form the Norwegian Labour and Welfare Administration, and established partnership arrangements between the new NAV and local government social services to formalize collaboration. Subsequently, the Coordination Reform was rolled out in 2012, to integrate and facilitate a shift from hospital-dominated treatment to prevention and general healthcare (Feiring 2012; Røberg et al. 2016). A key element of this reform was the introduction of municipal co-financing for residents' hospitalization following discharge from a specialized hospital (Ministry of Health and Care Services 2009, pp. 8–9).

Both countries have implemented management-inspired governing programmes and post-New Public Management logics, including the introduction of purchaser-provider arrangements, so as to create an internal market for rehabilitation services (Olsen 2008; Bonfils and Berger 2010; Byrkjeflot 2011). Their respective national reforms aimed to promote the integration of rehabilitation across different levels of the service structure, that is, state, regions, and municipalities. They have also led to new modes of governing that can be termed 'decentralized centralization' or 'government at a distance' (Rose 1999). Both governments have produced new standards, procedures, guides, and guidelines to standardize and monitor the efficiency and efficacy of regional and local authorities.

This study analyses five policy documents published by the national health authorities in Denmark and Norway. Three of the documents are guidelines concerning brain-injured persons, founded on international evidence-based research, while the other two documents are service guides promoting advice to support national rehabilitation practices more generally (see Sect. 5.3 for details of the five documents). By studying political technologies through document analysis, we aim to reveal how government programmes frame, construct, and monitor rehabilitation practices.

Adopting the framework of critical discourse analysis (CDA), we undertake a comparative study of central policy documents regulating neurorehabilitation practices in the two countries. We apply two analytical concepts: 'intertextuality', for identifying the relationship between the key documents and other relevant texts, and 'interdiscursivity', for identifying whether the diverse documents construct a mixture of styles, genres, and discourses in a rehabilitation context. According to Fairclough (2003), social practices undergoing transformations are often characterized by strong elements of intertextuality and interdiscursivity. Because rehabilitation is a service of great importance to chronically ill and disabled persons, it is crucial to analyse the main written recommendations, advice, and support provided by the health authorities in clinical guidelines and service guides. Our aim is to elaborate on how clinical guidelines and service guides, seen as political technologies, regulate neurorehabilitation practices in Denmark and Norway.

5.2 A Theoretical and Methodological Framework

This chapter draws on the theoretical and methodological frameworks of Norman Fairclough (2000, 2003) and Nikolas Rose (1999, 2006) to analyse the production of political technologies supporting rehabilitation practices in the two countries. Following Fairclough (2003, p. 133), we understand discourse as 'language in use' in a social context or 'ways of representing the social world', and we apply a combination of textual and social analysis.

In our study, we follow Rose who identifies three transformations embedded in what he terms advanced liberal democracies. First, the relationship between government and knowledge (politics and expertise) is shifting, entailing more accounting and management and a more regulated autonomy for knowledge-groups. Second, there is increasing use of political technologies, understood as programmes, documents, and procedures deployed for defining, guiding, assessing, and standardizing in order to effect governmental strategies. Third, there is increasing governing of the citizens as subjects, with a new role intended for the subjects involving a more active and regulated citizenship (Rose 2006).

In the language of Fairclough (2003), a reconstruction of relations between social, political, and economic domains is taking place, as well as a rescaling of relations between the global, national, regional, and local levels of social life. Our research investigates how such reconstruction and rescaling processes are articulated in policy documents governing rehabilitation practices today. As mentioned above, we use the twin textual analysis tools of *intertextuality* and *interdiscursivity*. We use *intertextuality* to identify the relationship between the studied documents and other texts (related laws and regulations, etc.). As a type of 'constitutive intertextuality', *interdiscursivity* helps us to see articulations of different genres, styles, and language representations in the key documents. For example, the right of a service recipient to an individual care plan, as regulated under several legal acts, is rearticulated into the language of science in clinical guidelines. We are interested in exploring and understanding this type of translations.

5.3   Collecting Documents

To identify relevant documents, we set two alternative criteria for selection: (1) central policy and administrative service guides to rehabilitation in general; or (2) specific clinical guidelines for neurorehabilitation. Because the political and administrative systems in Denmark and Norway employ different types of documents for administrative purpose, we selected documents that represent both categories (i.e. guides and guidelines). However, they differ in genre and style. We selected five documents altogether: three from Denmark and two from Norway.

The three Danish documents are as follows: *Guide to municipal rehabilitation* (hereafter 'DK Service Guide'; Ministry of Internal and Health Affairs et al. 2011); *Brain injury rehabilitation—a health technology assessment: Summary* (hereafter 'HTA'; National Board of Health 2011a); and *Disease management programme for rehabilitation of acquired brain injury* (hereafter 'DMP'; National Board of Health 2011b). The first document is selected according to the first criterion, as a general guide to services targeting rehabilitation at the municipal level. The other two documents meet the second criterion. The HTA is a report based on both evidence- and experience-based knowledge to regulate the development of neuro-rehabilitation in general, while the DMP articulates evidence-based practices, management logic, and legal language. Both are key documents in current policy strategy for the rehabilitation of brain injury in Denmark.

The two Norwegian documents were both updated in 2017: *Guide to rehabilitation, habilitation, individual care plan and coordinator* (hereafter 'NO Service Guide'; Directorate of Health 2017b); and *National clinical guideline for treatment and rehabilitation after stroke* (hereafter 'NCG'; Directorate of Health 2017c). The first document was selected under the first criterion and is a general service guide to rehabilitation in institutional and municipal practice. The second document meets the second criterion, with clinical guidelines representing evidence-based knowledge; as such, it mainly resembles the HTA in Denmark. The two selected documents are key texts regulating rehabilitation after stroke in Norway.

The two service guides (and the DMP) outline the principles underpinning the organizing of rehabilitation services, while the NCG and the

HTA (and parts of the DMP) recommend interventions based on evidence. The latter is seen as a strategy to create uniform services of high quality across the country. However, in both countries, the selected documents are interlinked with each other and with other texts.

5.4 Analysing Documents

To analyse the five key documents in more detail, we follow Fairclough's CDA approach, exploring three sociolinguistic dimensions: textual level, societal level, and social practices. At the textual level, written language defined as text is analysed as a social event or a network of such events. At a societal level, language is analysed as the semiotic aspect of larger social structures; in this understanding, the social order delimits what is possible, given different economic, political, and social circumstances. Fairclough (2003, p. 223) places social practices between the textual and societal levels; in this study, both the political and clinical rehabilitation practices exemplify this dimension.

The textual *social event* is the production of governmental service guides for rehabilitation and the NCG, HTA, and DMP, proposing evidence-based practices, while the social structures (such as Denmark's Structural Reform of 2007 and Norway's Coordination Reform of 2012) form the social order determining what is possible or achievable. Rehabilitation is a social practice and a product of the textual events and social reforms.

All five of the selected policy documents are understood as political technologies for designing and redesigning rehabilitation practices between 2010 and 2018. The two service guides aim to direct practice in a desired direction, while the three professional guideline documents aim to ensure consistent, high-quality treatment in neurorehabilitation by recommending specific courses of action. We undertake a close reading of the HTA/DMP for Denmark and the NCG for Norway to analyse rehabilitation as complex social practices. We are interested in how the authorities redesign the technologies of governing, such as service guides, management programmes, clinical guidelines, and health technology assessments, to increase efficiency and quality in rehabilitation services for brain-injured persons. In this context, rehabilitation is seen as a product of political, professional, and administrative structures and practices.

We address the key documents, or more precisely the programmes, procedures, and devices they propose, as elements of what we term governmental technologies. First, we contextualize and intertextualize the documents from each country, and analyse their links and references to other documents in order to identify relationships between these and other texts. Second, we look for interdiscursivity or how intertextuality is constitutive in the key documents, as for example, a mixture of genres, styles, and representations in the actual technologies regulating rehabilitation practices.

5.5   Intertextuality in Guides and Guidelines

Intertextuality concerns how the documents enter into dialogue with one another and with other relevant documents, either by explicit referencing or by implicitly drawing on other texts. On the one hand, the political authorities in Denmark and Norway are responsible for issuing laws, regulations, and service guides for policy areas like rehabilitation. On the other hand, they produce the NCG, HTA, and DMP, the latter of which is the most recently introduced. The NCG, HTA, and DMP provide empirical examples of increasing international emphasis on using evidence-based knowledge.

5.5.1   The Danish Documents

The three different documents were published just a few years after the 2007 Structural Reform (Ministry of Internal and Health Affairs et al. 2011; National Board of Health 2011a, b). We will refer to the production of the three documents as interlinked social events, following Fairclough's (2003) terminology, and as political technologies of governing, according to Rose's (2006) concept.

After being initiated in 2009, the HTA was published two years later as a systematic and comprehensive presentation and assessment of neurorehabilitation research. Its main purpose was to support the working group preparing the DMP, with evidence-based professional advice on rehabilitation after brain injury. The HTA comprises seven main chapters, the second of which is this study's main focus, although Chaps. 3, 4, 5, and 6 are also analysed (National Board of Health 2011a). The approach applied to find evidence on brain injury rehabilitation is described as a systematic literature review. It follows critical steps, which are meant to ensure the inclusion of studies, as explained by the Levels of Evidence and Grades of Recommendation for quantitative studies of the Oxford Centre for Evidence-Based Medicine (Oxford CEBM), while similar steps are applied for the evaluations and qualitative studies.

The HTA is intended to provide managers and professionals with knowledge-based advice on how to approach brain injury rehabilitation. Its recommendations are presented as research-based and oriented towards practical application. Published by the National Board of Health, the HTA's four editors combine expertise in neuropsychology, public health, health science, and nursing, while the authors of the different chapters are experts in neurology, neuropsychology/psychology, occupational therapy, physiotherapy, health science, anthropology, sociology, and economy. The report's reference group included representatives from state, regional, and municipal authorities; researchers, teachers, professors, and professional societies; and users' associations, individual users, and relatives. This indicates that the HTA was developed by multidisciplinary actors on the basis of broad evidence (National Board of Health 2011a).

The DMP prescribes a system and procedure for proactively organizing rehabilitation services for adults with acquired brain injury in multidisciplinary, multicomponent programmes, using evidence-based standards of care. The health authority committee that formulated the DMP was charged with following up on the HTA's conclusions (National Board of Health 2011b, p. 3). The DMP's main authors are the health authorities. In developing the DMP, both the professional working group and the reference group comprised representatives of the authorities, professional societies and associations, and two user organizations. The DMP is a national undertaking and encourages regional and municipal authorities to adopt its programme as part of their local practices and organization of brain injury rehabilitation.

Also published in 2011, the DK Service Guide followed up on the assignment to municipalities of primary responsibility for general rehabilitation in the 2007 Structural Reform. It has links to six legal acts: the Health Act, the Employment Initiatives Act, the Act on Active Social Policy, the Social Services Act, the Special Education Act, and the Act on Upper Secondary Education for Young People with Special Needs (National Board of Health 2011b, p. 3). There is no guide for specialist rehabilitation services in Denmark, but the DMP provides a common frame of reference.

The DK Service Guide offers general advice and an overview of the legal framework for directing the practices of all local rehabilitation services, focusing specifically on municipal responsibilities. It was produced by four ministries—Ministry of Internal and Health Affairs, Ministry of Social Affairs, Ministry of Employment, and Ministry of Education—and published in June 2011. The text does not mention using an external reference group. The primary purpose of the guide is 'to inspire and support the efforts that take place in the municipalities and to ensure cooperation and coordination between the professional and management areas responsible for the coherence and quality of the individual citizen's pathway' (Ministry of Internal and Health Affairs et al. 2011, p. 4). The DK Service Guide is structured into five chapters; we focus especially on Chap. 2, concerning legal regulations, and Chap. 4, on responsibility, coordination, and cooperation in rehabilitation pathways (Ministry of Internal and Health Affairs et al. 2011).

5.5.2 The Norwegian Documents

Work on the NO Service Guide was initiated in 2013, one year after the Coordination Reform; it was then published in 2015 and updated in 2017. As its title conveys, the guide is interlinked with the legislative 'Regulation on rehabilitation, habilitation, individual care plan and coordinator', implemented in 2012. The NO Service Guide has broader scope than the DK Service Guide, as it includes both municipal and specialist services.

As the NO Service Guide's main author, the Directorate of Health formulated its aim thus:

> to help managers and professionals to work better together on rehabilitation, habilitation, learning, coping and coordination. The Directorate of Health wishes to contribute to common understanding and unified guidance on key questions both related to content in services and interaction. (Directorate of Health 2017b, p. 2)

Therefore, the guide is primarily intended to advise and help managers and professionals in rehabilitation and habilitation services, rather than clients or patients. The document was written by an internal working group with a secretariat and project manager from the Directorate of Health, in consultation with an external reference group. Health professionals dominated the internal group, while the external reference group had a broader composition, with representation from the authorities, private institutions, educational institutions, professional associations, and user organizations.

The second Norwegian document, the NCG, represents quite a different genre to the guide. It classifies itself as a norm for professional treatment and interventions regarding rehabilitation after stroke (Directorate of Health 2017c). The NCG is stated to be based on knowledge-based practices. This means that 'research, clinical experience and user experience are included in the assessment of the desired and undesirable consequences of the proposed interventions. The consequences are related to values, resources, prioritization criteria, laws and regulations' (Directorate of Health 2017a, p. 10).

When published in 2017, the NCG replaced previous guidelines for treatment and rehabilitation after stroke (in force since 2010), in order to adapt to new knowledge and new routines devised for treating and rehabilitating stroke patients. Fundamentally, the NCG simplified the 2010 guidelines, introducing the GRADE (Grading of Recommendation, Assessment, Development, and Evaluation) method in place of the SIGN (Scottish Intercollegiate Guidelines Network) method. However, for recommendations from the 2010 guidelines repeated in the NCG, the SIGN method is retained.

The main working group behind the NCG's chapter on rehabilitation (Chap. IV) comprised seven professionals: four medical doctors and three therapists. The broad reference group comprised clinicians and representatives from: user organizations; professional associations of occupational therapists, physical therapists, nurses, doctors, psychologists, and ambulance drivers; regional health authorities; and the Norwegian Association of Local and Regional Authorities. The target audience for the NCG is health service professionals, and it covers all stages of the treatment chain from pre-hospital care to post-stroke rehabilitation (i.e. long-term management).

5.5.3 Summing-Up

We analysed five documents produced in Denmark and Norway between 2011 and 2017. The documents were devised to monitor rehabilitation practices, improve the efficiency of clinical interventions, and increase the quality of services in general. The two service guides—in contrast to the NCG, HTA, and DMP—do not concern a specific diagnostic group, but provide advice on general rehabilitation services, based on legal and political strategies. We identified close links to legal documents and other relevant policy texts throughout both key documents. The NO Service Guide covers both specialist and municipal levels, whereas the DK Service Guide only concerns municipal rehabilitation services. However, the latter refers more to sectors other than healthcare, including the social, employment, and pedagogical areas.

In both countries' key documents, we observe intertextuality between the two service guides on rehabilitation (NO Service Guide and DK Service Guide) and the recommendations for evidence-based practices (the NCG for stroke in Norway, and the DMP and HTA for brain injury in Denmark). The NCG, HTA, and DMP all provide recommendations on neurorehabilitation grounded in evidence-based knowledge. The HTA has a broader view on research than clinical guidelines, including qualitative studies, evaluations, organizational studies, and economic assessments; however, it privileges evidence based on randomized control trials.

There are various assessment methods, or ranking systems, for evidence-based practices in use. The Norwegian authorities have used SIGN (in 2010) and GRADE (in 2017), while the Danish authorities have applied the Oxford CEBM. The GRADE method is also used by the WHO, and to achieve simplicity, it classifies evidence into four levels of quality: high, moderate, low, and very low.

The discourse on rehabilitation articulated in the NCG, HTA, and DMP is broader in scope than a purely biomedical discourse. We can conceive this broader discourse as biopsychosocial (i.e. interdisciplinary) and inclusive in the sense that it incorporates patients' wishes. Thus, we interpret these documents as representing a composite view on knowledge. Compared to the Norwegian clinical guideline, the Danish HTA concerns a broader client group (acquired brain injury), concentrates only on post-acute rehabilitation, and has a broader view on knowledge and research-based evidence. In other words, patients with acquired brain injury (in the Danish document) are a broader client group than stroke patients (in the Norwegian document). While the HTA and the DMP encompass broader research knowledge, involving wider ethical and economic issues, the NCG concerns a broader patient pathway, including the acute stage, intensive examination and treatment, and rehabilitation interventions.

5.6 Interdiscursive Analysis of Language of Coordination in Guides and Guidelines

We apply interdiscursivity as an analytical lens for identifying combinations of diverse language conventions in the five documents. Where guides principally base recommendations on political decisions and legal acts, guidelines cite scientific evidence. We ask how their respective genres and styles intermix. What type of combinations of language representations, such as evidence, legal obligations, and patients' wishes are identified? Finally, how does this new mixture of language articulate hybridity in neurorehabilitation?

In this section, we analyse the five documents for different representations of coordination strategies in clinical recommendations and service directions regulating transfer of patients from specialist to local services. To accomplish this, we look for: (i) mixtures of different languages in the five documents; and (ii) how the different languages are interlinked and form a network of coordination strategies.

To contextualize and identify different representations of coordination, we closely read the sections concerning transitions between hospital and home in the DK Service Guide and NO Service Guide. In the Danish document, the relevant section is titled 'Responsibility, coordination and cooperation on rehabilitation processes' (Ministry of Internal and Health Affairs et al. 2011, pp. 34–42). In NO Service Guide, the relevant section is titled 'Clarification of responsibilities and tasks between the municipality and the specialist service within rehabilitation' (Directorate of Health 2017a, pp. 62–95). We then searched the HTA and NCG for commitments to truth or to obligation (modalities), such as 'evidence to recommendations' or 'references to legal acts' in descriptions of coordination procedures on discharge from hospital to municipal rehabilitation (Directorate of Health 2017c; National Board of Health 2011a).

The language of coordination (coordination strategies) is identified at several levels and in different contexts: between hospitals and municipalities, between multiple professions, and between individual clients and their professional helpers. We categorized them as: (a) *inter-institutional coordination*, such as formal or informal agreements between hospitals and municipalities, early discharge teams, and coordinating units at both levels; (b) *interprofessional coordination*, such as electronic communication between experts in different teams, discharge dialogues, and a discharge coordinator; and (c) *individual–client-centred coordination*, such as rehabilitation plans or individual care plans (see Table 5.1).

In Table 5.1, the different coordination strategies are identified in the first column.[1] We searched the documents for different language

---

[1] The DMP is not included in the part on interdiscursivity, in order to simplify the presentation and clarify the argumentation.

Table 5.1 Interdiscursivity between three strategies for coordination of rehabilitation practices

Coordination strategies	Denmark		Norway	
	Health technology assessment	DK Service Guide	National clinical guideline	NO Service Guide
Inter-institutional	Need for improving coordination Based on systematic review and other studies (p. 12)	*Health agreements* (municipal authorities) *Frame agreements* (municipal authorities) (ch. 4.2.1 & 4.2.2, pp. 34–39)	Strong evidence for interaction across administrative levels (SIGN: A1a) (p. 148)	*Cooperation agreements* (legal regulation) (ch. 10–11)
Interprofessional	Need for internal communication across professions Limited evidence based on different contexts (p. 12)	*Electronic communication* (legal regulation) (ch. 4.2.5, p. 55)	Strong evidence for procedures of interprofessional communication on discharge (SIGN: A1a) (pp. 147–149)	*Electronic communication* (legal regulation) (p. 37)
Individual client-centred	Limited research on rehabilitation plans (p. 11)	*Rehabilitation plan*[a] (legal regulation) (Summary, p. 54)	Weak evidence for individual planning documents (SIGN: D4) (p. 160) *Rehabilitation plan* (p. 165)	*Individual care plan* (legal regulation) (ch. 13)

[a]In Danish, 'genoptræningsplan' according to the Health Act

representations in the recommendations based on science and evidence and those based on politics and legal obligations or rights.

In the Danish HTA (second column), the text on *inter-institutional coordination* is headed 'Need for improving coordination', and states that 'Coordinating efforts across hospitals and municipalities and across municipal administrative units is a fundamental part of establishing coherent rehabilitation programmes'. This recommendation is based on barriers identified in both a systematic literature study and national and international research on the organization of rehabilitation for people with acquired brain injury (National Board of Health 2011a, p. 11).

Interprofessional coordination, such as electronic communication for knowledge transfer between hospitals and municipalities, seems to be recommended based on the same studies. The analysis behind recommending this procedure emphasizes 'the need for internal communication across professions and especially across the municipal administrative units', in order to coordinate appropriate care at the relevant time and place (National Board of Health 2011a, p. 12). The evidence on inter-institutional and interprofessional coordination is addressed as limited. In our view research on this issue must be studied to capture the diverse institutional and national contexts. However, electronic communication platforms are seen as effective for transferring information and knowledge between professions as well as institutions (National Board of Health 2011a, pp. 12, 157).

The DK Service Guide (third column) describes obligatory health agreements and coordinating committees at institutional level, alongside several informal voluntary procedures (Ministry of Internal and Health Affairs et al. 2011, pp. 37–38). The guide also cites § 205 of the Health Act (Ministry of Internal and Health Affairs 2008) to define the minimum content of health agreements between the regions and municipalities. On electronic communications, the recommendations are developed by KL (Local Government, Denmark), the Medical Association, and the Danish Health Authority (Ministry of Internal and Health Affairs et al. 2011, p. 62).

Both the HTA and the DK Service Guide base their recommendations to improve coordination at institutional and professional level on scientific evidence and legal obligations and rights. While the HTA cites both evidence and legal obligations, the DK Service Guide has fewer references to research and evidence.

The Norwegian clinical guideline (fourth column) confirms that there is strong evidence for coordinated services: 'Interaction across levels of administration seems to be of particular importance for success in the rehabilitation of stroke patients' (Directorate of Health 2017c, p. 148). The evidence to recommendations (SIGN: A1a) is based on one systematic review of services for reducing the duration of hospital care for acute stroke patients, which is assessed to be high quality. The NCG refers to electronic patient journals on discharge as a device for interprofessional communication: 'when [the patient is] discharged from the specialist health service, the transfer of necessary information and coordination for the further course shall be ensured' (Directorate of Health 2017c, pp. 147–148). Strong evidence for this procedure is cited (SIGN: 1a), referring to the aforementioned high-quality systematic review (Directorate of Health 2017c, pp. 147–148). The evidence to recommendations in the NCG is stronger than that in the HTA, referring to the recommendations as truth.

According to the NO Service Guide (fifth column), both the regional and local health authorities have a duty to establish coordination and cooperative agreements between hospital and municipalities, based on several legal acts and earlier policy processes (Directorate of Health 2017b, pp. 68–69). In addition, the guide states that 'the coordinating unit in the municipalities … shall have procedures for handling electronic messages referring to the Health Care Act, § 16' (Directorate of Health 2017b, p. 37).

While the NCG supports its recommendations with strong scientific evidence, the NO Service Guide primarily refers to legal obligations and personal rights. Both documents have the same author (Directorate of Health) and refer to the same legal basis (the Health and Care Act, § 12–5). The Service Guide states: 'NCG and guides describe how practice should be based on research-based knowledge. Choice of solutions that differ significantly from the guidelines should be justified and documented' (Directorate of Health 2017b, p. 14).

In the final part of this section, we will examine more closely the third type of coordination identified in Table 5.1 (bottom row), named 'rehabilitation plan' in Denmark and both 'rehabilitation plan' and 'individual care plan' in Norway. In the Danish HTA, 'A rehabilitation plan includes information on a person's total needs for multidisciplinary rehabilitation after discharge from the hospital and is essential for ensuring referral to relevant and high-quality rehabilitation services' (National Board of Health 2011a, p. 11). The HTA concludes that rehabilitation plans 'need to be further developed and all relevant aspects of the need for rehabilitation of people with acquired brain injury are described, including physical, emotional, cognitive, communication and social dimensions'. It also emphasizes that people in outpatient rehabilitation programmes or who are not hospitalized may also need a rehabilitation plan (National Board of Health 2011a, p. 11). The main language used relates to the needs and experiences of patients.

The DK Service Guide confirms that rehabilitation plans are regulated by § 84 and § 140 of the Health Act. The text section continues:

> All patients discharged from hospitals and in need of further rehabilitation should be offered a rehabilitation plan. Patients who have been hospitalized or have been in contact with the emergency room or hospital office should, at the time of discharge, be offered a rehabilitation plan if there is a medical need for rehabilitation. (Ministry of Health and Care Services 2011, p. 12)

The Norwegian clinical guideline states that 'Rehabilitation goals should be defined in a rehabilitation plan[2] and should be worked out with patients and relatives based on a comprehensive multidisciplinary assessment' (Directorate of Health 2017c, p. 165). It recommends drawing up a rehabilitation plan based on goals agreed with patients, users, and relatives. The evidence for recommendation is classified as SIGN: C3, meaning that there are solid descriptive and observation studies (Directorate of Health 2017c, p. 165). Compared to the evidence on 'information and coordination at discharge from hospital after brain injury' the scientific proof is weaker. In order to provide an adequate rehabilitation process, the guideline holds, anyone affected by stroke should be offered contact with the municipality's rehabilitation service.

---

[2] The NCG applies both the terms 'rehabilitation plan' and 'individual care plan' (Directorate of Health 2017c, p. 165).

'It should be considered if the patient needs or wishes a coordinator and an individual care plan' (Directorate of Health 2017c, p. 148). In these statements, the guideline refers to the individual care plan as both a legal right and as something, which can be dispensed upon personal wishes. The evidence to recommendations is strong using the expression 'should be'.

Finally, the Norwegian guide to rehabilitation states:

> Patients and users with a need for long-term and coordinated health and care services have the right to get an individual care plan [cf. section 2–5 of the Patient and User Rights Act]. They have the right to participate in the work on their individual care plan and this has to be arranged [cf. section 3–1 of the Patient and Users' Rights Act]. Relatives shall be included in the work if the patient or the user wishes. (Directorate of Health 2017b, p. 84)

In Norway, a person has a right to ask for an individual care plan, but there is not strong evidence-based recommendation for the scheme. This is an example of what we term hybridity between legal and personal language. The mixed language is more common, when the scientific evidence is weak. Comparing the texts on individual planning documents, a rehabilitation plan in Denmark is a medical concern initiated at the hospital, while an individual care plan in Norway is the responsibility of the municipal authorities. In both countries, an individual care/rehabilitation plan is a legal right for persons after brain injury and in need of coordinated rehabilitation services, however there is a stronger emphasis on medical need in Denmark and personal right in Norway. Both the clinical guideline and the HTA articulate a mixture of legal and scientific language. The recommendations for individual planning in the two service guides are referred to as a legal obligation and a personal right when certain conditions are met. In Denmark, the rehabilitation plan is regulated by the Health Act, and the condition is a medical need for rehabilitation. By contrast, the individual care plan is obligatory in Norway under the Patient and User Rights Act, and the individual has a right to decide how to participate in developing plans.

5.7   Discussion

The choice of words differs in the documents. The Danish HTA refers to the health technical assessments as 'analyses', including randomized control trials and qualitative interviews with patients and relatives. Invoking an even stronger term, the Norwegian clinical guideline uses the word 'evidence'. 'Analysis' usually refers to research processes that systematically study or examine a phenomenon, whereas 'evidence' serves to prove whether something is true.[3]

The language on individual care/rehabilitation plan hybridizes scientific evidence, legal obligations and rights, and personal needs and/or wishes. The two service guides refer to the individual care/rehabilitation plan as a legal right, while the NCG and HTA inform that using this type of planning has only a moderate-to-weak effect on recovery. The NCG recommends an individual care plan based on 'solid evidence' (moderate to weak, SIGN: C). For both clients and professionals, the basis for the NCG or HTA recommending an individual care/rehabilitation plan may not be clear. The mixture of language to recommend using individual service planning tools can be considered as 'attempts at governing' (Rose 1999, p. 4). In all the documents analysed, there are a mixture of representations (evidence and rights) and styles (language of truth and of obligations, including use of auxiliary verbs such as 'should do' or 'can do').

All three coordination strategies are described in the same text section in the documents—cooperation agreements, electronic communication, and individual care/rehabilitation plans—and they are integrated within a 'coordination network'. The following extract from the NCG is illustrative:

> The cooperation agreements between municipalities and health regions/ hospitals should emphasize that the collaboration should have a patient-oriented focus and involve professionals working close to the users. Routines for rapid electronic messages should be established between all parties involved. The coordinating unit for rehabilitation in the municipality or the rehabilitation team/unit should be those responsible for

---

[3] https://dictionary.cambridge.org/dictionary/english/evidence

coordinating rehabilitation plans or individual care plans. (Directorate of Health 2017c, p. 148)

What does this indicate? First, the coordinating agreements, electronic communication devices, and coordinated individual planning are all described in the same chapters of the documents and in the same text section. The coordinating strategies are interlinked, and if one is weak, then the coordination network is fragile. Second, these three coordination strategies are very different, and are located in various objects, procedures, and places; they are embedded in different environments, situations, contexts, objects, and procedures. Third, these diverse coordination strategies are all dependent on personal competence; in other words, success depends on a human factor. Thus, these components make coordination a composite and complex issue.

This tells us that it is difficult to turn composite organizational and professional issues into technical ones to be solved by evidence-based research (Greenhalgh and Russell 2009; Greenhalgh et al. 2015). Following Hammersley (2001), this might lead to the neglect of democratic policy processes, including practical wisdom and experience-based knowledge. Obligatory cooperative agreements, the advice to use electronic communication between institutions and professionals, and the development of individual care/rehabilitation plans are all products of political processes, including parliamentary legislative processes. The evidence to clinical recommendations is supported by legal language of obligations and rights.

5.8 Conclusion

Denmark's Structural Reform and Norway's Coordination Reform are political transformations reframing and redesigning health services, including rehabilitation, into new practices. This study has shown that dominant political rationalities and knowledge practices are being interwoven in new ways, creating more composite and complex rehabilitation practices.

We have investigated how the governmental technologies, such as guidelines and guides applied in rehabilitation display features of both intertextuality (entering into dialogue with one another and with other relevant texts) and interdiscursivity (mixing different uses of language, i.e. of scientific evidence, management, citizenship rights, and citizens' wishes). By conducting a textual analysis of key documents, we examined how Danish and Norwegian authorities have redesigned rehabilitation practices. More concretely, these documents support a design towards intersectoral, interprofessional, and client-centred arrangements. The general aim of these efforts is to improve the efficiency of the clinical interventions and increase the quality of services, under new government structures. The key documents are using a mixed language of legal rights, scientific evidence, and patients/users' wishes. The technologies of governing represented by the clinical guidelines and service guides indicate a shift in the relationship between political and scientific knowledge. Management logics, evidence-based guidelines, and person-centred care represent a shift towards a new plurality of technologies for regulating rehabilitation practices. Amidst this multitude of technologies, the experience-based knowledge of citizens and patients may come under pressure.

Another shift is the increased focus on coordination strategies in governmental policies and professional practices. Coordination is addressed as a core problem in today's rehabilitation practice. Policies frame solutions at multiple levels and through multiple measures, such as legal obligations and patients' rights, and evidence-based practices. A new coordination discourse, understood as new language in use in a rehabilitation context, has evidently emerged, placing health authorities and professions under pressure when advised to find simplified solutions to composite situations.

References

Bonfils, I. S. (2003). Historiske spor og nutidige udfordringer i handicappolitikken [Historical paths and contemporary challenges in disability policy]. In S. Bengtsson, I. S. Bonfils, & L. Olsen (Eds.), *Handicap, kvalitetsudvikling og brugerinddragelse* [Disability, quality development and user involvement] (pp. 13–36). København: Anvendt KommunalForskning.

Bonfils, I. S., & Berger, N. P. (2010). *Specialiserede tilbud til borgere med handicap—efter reformen* [Specialized services for people with disabilities—After the reform]. København: AKF Forlag.

Bowen, A., James, M., & Young, G. (Eds.). (2016). *National clinical guideline for stroke*. Prepared by the Intercollegiate Stroke Working Party. London: Royal College of Physicians.

Byrkjeflot, H. (2011). Healthcare states and medical professions: The challenges from NPM. In T. Christensen & P. Lægreid (Eds.), *The Ashgate research companion to new public management*. Farnham: Taylor and Francis.

Directorate of Health. (2017a). *Veileder for utvikling av kunnskapsbaserte retningslinjer* [Guide to the development of knowledge-based guidelines] (IS-1870). Oslo: The Directorate of Health.

Directorate of Health. (2017b). *Veileder om rehabilitering, habilitering, individuell plan og koordinator* [Guide to rehabilitation, habilitation, individual care plan and coordinator]. Oslo: The Directorate of Health.

Directorate of Health. (2017c). *Nasjonal faglig retningslinje for behandling og rehabilitering ved hjerneslag* [National clinical guideline for treatment and rehabilitation after stroke]. Oslo: The Directorate of Health.

Fairclough, N. (2000). Discourse, social theory, and social research: The discourse of welfare reform. *Journal of SocioLinguistics, 4*(2), 163–195.

Fairclough, N. (2003). *Analysing discourse: Textual analysis for social research*. London: Routledge.

Feiring, M. (2012). Rehabilitation—Between management and knowledge practices: An historical overview of Norwegian welfare reforms. *Policy and Society, 31*, 119–129.

Feiring, M. (2016). Rehabiliteringsfeltet i Danmark—En begrebshistorie [The field of rehabilitation in Denmark—A history of concept]. *Tidsskrift for professionsstudier* [*Journal for Professional Studies*], *24*(1), 86–97.

Greenhalgh, T., & Russell, J. (2009). Evidence-based policymaking: A critique. *Perspectives in Biology and Medicine, 52*(2), 304–318.

Greenhalgh, T., Snow, R., Ryan, S., Rees, S., & Salisbury, H. (2015). Six 'biases' against patients and carers in evidence-based medicine. *BMC Medicine, 13*(1), 200.

Hammell, K. W. (2006). *Perspectives on disability & rehabilitation: Contesting assumptions; challenging practice*. Edinburgh: Churchill Livingstone/Elsevier.

Hammersley, M. (2001, September 13–15). Some questions about evidence-based practice in education. *The annual conference of the British Educational Research Association: Evidence-based practice in education*. Paper presented at the symposium on University of Leeds.

Ministry of Health and Care Services. (2009). Report no. 47 (2008–2009) to the Storting: The coordination reform—Proper treatment—At the right place and right time. Oslo: The Ministry.

Ministry of Health and Care Services. (2011). ACT 24/06/2011 no. 30: ACT relating to municipal health and care services etc. Health and Care Services Act. Oslo: The Ministry.

Ministry of Internal and Health Affairs. (2008). Sundhedsloven [The health act]. Copenhagen: The Ministry.

Ministry of Internal and Health Affairs, Ministry of Social Affairs, Ministry of Work, & Ministry of Education. (2011). Vejledning om kommunal rehabilitering [Guidance on municipal rehabilitation]. Copenhagen: The Ministries.

National Board of Health. (2011a). Hjerneskaderehabilitering—en medicinsk teknologivurdering [Brain injury rehabilitation—A health technology assessment: Summary]. Copenhagen: The National Board.

National Board of Health. (2011b). Forløbsprogram for rehabilitering af voksne med erhvervet hjerneskade [Disease management programme for rehabilitation in adult acquired brain injury]. Copenhagen: The National Board.

Olsen, L. (2008). Ny kommunal struktur og opgavefordeling—en vej til lige muligheder? [New municipal structure and division of tasks—A path to equal opportunities?]. In S. Bengtsson, I. S. Bonfils, & L. Olsen (Eds.), Handicap og ligebehandling i praksis [Disability and equal opportunities in practice] (pp. 63–83). København: Socialforskningsinstituttet.

Røberg, A.-S., Feiring, M., & Romsland, G. (2016). Norwegian rehabilitation policies and the coordination Reform's effect: A critical discourse analysis. Scandinavian Journal of Disability Research, 19(1), 56–68.

Rose, N. (1999). Powers of freedom: Reframing political thought. Cambridge: Cambridge University Press.

Rose, N. (2006). Governing "advanced" liberal democracies. In A. Sharma & A. Gupta (Eds.), The anthropology of the state: A reader (pp. 144–162). Malden: Blackwell.

Rose, N., & Miller, P. (2010). Political power beyond the state: Problematics of government. British Journal of Sociology, 61(S1), 271–303.

WHO. (2017). Rehabilitation in health systems. Geneva: World Health Organization.

6

Rehabilitation as a Reformed Governance Technology: Freedom, Constraint, and Concealment

Anne-Stine B. Røberg

6.1 Introduction

Rehabilitation is predicted to become a key global health strategy of the twenty-first century (Stucki et al. 2017). The term 'rehabilitation' describes a range of responses to disability and chronic conditions: from early interventions to improve body function, to later, comprehensive measures to promote and coordinate disabled peoples' well-being, inclusion, and participation in society. As a concept and practice, it is anchored in the social engineering visions of European welfare states, particularly as a remedy to curb increasing numbers of people unable to work (Kildal and Kuhnle 2012; Hanssen and Sandvin 2003). Accordingly, new knowledge about rehabilitation continues to be produced, circulated, and applied, in turn contributing to the transformation of what rehabilitation entails. Focusing on Norway, this chapter contributes by critically investigating changes in

A.-S. B. Røberg (✉)
TRS National Resource Center for Rare Disorders, Sunnaas Hospital,
Oslo, Norway
e-mail: Anne-Stine.Roberg@sunnaas.no

© The Author(s) 2019   **121**
I. Harsløf et al. (eds.), *New Dynamics of Disability and Rehabilitation*,
https://doi.org/10.1007/978-981-13-7346-6_6

the forms of interaction around political and social processes concerning rehabilitation.

In contrast to more conservative Continental welfare systems, the Norwegian state plays a dominant role in distributing resources, with the aim of promoting the highest standards of equality (Esping-Andersen 2013). Based on principles of universalism, the Norwegian welfare state has developed as a comprehensive and generous social security system, protecting the entire population against social risks, including unemployment, disability, and illness. Nevertheless, like other welfare systems, its context is moulded by certain principal rationales: first, the legal context that, through growing juridification, drives the progressive realization of human rights; second, the psychosocial context that ensures autonomy, empowerment, and involvement of the people concerned, and targets genuine sensitivity to differences in human situations; and, third, the market-oriented context that structures economic prioritizing and promotes accountability and activation in citizens (Mik-Meyer and Villadsen 2013; Kvist 2016; Bickenbach 2014). These rationales pertain to each other and their discourses exhibit mutual relationships that are exposed to various types of influences.

On the one hand, for people living with disabilities or chronic conditions in Norway, various strong non-governmental organizations (NGOs) have, 'from below', forced a reorientation that secures more social rights and emancipates from oppressive exercises of state power and economic dependability. Their critical power has helped to shift attention from the needs of people with disabilities to issues of justice: from the traditional, medically informed rehabilitation approaches to social and environmental structures, with growing attention towards psychosocial perspectives and therapies based on holistic processes (Oliver 2013; Gibson 2016). Today, expanded conceptualizations of objectives in rehabilitation services encompass social perspectives such as quality of life, human rights, equal opportunities, and (not least) individuals' freedom of will.

On the other hand, demographic and epidemiological trends suggest accumulating burdens on the system, and that Norwegian society will increasingly need to attend to peoples' functioning and capabilities. Thus, despite stronger policy emphasis on the perspectives and preferences of individual users, the system faces political pressure 'from above', with demands for smaller government and for more constrained and rational uses of public resources (Harvey 2006). Healthcare budgets, including those for rehabilitation, depend on intensive and effective treatments, and are based on stronger political prioritizing and reforms of the healthcare sector (e.g. Kvist 2015, 2016; Harvey 2006; Grimsmo and Magnussen 2015).

This chapter discusses strategies embedded in the Norwegian healthcare reform implemented in 2012, which institutes changes affecting all healthcare stakeholders. Called the Coordination Reform, its strategies include a particular emphasis on rehabilitation. A core objective is to improve management of an increasingly care-demanding patient demography while also meeting budgetary constraints. The government's white (reform) paper that preceded the reform urged system and administration development to enhance health monitoring and public health investment. It also emphasized that professionals should be accountable for assessing individual patients and service users as subjects, focusing on proficiency in self-determination, independence, and the ability to care for themselves (Hagen and Johnsen 2013). Such political impulses are categorized as neoliberalism (e.g. Harvey 2006; Carter 2015; Rose 1999), which is defined as the dominant ideology guiding political economic practices in most Western states. As a mode of discourse, neoliberalist ideology contends that human well-being is best advanced by less state intervention and the maximization of organizational and individual liberty, with active citizenship. It represents a partial transfer of responsibility for well-being to individuals and their families (Harvey 2006, p. 7; Kivelä 2018). Relatedly, neoliberal values affect the professionals' room for 'manoeuvre', not by completely removing professionals and their particular practices, but by promoting an authorized assumption about the responsible and autonomous individual (Mik-Meyer and Villadsen 2013, p. 4; Villadsen 2007).

This chapter applies a critical discourse analysis (CDA) to examine two different sets of empirical materials. First, it analyses a policy document identified as important for examining specific features of political strategy development in Norway: Report No. 47, 'Coordination Reform. Proper Treatment—At the Right Place and the Right Time' (Norwegian Ministry of Health and Care Services 2009; hereafter the 'Reform Paper').

Second, to support and contrast the documentary analysis, interviews with professionals working in different rehabilitation services are also analysed. The purpose of including interviews to the analysis is based on the assumption that social change is mediated by discourse (Laine and Vaara 2007). Policy strategy discourse might transform professionals into subjects, whose sense of meaning and reality become tied to their participation in the discourse. The analysis, thus, focuses on how the reform strategies aim to achieve changes in the structures and practices of rehabilitation and on the ways that rehabilitation professionals, at an 'overall level', make meaning of rehabilitation. The following critical question is discussed: how do linguistic categories present in the document and interview discourse construe rehabilitation?

6.2   Research Theory and Methodology

Regarding Saussure's conception of the arbitrary connection between linguistic categories and reality, an important development is the claim that language in use—discourses—construes social relations and knowledge about reality (Jäger and Maier 2009; Fairclough 2013). Knowledge, in such terms, sets the frames of meaning within which individuals and groups act (Fairclough 2003; Foucault 1972). Foucault (1977, 1978) posited that discourses produce a fundamental link between power relations and knowledge. Drawing on Foucault's work and adopting a more complex model of interpretation and meaning (Mills 2011, p. 119), Fairclough (1992, p. 71; 2003, 2013) has developed a CDA framework for connecting the detail of texts with broader social structures, on the premise that 'ideologies reside in texts'. Ideology is defined, here, as a representation of aspects of the world with the force to establish, maintain, and change social power relations (Fairclough 2003, p. 9).

This chapter discusses findings from the author's PhD thesis, which has yielded three published articles (Røberg et al. 2017a, b, 2018). It attempts to deconstruct covert ideologies hidden in written and spoken language. The chapter investigates possible interrelatedness of textual properties and power relations, aiming to link social structures and language use, as well as relationships of discourse in the documentary and interview material (Fairclough 2013; Van Dijk 1993, p. 254; Howarth 2005; Barnett-Page and Thomas 2009, p. 2). It is based on a textual analysis of the Reform Paper: a policy document acknowledged to contribute to major changes in the organization and service provision of Norwegian healthcare. For further insight into rehabilitation discourse, the chapter analyses language use among rehabilitation professionals working in various services at different levels of the Norwegian healthcare system (Røberg et al. 2017a, b). Data comprise 176 pages of iteratively transcribed interviews, focusing on similarities and variation in ways of discussing rehabilitation among 19 professionals with different professional backgrounds: nurses, nurse assistants, physicians, occupational therapists and physiotherapists, and social workers. The participants were affiliated to one public and one private specialized rehabilitation hospital, two general hospital rehabilitation units, three municipal inpatient rehabilitation units, two municipal ambulatory teams, and two municipal outpatient rehabilitation services. Against the background of discourses identified in the Reform Paper, the aim is to identify if and how the participants' ways of construing rehabilitation relate to macro-context (political) discourses (Matheson 2008; Rapley 2006; Wodak and Meyer 2002). The interviews were conducted by the author in 2015, three years after the reform's adoption. In keeping with the CDA framework, it is assumed that rehabilitation professionals' thoughts and actions fit within certain discursive frameworks (Fairclough 2013), which demarcate the boundaries within which the meaning of rehabilitation can be negotiated. As such, the chapter adopts a 'strategy-to-practice' perspective which, in line with Laine and Vaara (2007), involves investigating both policy texts and interview texts to examine rehabilitation discourses and social processes of strategic development.

The synthetic product is two nodal discourses which subsume and articulate, in particular ways, the constituent discourses of the policies and interviews. One nodal discourse approaches rehabilitation as a clinical practice. It is based in traditional medical science as a means for political action, and considers the body as an object of government policies and practices. The other nodal discourse concerns rehabilitation as a management practice, regarding the individual as a subject of life regulation governance. According to Fairclough (2005, p. 14), nodal discourses constitute selective representations—'simplifications' and 'condensations'—of complex economic, political, social, and cultural realities, in the sense that they subsume and articulate, in particular ways, the other constituent discourses. The nodal discourses shift across structural boundaries of policies and of language used by rehabilitation professionals; from being 'construal' to being 'constructions'. Social change emerges when policy imaginaries and representations are having transformative effects on the social reality of rehabilitation professionals. As described by Fairclough (2003, p. 208): enacted as new ways of interacting in the rehabilitation field; inculcated in new ways of being and forming the identities of rehabilitation professionals and those experiencing disabilities, injuries, or functional deficits; and materialized in new techniques of offering and organizing rehabilitation services. The following section provides insight into the Norwegian Coordination Reform.

6.3   Reforming Health Policies: Ambiguities and Contradictions

The Norwegian healthcare system is divided into a general (municipal) and a specialized level. General health services provide care, treatment, health promotion, and health preventive efforts for all inhabitants. The specialist level includes public hospitals, polyclinics, emergency and ambulance services, and some medical rehabilitation facilities. Accordingly, the specialized healthcare level is structured by differentiated medical specialties, numerous professions, and great numbers of organizations providing services. These specialities, professions, and organizations form the basis for extensive relationships among actors both within and at the municipal level, including services outside the healthcare system (Hagen and Johnsen 2013).

The Reform Paper recontextualized policies detailed in Norwegian public documents in recent decades (e.g. Christensen and Lægreid 2007; Byrkjeflot et al. 2016; Sandvin 2012). It is claimed to target a persistent mismatch between the very large national cost for health and what Norwegian society receives in the form of health benefits, particularly emphasizing the lack of coordination in service provision.

The Coordination Reform was implemented in 2012 with the over-arching ambition to reverse allegedly unsustainable growth in national health costs (Monkerud and Tjerbo 2016). In line with international trends, the reform aims to foster better health service integration and empowerment of service recipients, thus forming the basis for an effective system of patient transference throughout the system, with rapid discharge and shorter hospital stays (Kirchhoff and Ljunggren 2015). The goal is to achieve a shift from hospital-dominated treatment to preventive or municipal healthcare (Byrkjeflot et al. 2016). According to Hagen and Johnsen (2013, p. 46), the reform rhetoric expects all involved professionals to embrace the overall objective of coherence and coordination, motivated by shared, societal interests. They should also adopt these objectives as the basis for their actions, rather than merely their own (professional) interests. Professionals' effort should be based on users' individual goals, presupposing accountability and effort to actively engage in health-related processes (Røberg et al. 2017a, b, 2018).

Such policy strategies might lead to an unclear conceptualization of rehabilitation (Røberg et al. 2017b). Indeed, close readings uncover numerous ambiguities and contradictions in the Coordination Reform's rehabilitation policy rhetoric. The Reform Paper promotes coordination in rehabilitation because 'all its elements must interact for rehabilitation to achieve sufficient results' (Norwegian Ministry of Health and Care Services 2009, p. 62). This forms the basis for the Reform Paper's approach to redefining rehabilitation. When individuals' needs require the involvement of several actors with different standpoints and competencies, the authorities and professionals are responsible for coordination and cooperation across professional and administrative demarcations. Rehabilitation processes indicate, in this line of thought, professionals' mercantile tasks.

Establishing the concept of rehabilitation, the Reform Paper clarifies that it differs from training's limited focus: rehabilitation is not 'just to recover a functional ability or to train a wounded body part' (Norwegian Ministry of Health and Care Services 2009, p. 62). The Reform Paper thereby rejects the reductive effect of treating body parts as informed by a medical scheme. However, it suggests that training might be seen as 'one of the important elements of a rehabilitation process' (Norwegian

Ministry of Health and Care Services 2009, p. 62), indicating that rehabilitation comprises several coordinated elements. Rehabilitation is, thus,
projected as departing from medical treatment and constituting different
sets of services coherently provided to individuals: 'Rehabilitation measures are *parallel* to medical treatment' (Norwegian Ministry of Health
and Care Services 2009, p. 62, author's emphasis). Hence, the Reform
Paper has established that rehabilitation is distinguished from both training and medical treatment. In this instance, rehabilitation is framed in a
discourse of services that are *reactive* to occurred conditions upon which
eligibility is defined.

The Reform Paper next suggests that '[f]or many patients, the goal [of
rehabilitation] is to improve levels of functional ability to become able to
dwell in private homes. To enable dwelling in private homes, training and
retraining in everyday activities are crucial measures' (Norwegian Ministry
of Health and Care Services 2009, p. 62). Promoting the concept of independence, the reform policy emphasizes municipal physiotherapy or
occupational therapy as two central interventions provided for patients
that 'will be *training* [their] function to manage everyday life' (Norwegian
Ministry of Health and Care Services 2009, p. 62, author's emphasis).
This contradicts the originally established concept that training alone is
not rehabilitation, instead construing rehabilitation as a means to recover
bodily functioning by activating individuals, with the outcome goal of
independence. The Coordination Reform thereby promotes individuals as
active partners in achieving national economic goals by utilizing individuals' and common resources more efficiently. For example, it states
that '[i]ndividuals' approaches must be goal oriented … as to train after
a car accident, to get rid of a painful arm tenosynovitis [*musearm*] so that
one can return to work, or to manage being home after a hip fracture'
(Norwegian Ministry of Health and Care Services 2009, p. 63). In these
instances, rehabilitation is framed as proactive efforts which might prevent the need for and uses of specialized services. This perspective of rehabilitation values individuals as active partners, accountable for making
sufficient effort and cooperating with the public to succeed in their
rehabilitation processes. Their contribution is to limit their need for services and, as such, reduce health costs.

In sum, the reform endorses coordination of professional efforts and cooperation amongst actors to support individual processes and accountability, and expands the range of rehabilitation to include all parts of health and social policy. The Reform Paper construes rehabilitation in an ambiguous way, with rhetorical contradictions such as articulating rehabilitation as both complementing and diverging from training and medical treatment; both limited to and exceeding focus on function ability; and both reactive therapy-related services and proactive preventive efforts. Sandvin (2012, p. 63) suggested that such ambiguous policy development contributes to making rehabilitation unclear and invisible to the actors involved. An additional confounder in comprehending rehabilitation is the transfer of responsibility for health to the individual citizen, blurring the line between public and individual obligation. The following sections critically analyse and discuss the two identified nodal discourses: rehabilitation as a clinical practice and rehabilitation as a management practice.

6.4 The Discourse of Rehabilitation as a Clinical Practice

Based in the discourse of medical knowledge, the nodal discourse of rehabilitation as a clinical practice represents individuals as eligible for rehabilitation services based on their physical or mental conditions. Hence, they are regarded as the objects of a multiplicity of professionals who are presumed to have the power and knowledge to define and provide rehabilitation services. Rehabilitation is construed as interventions decided by rehabilitation professionals' assessment and provided as services reactive to occurred disease or injury. From this perspective, the policy strategy of the Coordination Reform specifies the positioning and responsibilities of rehabilitation professionals' particular contributions:

> The goal must be for patients and users to meet a holistic health service provision that is thoroughly coordinated, characterised by continuous and holistic *treatment and patient courses* that provide *sufficient treatment quality* regardless of levels of services. This is especially important for individuals

with long-term and complex conditions, such as older persons with multiple illnesses, ill children and youth, patients with chronic conditions, with psychiatric conditions, drug addicts, and terminally ill patients. (Norwegian Ministry of Health and Care Services 2009, p. 48, author's emphases)

The phrase 'treatment and patient courses' reflects policy strategies that encourage effective transference between levels of professional practices, while 'sufficient treatment quality' reflects the knowledge basis and, as such, the significant role assigned to professionals who provide the services. Relating to large, non-homogenous groups of patients who have been diagnosed with disabling conditions, the policy frames rehabilitation processes as professionals cooperating in intervention-based and medical scientific therapies that are responsive to 'disruptive' events (Bury 2005), including injuries, illnesses, or decline in function. Relating to the rehabilitation professionals' responsibilities, the Reform Paper emphasizes the significance of early interventions and high doses of therapies as municipal-level strategies to improve patient functioning and self-management:

Physiotherapy and occupational therapy are central services for patients that must retrain their functioning to manage their lives. Tight follow-up and intensive training is often necessary to reach optimal outcomes. If the patient has a simultaneous need for nursing, then this should be an integrated part of the training. Resources must be allocated at an early stage to avoid admittance or re-admittance to hospitals. (Norwegian Ministry of Health and Care Services 2009, p. 62)

The words used—'therapies', 'patients', 'functioning', and 'outcomes'—connect rehabilitation to the medical glossary (Dijkers et al. 2014). The word *must* in the last sentence builds on the conception that, without rehabilitation services, patients might experience escalating illness and the need for hospital services. Moreover, the extract reflects that services provided promptly are assumed to prevent readmittance (Skempes et al. 2018; Rose et al. 2009; Flynn 2002). The implicit assumption is that rehabilitation services induced by interdisciplinary collaborating professionals might be more beneficial, at both the individual and the collective level, than sole medical treatment. The statement accentuates the notion that hospital services might be averted by implementing rehabilitation interventions at an early stage, to *prevent* illness or a decline in function from developing. Applying the reactive rehabilitation discourse gives priority to early induced treatment after a medical cure as a means to prevent health deterioration, and separate (expensive) hospital services from general-level rehabilitation. The Norwegian governing strategies which manage human life processes under regimes of authority over knowledge, institutions, and administration are, as pinpointed by Foucault (1977, 1990), extending domains of human social and biological existence and conceiving health in economic terms.

In searching for interdiscursive connections across the policy and interview genres (Fairclough 2005), interviews with rehabilitation professionals recontextualize elements from the clinical practice discourse identified in the reform policies. When approaching rehabilitation as a professional service, the professionals reflect upon their expertise in making clinical decisions and upon ways to systematize and frame their interventions to achieve improvement in a patient's physical functioning:

Systematically screening levels of functioning helps to choose interventions that give the best measurable results. The sooner we start working, the better the chances to regain patients' abilities. (Physiotherapist, specialised rehabilitation hospital)

This statement is interesting for several reasons. First, it reveals how a rehabilitation professional supports the concept that early induced therapeutic interventions are more effective in terms of outcome. The statement conveys rehabilitation as interventions that record and embrace health perspectives and that focus on problems in functioning. Rehabilitation is accordingly construed as interventions applied to return patients' functional abilities to a prior condition: that which existed *before* the disruptive event. Further, this perspective implies that rehabilitation, as a clinical practice, is informed by retrospective conceptual comparisons with the 'normal' past, achieved by proximal, short-term, measurable goal approaches, defined and assessed by rehabilitation professionals and targeting physical abilities: 'We want rehabilitation to be a distinct effort. We want it to be time limited and reflect measurable outcomes of regained functioning' (Nurse, municipal inpatient rehabilitation unit). Professional-driven rehabilitation interventions might accordingly structure social practices as retraining, returning, recovering, or re-evaluating the ability to function and bodily attributes (Gibson 2016; Stiker 1999).

According to Foucault (1972), such 'general politics' and 'regimes of truth' are the results of scientific discourse and institutions, and are reinforced and redefined constantly through the healthcare system and the flux of political and economic ideologies. Foucault's ideas about people's actions are concerned with their capacities to recognize socialized norms and constraints. The interviews reflected that resources, including the time allocated to rehabilitation, have been significantly reduced. Thus, in a discourse of resource availability, the professionals talked in different ways about how they scale down and ration their interventions and effort:

> There is limitation in what we manage to achieve within such short stays. Sometimes, now, there is only time for one consultation. Ironically, we can still document that we attend to our core responsibilities. (Social worker, general hospital rehabilitation unit)

Thus, under these constraints, professionals have the power to define practice criteria; however, their tasks are as stated in the policy, to achieve goals within limits set by fiscal disciplining authorities (Harvey 2006). In other words, rehabilitation is a constitutive condition for how the authorities and professionals best act and exert power for a specific politico-economic organization of health services, as introduced in current health policies, specifically the Coordination Reform.

A key point about Foucault's approach to power is that it transcends politics and is present as an everyday, socialized, and embodied phenomenon. Foucault explains this as the reason why power struggles do not always lead to change in the social order: power is, rather, a mode of action upon the actions of others (Foucault 1999). The discourse of constraint, time limits, and practices of rapid transference poses certain ethical challenges for the professionals' practices (Røberg et al. 2017b). In this instance, a discourse of individual's meaningful living is invoked in rehabilitation professionals' language use: the outcome of patients' improved abilities is thought to be dependent on adequate interventions related to their everyday situation and prosperity in life. As services are constrained, patients discharged from hospital might then be deprived of opportunities to reach an optimal functional state and possibilities to participate in meaningful activities:

> It's a new situation that hospitals now discharge patients very early and that the municipal rehabilitation units are occupied with patients with great need for medical treatment. Often these patients are discharged to their home before any rehabilitation process is sufficiently implemented. The result is that patients more often become isolated and lonely, and I feel that the system is responsible for their poor conditions. (Occupational therapist, municipal inpatient rehabilitation unit)

In response to constrained resource availability, the interviews reflected that rehabilitation as a clinical practice includes limited professional involvement and the transfer of responsibility from professionals to individuals regarding their future prospects:

> In rehabilitation, our object is to raise awareness in the service users of the factual problem limited to functional abilities and the very short here-and-now therapeutic situation, and to provide them the tools they need for the processes that start after discharge. (Physiotherapist, municipal ambulatory team)

The discourse of rehabilitation as a clinical practice distinguishes between what can be assessed by rehabilitation professionals (physical functioning) and what might be given less priority (psychosocial conditions). Accordingly, the system in which the content and duration of services are defined by the authorities undermines efforts of patient-centred, socio-psychological approaches in rehabilitation. Patients are admitted according to a system that identifies those likely to benefit from services to help them become independent; however, as reflected by Flynn (2002), the same system hinders the possibility of becoming independent by constraining service availability and limiting professionals' options in making clinical decisions. Accordingly, though based on the neoliberal concept of individual freedom, the strategies of the Coordination Reform reflect a kind of physical constraint of individuals' actions. Such constraint, Foucault claimed (1990, p. 790), reflects how freedom disappears everywhere power is exercised.

6.5   The Discourse of Rehabilitation as a Management Practice

The discourse of rehabilitation as a management practice is also rooted in reform strategies of effectiveness and decreasing health costs. It emphasizes that organizations and individual actors within government should be made more accountable for their actions. However, as opposed to developing or restraining certain clinical rehabilitation practices, this particular discourse structures rehabilitation as a management of social processes. Applying this discourse, the reform frames rehabilitation as approaches directed towards social—in addition to physical and mental—conditions in individuals. Rehabilitation processes, thus, depend on individual users' subjective accountability accompanying professionals' responsibilities, which implies a patient-centred approach by service providers. The following statement is from the Reform Paper:

> In many areas of health and care services the goal of the services exceeds healing in medical terms. Their task is fulfilled only if they have sufficiently facilitated for the patients self-management of the totality of their life situation challenges. Developing social networks is an important element in this work. (Norwegian Ministry of Health and Care Services 2009, p. 143)

This statement refers to the authorities' management of overall healthcare. Rehabilitation, hence, involves structural and administrative features comprising institutions and professionals who provide and coordinate services, and as such enact political programmes (Hanssen and Sandvin 2003; Christensen and Lægreid 2007; Rose and Miller 1992, p. 184). The quoted statement exhibits a belief in the potential of investment in individuals in order for them to become active and less in need of help. The policy emphasizes 'independent management' and focuses on approaches to limit the need for healthcare for individuals with chronic diseases and reduced functional abilities:

> We must develop new approaches and technological innovations as aids for patients and their relatives. ... For instance, the project SafetyNet [*TrygghetsNett*] is intended to have a preventive effect as the uses of information and communications technology will contribute to increased knowledge and competence in patients and their relatives to manage everyday life. The goal is to prevent and postpone patients' admission to institutions and to prevent burn-out and exhaustion in relatives, and also to facilitate social networks. (Norwegian Ministry of Health and Care Services 2009, p. 133)

The discourse of activating individuals thus relates rehabilitation to social processes of coping (Røberg et al. 2017a). Words in the policy statement, such as 'knowledge', 'competence', 'management', and 'everyday life', connect rehabilitation to a psychosocial glossary (Marini 2011). Furthermore, the statement alludes to individuals' (and their relatives') responsibility for their own health. Reflecting the burden of such care, it suggests that increased knowledge and competence in relatives will secure their resilience. The presence of a 'lifeworld discourse' reflects the perspectives of those involved in services (Fairclough 1992, p. 203), and signifies that the individuals concerned are conveyed as empowered, and not inferior citizens (McLaughlin 2009). The policy strategy evidently prompts investment in individuals by offering new technological solutions for them to apply in their health processes. Thus, within this discourse, the reform strategies do not portray rehabilitation as interventions in medical terms; rather, a presupposed semantic relationship between rehabilitation, knowledge, and competence instructs a change in professionals' responsibility to add economic sustainability to concern for individual functioning (Røberg et al. 2017a, p. 64). Within the discourse of rehabilitation as a management practice, rehabilitation is related to processes in which the general population of disabled or chronically ill might be situated: treatment ends at the point of hospital discharge and the public responsibility is to create further opportunities for self-managing subjects to interact with technological aids. Accordingly, rehabilitation is related to future-oriented processes beginning after disruptive events and extending beyond initial medical treatment, which obscures or *conceals* services' responsibilities.

Analysing interdiscursive interactions across the policy and interview genres revealed that the discourse of action was recontextualized in the interviews. The language used by interviewees about professional clinical performance and limited resource availability construed rehabilitation as a way of providing certain interventions and clinical practices. By contrast, the discourse of rehabilitation to achieve independence construed rehabilitation as psychosocial elements *excluded* from clinical practices:

> Patients need time to adjust. My responsibility is to approach their initial impairments. They must themselves get a grip of their new life circumstances. (Nurse, municipal inpatient rehabilitation unit)

This statement displays an interdiscursive relationship with policies based on the shared appropriations of activated individuals' social processes of coping and adjustment. It also reflects the concept that rehabilitation involves changes in individuals' attitudes towards life circumstances. Thus, the importance of bodily functioning (or dysfunctioning) to achieve independence is obscured. As such, interviews applying the policy discourse of action emphasize the individual's adaptability in rehabilitation processes. Accordingly, the discourse of rehabilitation as a professional clinical performance is embedded with elements other than what is done *to* or *with* the patients:

> There is a development towards a 'rehabilitation attitude' at our work place. There is so much in the tradition of nursing and care that deprives people of the opportunity to do things by themselves. People are able to do things by themselves! Yes, this is about professionals walking that road along their side, rather than giving help. (Nurse, municipal outpatient service)

This statement signifies the professionals' assumption that compensating care can, in some cases, prevent the patient from becoming self-reliant. Hence, language use by rehabilitation professionals might adapt to the reform strategies of activating individuals. Recontextualized, the interview discourse of resource availability in rehabilitation services comprises ways for professionals to legitimize the rapid transference of patients from institutions to their homes. The statement displays how rehabilitation discourses give form to the resources that professionals use with patients and the ways professionals seek to change how they relate to patients. Contrary to construing rehabilitation as clinical interventions that return abilities to their original state, the discourse of constraint herein relates rehabilitation to individuals' future-oriented adjustments to their surroundings with little, or no, support from the authorities, if possible. Evidently, even nursing and care are conceived to inhibit making individuals independent: 'The absolute best course is for individuals to manage independently, to have the ability to manage everyday life on their own, not being dependent upon any support' (Social worker, general hospital rehabilitation unit). Hibbard and Greene (2013, p. 210) show that interventions aiming to increase individuals' activation levels seek to change the social environment, thereby facilitating changes in people's beliefs, social norms, skills, and opportunities to encourage healthy behaviour. By accentuating the everyday arena and reflecting ideology concealing the state's role (Foucault 1994), the nodal discourse of rehabilitation as a management practice aims to opt out of the institutional environment. Rehabilitation professionals in the interviews recontextualize the emphasis on individual accountability to everyday-life independence in the rehabilitation processes, and apparently reflect disciplinary practices (Røberg et al. 2017b). As discussed in this chapter's opening section, the Norwegian welfare system is arguably undergoing substantial change: emphasis is shifting from protecting citizens against social risks through rehabilitation services to changing people's behaviour to make individuals help themselves.

6.6   Conclusion

This chapter explored ongoing changes in the Norwegian welfare system through a critical investigation of how policy strategies in the Norwegian Coordination Reform make meaning of rehabilitation. It has particularly emphasized how the linguistic categories in current discourses construe rehabilitation. Reflecting a strategies-as-practice perspective by including interviews with rehabilitation professionals in the analysis (Laine and Vaara 2007), the chapter increases knowledge of the social and, hence, discursive processes of reforming rehabilitation policies. Applying the CDA framework, the analysis used concrete examples of how texts work to create power relations and the mechanics of particular discursive processes.

The Reform Paper construes rehabilitation in ways which reflect ambiguities and contradictions; both complementing and diverging from training and medical treatment; both limited to and exceeding focus on function ability; and both reactive therapy-related services and proactive preventive efforts. Notwithstanding, the analysis indicates that the Norwegian reform attempts to reorganize internal spaces and social relations within the organization of rehabilitation in order to save health costs. The reform contributes to reshaping the behaviour and characteristics of professionals providing services and of those experiencing disabling conditions, in accordance with the dominant political force: the neoliberalization of health (Carter 2015). Rehabilitation policies, as expressed in the Coordination Reform, might be seen as a shift from the top-down biopolitics of the population (Foucault 1977) to the bottom-up ethico-politics in the sense of giving the power and moral right to individual self-government (Rose 1999; Kivelä 2018; Carter 2015).

As advocated by Kildal and Kuhnle (2012, p. 67), when observing the Norwegian welfare system, one should pay critical attention to whether the aim of protecting citizens against social risks (by providing rehabilitation services) is being sidelined by the current aim of changing people's behaviour in ways to make individuals help themselves (perhaps regardless of capacity). By drawing on a logic that pertains to the environmental structures and psychosocial perspectives in rehabilitation, the Norwegian authorities might legitimize reform strategies of 'fiscal austerity' and constrained services. Under such terms, and being offered as life-saving and therapy-related care, rehabilitation might be seen as a kind of political rationality on how modern society can regulate, control, and define while also liberating the subject.

In sum, the nodal discourse of rehabilitation as a clinical practice provides a way—a technology—for the authorities to constrain certain public activities through resource allocation. Arguably, regulation of the tasks of professionals strengthens public control and restricts rehabilitation professionals' autonomy regarding clinical decisions (Harvey 2006). Drawing on Foucault (1988), both rehabilitation professionals and individuals involved as patients or service users (the 'subjects') can be seen as 'objects' of a particular kind of authorial power: that of the clinic. Such strategies are suggested to contribute to frugal and effectively cooperating professionals, as well as regulating expectations of services in the population. It might be that self-technologies, still construed as an expression of freedom of will (Carter 2015), work as a technology of subjectification designed to construct 'desirable' citizen-subjects (Kivelä 2018). There is a particular powerful rationality in the nodal discourse of rehabilitation as a clinical practice, as it invokes an end-and-means consideration of profitability in terms of outcome and cost. It might be questioned whether this discourse actively creates an asymmetrical power relation between governing professionals and governed individuals. The political rationalization of healthcare availability seems to be preserving the determinant role of the state as healthcare director, affecting the involved individuals' practices and capacities.

Correspondingly, in the nodal discourse of rehabilitation as a management practice, embedded elements of professionals' constrained involvement and individuals' accountability are found to be interrelated, as the assumed potential in activating individuals anticipates less need for services. Following Foucault, the term 'governmentality' encompasses modes of government designed to produce docile individuals (Foucault 1988). The production of disciplinary practices—evident in this nodal discourse as limits on possible conduct—might be interpreted as a concealing discourse (Wandel 2001; Foucault 1999) attributed to an anti-medical discourse (Grue 2017). Thus, in making administrative, management-related decisions in rehabilitation and concealing the norms of the medical discourse (or the role required thereof), a model of the activated and self-governed individual is constructed (Foucault 1972). Hence, concealment is what allows the naturalization and legitimation of construing rehabilitation as a management practice.

To conclude, this chapter's inquiry into how linguistic categories in current discourses construe rehabilitation highlights that the Norwegian authorities govern professionals and individuals at a distance (cf. Rose 1999), through political rationales and programmes intended to reduce the use of costly services and increase individuals' activation and self-realization.

References

Barnett-Page, E., & Thomas, J. (2009). Methods for the synthesis of qualitative research: A critical review. *BMC Medical Research Methodology, 9*, 59.

Bickenbach, J. (2014). Universally design social policy: When disability disappears? *Disability and Rehabilitation, 36*(16), 1320–1327.

Bury, M. (2005). *Health and illness*. Cambridge: Polity Press.

Byrkjeflot, H., Christensen, T., & Legreid, P. (2016). Accountability in multi-level health care services: The case of Norway. In P. Mattei (Ed.), *Public accountability and health care governance*. London: Palgrave Macmillan.

Carter, E. D. (2015). Making the blue zones: Neoliberalism and nudges in public health promotion. *Social Science and Medicine, 133*, 374–382.

Christensen, T., & Lægreid, P. (2007). The whole-of-government approach to public sector reform. *Public Administration Review, 67*, 1059–1066.

Dijkers, M. P., Hart, T., Tsaousides, T., Whyte, E. J., & Zanca, J. M. (2014). Treatment taxonomy for rehabilitation: Past, present, and prospects. *Archives of Physical Medicine and Rehabilitation, 95*, S6–S16.

Esping-Andersen, G. (2013). *The three worlds of welfare capitalism*. Cambridge: Polity Press.

Fairclough, N. (1992). Discourse and text: Linguistic and intertextual analysis within discourse analysis. *Discourse and Society, 3*, 193–217.

Fairclough, N. (2003). *Analysing discourse: Textual analysis for social research*. New York: Routledge.

Fairclough, N. (2005). Peripheral vision discourse analysis in organization studies: The case for critical realism. *Organization Studies, 26*(6), 915–939.

Fairclough, N. (2013). *Critical discourse analysis: The critical study of language*. New York: Routledge.

Flynn, R. (2002). Clinical governance and governmentality. *Health, Risk and Society, 4*, 155–173.

Foucault, M. (1972). *Archaeology of knowledge*. New York: Routledge.

Foucault, M. (1977). *Discipline and punish: The birth of the prison.* London: Allen Lane.

Foucault, M. (1978). *The history of sexuality.* London: Penguin.

Foucault, M. (1988). Technologies of the self. In L. H. Martin, H. Gutman, & P. H. Hutton (Eds.), *Technologies of the self: A seminar with Michel Foucault* (pp. 16–49). London: Tavistock.

Foucault, M. (1990). The subject and power. In H. Dreyfus & P. Rabinow (Eds.), *Michel Foucault: Beyond structuralism and hermeneutic* (pp. 208–229). New York: Harvester Wheatsheaf.

Foucault, M. (1994). Truth and power. In J. D. Faubion (Ed.), *Essential works of Foucault* (pp. 1954–1984). New York: The New York Press.

Foucault, M. (1999). *Diskursenes Orden [L'ordre du Discours].* Oslo: Spartacus Forlag AS.

Gibson, B. (2016). *Rehabilitation. A post critical approach.* Boca Raton: CRC Press.

Grimsmo, A., & Magnussen, J. (2015). *Norsk Samhandlingsreform i et internasjonalt perspektiv* [Norwegian coordination reform from an international perspective]. Trondheim: Institutt for Samfunnsmedisin, NTNU, EVASAM, Norges Forskningsråd.

Grue, J. (2017). Now you see it, now you don't: A discourse view of disability and multidisciplinarity. *Alter – European Journal of Disability Research/Revue européenne de recherche sur le handicap, 11,* 168–178.

Hagen, R., & Johnsen, E. (2013). *Styring gjennom samhandling: Samhandlingsreformen som kasus* [Governing by coordination: The coordination reform as a case]. In A. Tjora & L. M. Melby (Eds.), *Samhandling for helse [Coordination for health]* (pp. 31–52). Oslo: Gyldendal Akademisk.

Hanssen, J.-I., & Sandvin, J. T. (2003). Conceptualising rehabilitation in late modern society. *Scandinavian Journal of Disability Research, 5,* 24–41.

Harvey, D. (2006). Neo-liberalism as creative destruction. *Geografiska Annaler: Series B, Human Geography, 88,* 145–158.

Hibbard, J., & Greene, J. (2013). What the evidence shows about patient activation: Better health outcomes and care experiences; fewer data on costs. *Health Affairs, 32,* 207–214.

Howarth, D. (2005). Applying discourse theory: The method of articulation. In D. Howarth & J. Torfing (Eds.), *Discourse theory in European politics: Identity, policy and governance* (pp. 316–349). London: Palgrave Macmillan.

Jäger, S., & Maier, F. (2009). Theoretical and methodological aspects of Foucauldian critical discourse analysis and dispositive analysis. In *Methods of critical discourse analysis* (pp. 34–61). London: Sage.

Kildal, N., & Kuhnle, S. (2012). Welfare principles and reform trends in Norway: Towards more conditional social rights? *Journal of Zhejiang University (Humanities and Social Sciences), 42*(2), 57–67.

Kirchhoff, R., & Ljunggren, B. (2015). Equality in partnerships. The Coordination Reform in Norway. *International Journal of Integrated Care, 15*(5), Annual Conference Supplement; URN:NBN:NL:UI:10-1-116943.

Kivelä, S. (2018). Active citizenship, public sector and the markets: Freedom of choice as state project in health care. *Geoforum, 91*, 160–169.

Kvist, J. (2015). A framework for social investment strategies: Integrating generational, life course and gender perspectives in the EU social investment strategy. *Comparative European Politics, 13*, 131–149.

Kvist, J. (2016). *Fighting poverty and exclusion through social investment: A European research perspective: A policy review.* Brussels: European Commission.

Laine, P.-M., & Vaara, E. (2007). Struggling over subjectivity: A discursive analysis of strategic development in an engineering group. *Human Relations, 60*, 29–58.

Marini, I. (2011). Theories of adjustment and adaptation to disability. In I. Marina, N. M. Glover-Graf, & M. J. Millington (Eds.), *Psychosocial aspects of disability: Insider perspectives and strategies for counselors* (pp. 133–168). New York: Springer.

Matheson, D. (2008). Critiquing the critical: A reflection on critical discourse analysis. *Communication Journal of New Zealand, 9*, 83–96.

McLaughlin, H. (2009). What's in a name: 'Client', 'patient', 'customer', 'consumer', 'expert by experience', 'service user' – what's next? *British Journal of Social Work, 39*, 1101–1117.

Mik-Meyer, N., & Villadsen, K. (2013). *Power and welfare: Understanding citizens' encounters with state welfare.* Oxon: Routledge.

Mills, S. (2011). *Discourse: The new critical idiom.* New York: Routledge.

Monkerud, L. C., & Tjerbo, T. (2016). The effects of the Norwegian coordination reform on the use of rehabilitation services: Panel data analyses of service use, 2010 to 2013. *BMS Health Services Research, 16*, 353.

Norwegian Ministry of Health and Care Services. (2009). Report no. 47 (2008–2009) to the Storting: The coordination reform – Proper treatment – At the right place and right time. Oslo.

Oliver, M. (2013). The social model of disability: Thirty years on. *Disability and Society, 28*(7), 1024–1026.

Rapley, T. (2006). Interviews. In G. Saele, J. Gobo, J. F. Gubrium, & D. Silverman (Eds.), *Qualitative research practices: Concise paperback edition.* London: Sage.

Røberg, A.-S. B., Feirinig, M., & Romsland, G. I. (2017a). Norwegian rehabilitation policies and the coordination reform's effect: A critical discourse analysis. *Scandinavian Journal of Disability Research, 19*, 56–68.

Røberg, A.-S. B., Hansen, H. P., Feiring, M., & Romsland, G. I. (2017b). Rehabilitation in momentum of Norwegian coordination reform: From practices of discipline to disciplinary practices. *Alter – European Journal of Disability Research/Revue européenne de recherche sur le handicap, 11*, 15–29.

Røberg, A.-S. B., Feiring, M., & Romsland, G. I. (2018). Rehabilitation, language, and power: Interdiscursive relationships between policy strategies and professional practices in Norway. *Critical Discourse Studies, 1.* https://doi.org /10.1080/17405904.2018.1546605.

Rose, N. (1999). *Powers of freedom: Reframing political thought.* Cambridge: Cambridge University Press.

Rose, N., & Miller, P. (1992). Political power beyond the state: Problematics of government. *The British Journal of Sociology, 42*, 173–205.

Rose, N., O'Malley, P., & Valverde, M. (2009). Governmentality. Sydney Law School research paper no. 09/94, 2. http://papers.ssrn.com/sol3/papers. cfm?abstract_id=1474131. Accessed 26 July 2016.

Sandvin, J. (2012). Rehabilitering som koordinering og samhandling [Rehabilitation as coordination and cooperation]. In P. Solvang & A. Slettebø (Eds.), *Rehabilitering. Individuelle prosesser, fagutvikling og samordning av tjenester* [Rehabilitation. Individual processes, professional development and coordination of services] (pp. 52–64). Oslo: Gyldendal Norsk Forlag AS.

Skempes, D., Melvin, J., von Groote, P., Stucki, G., & Bickenbach, J. (2018). Using concept mapping to develop a human rights based indicator framework to assess country efforts to strengthen rehabilitation provision and policy: The rehabilitation system diagnosis and dialogue framework (RESYST). *Globalization and Health, 14*(1), 1–96.

Stiker, H.-J. (1999). *A history of disability.* Ann Arbor: University of Michigan Press.

Stucki, G., Bickenbach, J., Gutenbrunner, C., & Melvin, J. (2017). Rehabilitation: The health strategy of the 21st century. *Journal of Rehabilitation Medicine, 50*, 309–316.

Van Dijk, T. A. (1993). Principles of discourse analysis. *Discourse and Society, 4*, 249–283.

Villadsen, K. (2007). Power and self-technology. Foucault's relevance for current welfare studies? *Tidsskrift for Velferdsforskning, 10*, 156–167.

Wandel, T. (2001). The power of discourse: Michel Foucault and critical theory. *Cultural Values, 5*, 368–382.

Wodak, R., & Meyer, M. (2002). Critical discourse analysis: History, agenda, theory, and methodology. In R. Wodak & M. Meyer (Eds.), *Methods of critical discourse analysis* (pp. 1–32). London: Sage.

7

Return to Work After Severe Traumatic Brain Injury in Diverse Labour Market and Welfare State Contexts

Lene Odgaard, Ivan Harsløf, and Peter W. Stubbs

7.1 Introduction

Survivors of severe traumatic brain injury (TBI) often experience lifelong physical and cognitive changes. These changes include attention deficits, impaired memory, and difficulties in problem-solving, decision-making, and impulse control (Sherer et al. 2000). Such deficits may particularly

L. Odgaard (✉)
Hammel Neurorehabilitation and Research Center, Aarhus University, Hammel, Denmark
e-mail: lene.odgaard@midt.rm.dk

I. Harsløf
Department of Social Work, Child Welfare and Social Policy, Oslo Metropolitan University, Oslo, Norway
e-mail: ivan.harslof@oslomet.no

P. W. Stubbs
Graduate School of Health, Discipline of Physiotherapy, University of Technology Sydney, Sydney, NSW, Australia
e-mail: Peter.Stubbs@uts.edu.au

© The Author(s) 2019
I. Harsløf et al. (eds.), *New Dynamics of Disability and Rehabilitation*,
https://doi.org/10.1007/978-981-13-7346-6_7

inhibit obtaining a stable foothold in the post-industrial, knowledge-intensive labour markets that increasingly characterize Northern Europe. Yet recent decades have seen strong reinforcement of employment-oriented measures targeting people with disabilities (OECD 2010a, b). Such efforts have been motivated by the significant financial burden of unemployment and the lack of employment opportunities on the individual, their family, and wider society (Access Economics 2009). Moreover, policymakers now increasingly acknowledge that missing the latent aspects of work, such as immersion in collegial communities, self-realization, and social identity formation, substantially increases the individual's burden (Griep et al. 2016).

This chapter's purpose is to assess the success and failure of labour market integration of severe TBI survivors, and how it may be affected by the larger socioeconomic contexts of disability and social security policies and labour market regulation and characteristics. We first analyse Danish return to work ('RTW') rates, using narrow and broad definitions of RTW, and considering a multitude of factors that may determine successful outcomes. We then review several studies from other countries. As each study relies on specific RTW definitions and methods, comparing RTW rates across countries proves notoriously difficult. For the purpose of comparative assessments, we group the countries by performance into rough categories, enabling discussion of how socioeconomic differences between countries may impact RTW. Such meta-processing is rarely performed in the field of quantitative health science, where the focus is usually on exact estimates. We deem it important to venture into such qualitative discussions to address policymakers' potential role in improving TBI survivors' RTW rates.

7.2   Analysing RTW in Denmark

Denmark is a comprehensive welfare state, reflected in the significant support for people with reduced work capacity, for example, through wage subsidies and supplementary cash benefits. This needs to be accounted for when determining 'successful RTW outcomes'.

Young et al. (2005) argue that there are different stakeholder perspectives on what constitutes a successful RTW outcome. For the purpose of this discussion, we consider two stakeholder groups: 'Payer' and 'Society'. The 'Payer' is interested in the citizen becoming economically self-reliant, that is, independent of any state-supported initiatives, or at least in a position where economic transfers are temporary and 'reproductive' (e.g. when studying or on maternity leave). By contrast, 'Society' has broader interests, such that the citizen receiving transfers while in the process of further labour market integration is considered a successful RTW outcome. This perspective includes positions supported through wage subsidies, activation, or vocational rehabilitation benefits. Given these constructs, 'Payer' and 'Society' respectively refer to narrow and broad perspectives of RTW, and are referred to as such in this chapter.

The Danish studies included in this chapter (Odgaard et al. 2017a, b, 2018) use both the narrow and the broad perspectives. They investigated patients admitted to highly specialized neurorehabilitation after surviving severe TBI between 2004 and 2012. Approximately 84% of the total population of these patients were included in the studies (Odgaard et al. 2015). Attrition due to death and emigration was between 4% and 12%, depending on the time point of follow-up. The studies also included matched controls from the general population. Matching was based on age, sex, pre-injury employment status, educational level, and residence municipality in the calendar year before the index date, that is, the date of injury.

RTW data in the Danish studies were retrieved from the Danish Register for Evaluation of Marginalization (DREAM register), a national administrative register containing weekly information on all public assistance benefits, that is, social benefits and other transfer payments (Hjollund et al. 2007). These data were extracted from nine weeks to five years after the index date. The first week of RTW following the index date was referred to as the 'date of first RTW attempt'. If a person had worked for at least one week from this date, they were deemed to have 'attempted to RTW'. The number of people that had attempted to RTW increased each week resulting in a weekly cumulative proportion (so long as people continued attempting to RTW). As such, the total number of people in the total population of TBI survivors that had attempted to RTW within the first year post-injury was the one-year cumulative proportion of a 'first RTW attempt'. In these analyses, cases of attrition were analysed as competing (i.e. death or normal retirement) or censored (i.e. emigration) events; therefore, loss to follow-up is considered in these analyses.

A 'first RTW attempt' may or may not be stable. For example, a person may find a job but only be able to keep it for a short period. To assess the stability of RTW, subjects were graded using a work participation score, which assessed the number of weeks per year in which a person was working (Biering et al. 2013). Working more than 39 weeks in the year following the 'first RTW attempt' was considered to represent a 'stable RTW'. The number of people with severe TBI that have stable RTW was calculated as a proportion of the total number of severe TBI survivors.

Finally, the working proportion of patients and general population matched controls were calculated at a specific time point (calculated weekly) after the index date. Estimates calculated for a specific time point are referred to as the 'point prevalence', which excludes weeks with retirement, death, or emigration. The point prevalence is the most frequently reported estimate of RTW in studies from other countries. Since only the Danish studies reviewed in this chapter reported estimates of attempts to RTW or subsequent work stability, the point prevalence is an important measure of RTW for international comparison purposes.

Finally, multivariable competing risk and logistic regression models were used to assess whether selected characteristics were associated with RTW, including stable RTW. These data were retrieved from registers at Statistics Denmark and from a national clinical quality database focusing on neurorehabilitation after severe TBI (Odgaard et al. 2015). The selected characteristics were:

1. Pre-injury characteristics, including socio-demographics (sex, age, educational level, pre-injury transfer incomes, cohabitation status) and comorbidity (Charlson Comorbidity Index);
2. Injury severity (duration of post-traumatic amnesia and length of stay in acute care);
3. Functional ability after injury (Early Functional Ability score (Hankemeier and Rollnik 2015) on admission to highly specialized neurorehabilitation and at discharge therefrom);

4. Rehabilitation trajectories (number of attended rehabilitation hospitals, calendar year of injury, and number of inhabitants in the patients'/controls' residence municipality).

Results: RTW After Severe TBI in Denmark

The first RTW attempt mainly occurred in the first two years following TBI. RTW outcomes varied according to narrow or broad perspectives of RTW. As such, RTW outcome is presented as a percentage range. Depending on the RTW perspective, 30–52% (40–64% among previously employed people) first attempted to RTW within the first two years after the injury, and 16–31% (22–39% among previously employed people) achieved stable RTW. The percentage of individuals working after severe TBI declined from 15–33% two years post-injury to 11–30% five years post-injury, whereas the corresponding percentage in the general population that matched controls was stable at over 70% (Fig. 7.1).

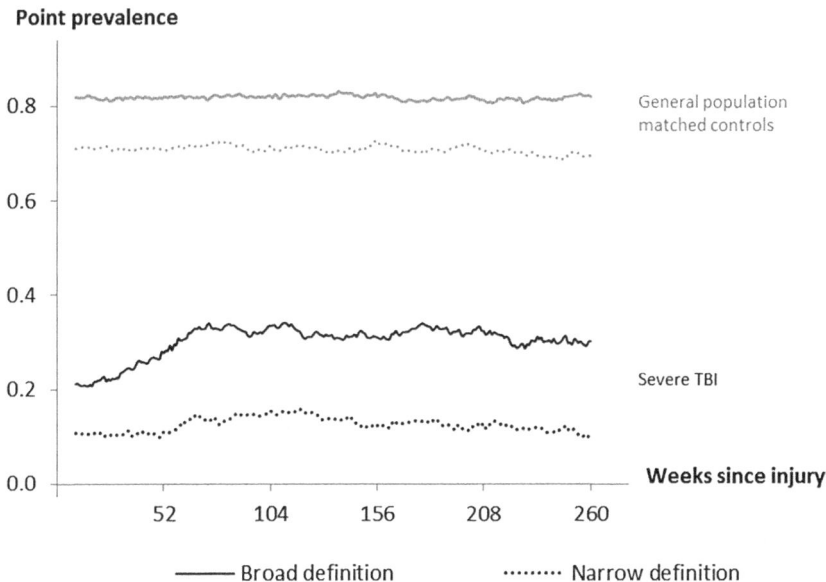

Fig. 7.1 Weekly prevalence of employment for the two definitions of work among general population matched controls and people with severe TBI

Characteristics associated with embarking on the RTW process (first RTW attempt) were younger age; higher education level; receiving no transfer income or receiving transfer income related to supported employment prior to injury; shorter stay in acute care; higher functional ability after injury on admission to highly specialized neurorehabilitation; and injury after 2009. The only significant predictor of stable RTW was younger age. Tested factors not associated with RTW or stable RTW following severe TBI were sex; cohabitation status; duration of post-traumatic amnesia; functional ability on discharge from highly specialized rehabilitation; and size of the residence municipality.

7.3   Comparing the Danish Results with RTW in Other Countries

This section reviews studies in other countries of RTW after severe TBI, thereby providing the basis for comparative assessment. To aid interpretation of the results, we provide the contextual detail of general unemployment rates between countries, and discuss methodological differences between the studies. In general, the estimates of RTW after severe TBI varied significantly (ranging from 15% to 63%), with Danish estimates at the lower end. Table 7.1 provides an overview of these studies. We also group the countries into rough categories of low, moderate, and high RTW performance, as summarized in Table 7.2. It should be noted that the assessment of RTW performance is non-normative: high RTW performance is not necessarily the ideal outcome or in the best interests of people with TBI (see Sect. 7.4).

7.3.1   Identifying Studies for Comparison

The studies for comparison were identified through PubMed, a search engine retrieving life sciences and biomedical research databases.[1] The

---

[1] We used the following search string: 'Craniocerebral Trauma' [MeSH] AND ('Employment, Supported' [MeSH] OR 'Employment' [MeSH] OR 'Return to Work' [MeSH] OR 'Rehabilitation, Vocational' [MeSH]).

Table 7.1 Overview of studies on the frequency of RTW following severe TBI

Country	General unemployment[a] at the time of injury	RTW estimates after severe TBI	RTW definition	Design	Study population	Reference
Denmark	2004–2008: 3.4–5.2% 2009–2012: 6.6–7.6%	1 year: ≤26% 2 years: ≤33% 3 years: ≤30% 5 years: ≤30% Pre-injury employed: First attempt to RTW within 1 year: ≤46% Stable RTW after first RTW within 1 year: ≤30%	*Narrow definition* Economic self-reliance (no public assistance benefits except leave and state educational fund grant) *Broad definition* Economic self-reliance and supported employment (wage subsidies/activation/ vocational rehabilitation benefits)	Close to population-based Register-based data	TBI acute care survivors 2004–2012 Attrition: 4–12% Severe TBI defined as GCS ≤8 within 48 hours of injury	Odgaard, Johnsen, Pedersen, and Nielsen (2017a); Odgaard, Johnsen, Stubbs, et al. (2017b)
Norway	1995–1996: 5.0–6.3%	10 years: ≤40%	*Narrow definition* Full-time employment/ studying *Broad definition* Full-time and part-time employment/studying	Population-based[b] Self-reported data	TBI acute care survivors 1995–1996 Attrition: 54% Excluded patients with neurological or psychiatric comorbidities and patients with associated spinal cord injury Severe TBI defined as GCS ≤8 on emergency admission	Andelic et al. (2009)

(continued)

Table 7.1 (continued)

Country	General unemployment[a] at the time of injury	RTW estimates after severe TBI	RTW definition	Design	Study population	Reference
France	2005–2007: 7.7–8.5%	1 year: 40%	*Broad definition* Paid or volunteer activities including studying	Population-based[b] Self-reported data	TBI acute care survivors 2005–2007 Attrition: 47% Severe TBI defined as GCS ≤8 before hospital admission	Jourdan et al. (2013)
The Netherlands	1999–2004: 2.1–4.7%	3 years: 54% 10 years: 47%	*Narrow definition* Paid activities Student status is not counted as RTW	Population-based[b] Self-reported data	TBI acute care survivors 1999–2004 Excluded patients with pre-injury neurological, oncological, or systemic impairments and patients who did not want to participate Attrition: 3 years: 17%; 10 years: 71% Severe TBI defined as GCS ≤8 within 24 hours of injury	Grauwmeijer et al. (2012) Grauwmeijer et al. (2017)

(continued)

Table 7.1 (continued)

Country	General unemployment[a] at the time of injury	RTW estimates after severe TBI	RTW definition	Design	Study population	Reference
USA	1984–1990: NA 1991–1994: 6.1–7.5%	1 year: 38%	*Narrow definition* Competitive employment Students were excluded from the USA2 and USA4 studies USA3 did not count student status as RTW, and USA1 provided no relevant information	Clinic-based Self-reported data	Pre-injury working TBI patients enrolled in randomized trials, injured 1984–1994 Attrition: 11% Severe TBI defined as GCS ≤ 8 within 24 hours of injury	USA1: Doctor et al. (2005)
	1999–2003: 4.0–6.0%	1 year: 54%			Pre-injury working TBI survivors 1999–2003 Attrition: 25–43% Severity defined with the Abbreviated Injury Scale (AIS) Head Region	USA2: Corrigan et al. (2007)
	1990: NA 1991–2000: 4.0–7.5% 2001–2009: 4.4–9.3%	1 year: 23%			Hispanic TBI acute care survivors 1990–2009 Attrition: 30% Severe TBI defined as GCS ≤ 8 on emergency admission	USA3: Ketchum et al. (2012)
	2009–2014: 6.2–9.3%	1 year: 15%			War veterans 2009–2014, TBI patients with no pre-injury work limitations, discharged alive Attrition: 21% Severe TBI defined as GCS ≤ 8 within 24 hours of injury	USA4: Dillahunt- Aspillaga et al. (2017)

(continued)

Table 7.1 (continued)

Country	General unemployment[a] at the time of injury	RTW estimates after severe TBI	RTW definition	Design	Study population	Reference
Brazil	2006–2011: 6.7–8.4%	1.5 years: 63%	*Narrow definition* Competitive employment No information regarding students	Clinic-based Self-reported data	TBI survivors 2006–2011 Excluded post-injury vegetative state patients Attrition: 28% Severe TBI defined as GCS ≤8	Diaz et al. (2014)

RTW return to work, *NA* not available, *GCS* Glasgow Coma Scale

[a]General unemployment rates according to the International Labour Organization (2016)

[b]The extent to which the study is truly population-based (i.e. representative) is unknown, as patients refusing to participate were excluded and attrition was high

Table 7.2 Qualitative assessments of RTW performance after severe TBI in selected countries

Low RTW	Moderate RTW	High RTW
Denmark	France	Brazil
Norway	Netherlands	
	USA	

Please note that the assessment of RTW performance is non-normative, that is, high RTW performance is not necessarily the ideal outcome or in the best interests of people with TBI

search was restricted to the period of January 2004–May 2018. The search revealed ten studies reporting the frequency of RTW after severe TBI in countries other than Denmark. One study was excluded as its attrition rate was 89% (Ponsford et al. 2014).

7.3.2 General Unemployment Rates When the Studies Were Conducted

The general unemployment rates in the different countries become a methodological concern when comparing RTW rates, since high (low) general unemployment plausibly reduces (increases) employment opportunities for people with severe TBI. Unemployment rates could, for instance, explain the differences in RTW between the Dutch studies (RTW 54% and 47% at 3 and 10 years and low unemployment of 2.1–4.7%) and the French study (RTW 40% at 1 year and high unemployment of 7.7–8.5%). Over the study period in Denmark, unemployment was 3.4–7.6%, which is comparatively lower than unemployment rates in other countries. Furthermore, if general unemployment affected RTW outcome, the higher unemployment rates in the study's later period (2009–2012) would have been accompanied by less people attempting to RTW. However, this was not the case, and those injured from 2009 onwards were actually more likely to RTW compared to those injured during 2004–2005, when unemployment rates were lower. Therefore, unemployment was not the reason for the relatively low RTW detected in Denmark.

Taking other methodological concerns into consideration (see Sects. 7.3.4 and 7.3.5), low RTW despite low general unemployment rates is also conspicuous in the Norwegian study (RTW 40% at 10 years and low unemployment of 5.0–6.3%) (see the OECD's (2006, 2008) general assessment of people with disabilities' RTW in Norway and Denmark).

7.3.3 The Time Point of Follow-Up

In the studies in other countries, the time point of follow-up varied from one to ten years post-injury, with most studies only including one time point (the point prevalence). As the Danish studies had data for the whole period up to five years post-injury, the Danish RTW estimates can be compared with the point prevalence estimates of other studies. This comparison generally revealed lower RTW in Denmark regardless of the time point post-injury. However, the time point could explain differences in RTW between some of the other studies. For example, it is likely that some people will RTW later than one year post-injury. Therefore, the French RTW estimate of 40% at one year post-injury would likely increase after the time point of follow-up and become close to the Dutch estimate of 54% at three years post-injury.

7.3.4 The Definitions of Successful RTW Outcome

Some studies, including all four US studies, used a narrow definition of RTW, solely considering the achievement of paid employment as a successful outcome. Some other studies used a broader definition of successful RTW, including voluntary activities (France) and studying (France and Norway). The only European study that used a narrow RTW definition was the Dutch study. However, if voluntary work had been included in the Dutch study, the Dutch RTW estimate may have been largely unchanged, as general unemployment was low during the study period. On the other hand, the inclusion of students in the Dutch definition of a successful RTW outcome would have increased the RTW estimate, since many patients with TBI are in education at the time of injury (as they tend to be young). Although RTW performance appears higher in the Dutch study than in the French study, both countries were assessed as exhibiting moderate RTW performance (Table 7.2) due to reasons related to study design.

The Danish studies used narrow and broad definitions of RTW. However, even when adopting the broad definition, which classifies a larger spectrum of outcomes as successful RTW, Denmark performs poorly compared to France, Brazil, the Netherlands, and the USA (based on the most representative US study, USA2) (see Sect. 7.3.5).

7.3.5   Study Design and Study Population in the Different National Studies

A major source of difference between the studies lies in design and population. The population- and register-based design used in the Danish studies entails a lower risk of bias or incorrect inferences, compared to the design of studies in other countries. First, non-register-based studies often have a large loss to follow-up. Since loss to follow-up is more common among pre-injury unemployed people compared to employed persons (Jourdan et al. 2016; Corrigan et al. 2003), studies with high attrition likely overestimate RTW. Also, while self-reported, retrospective employment data generally tend to have good validity (Dex and McCulloch 1998), data based on self-reporting, as used in all the studies but the Danish, are often biased, as people recovering from TBI may not be able to understand some survey questions or may not remember things correctly.

The French, Dutch, and Norwegian studies were confined to a defined geographical area. However, the extent to which these studies were truly population-based within their defined areas is unknown, as patients refusing to participate were excluded and attrition was high. Therefore, RTW numbers in these European studies are most likely overestimated. The overestimation was probably higher in the Dutch and the Norwegian studies than in the French study, since they excluded patients with pre-injury illnesses such as neurological and psychiatric diseases, known to decrease the likelihood of RTW.

Based on these considerations, together with general unemployment rates and the definition of RTW, the Dutch RTW estimates (54% and 47% paid activities at three and ten years post-injury) are likely only slightly higher than the French RTW estimate (40% paid/volunteer/ student activities one year post-injury), that is, both countries' RTW performance is moderate. Similarly, we assume that the Norwegian estimate (40% full-time/part-time/student ten years post-injury) is only slightly higher than the Danish estimates (≤30% five years post-injury), reflecting relatively low RTW performance (see Table 7.2).

When assessing the US studies, we should note that the attrition rate was high and studies were confined to the population of patients admitted to certain clinics. In the USA, patients that receive rehabilitation in clinics are predominantly young, with a pre-injury work record (Corrigan et al. 2012; Cuthbert et al. 2012): both factors are associated with high RTW.

One US study (USA2) specifically excluded people who were not working pre-injury and weighted loss to follow-up using a standard procedure. Therefore, the selection bias from the non-register-based design is minimized, and the study is largely representative of severe TBI survivors with a pre-injury work record in the USA. Comparing this study's estimate with the Danish estimates among TBI survivors working pre-injury reveals higher RTW in the USA (USA2 among pre-injury working: 54% at one year; Denmark among pre-injury working: ≤46% first RTW attempt within one year; ≤30% stable RTW after first RTW attempt within one year). Since the USA2 study included only people working pre-injury, its RTW estimate may be comparable to the French overall RTW estimate (40% paid/volunteer/student activities one year post-injury), that is, moderate RTW performance (see Table 7.2).

The studies USA3 and USA4 were restricted to specific populations with a known lower probability of RTW, that is, Hispanics (USA3), who do not have the same opportunities as the general population (Arango-Lasprilla et al. 2011), and war veterans (USA4). These studies had similar RTW estimates to the Danish RTW estimates, that is, low RTW performance. However, they focused on minority groups, which are unlikely representative of the severe TBI population in the USA. The study USA1 is relatively old, as it included patients injured from 1984 to

1994. Its low RTW estimate (38% among people working pre-injury) probably reflects the lack of rehabilitation opportunities during this time period. These patients' representativeness of the general severe TBI population in the USA during this period is also unknown. For these reasons, caution must be exercised when using the studies USA1, USA3, and USA4 to compare RTW performance between countries.

Finally, the Brazilian study had the same methodological weaknesses as those in other countries, including a non-register-based design, self-reported data, a relatively high attrition rate, and exclusion of patients in a persistent vegetative state, that is, groups with a known lower probability of RTW. The study demonstrated the highest RTW (63% 1.5 years post-injury); as such, Brazil has high RTW performance (Table 7.2).

A final difference between the study populations lies in their definitions of severe TBI. The most commonly used scale of injury severity was the Glasgow Coma Scale (GCS). However, the studies used GCS scores at different time points post-injury, and as GCS rapidly changes post-TBI, it is likely that the studies recruited slightly different patient cohorts. Furthermore, some studies used different scales to define TBI severity, such as the abbreviated injury scale (USA2). As such, the severity of patients' injuries might also differ between studies. Unfortunately, the impact of these differences on RTW estimates is unknown, and the definition of severe TBI is not considered in our assessment of RTW performance.

7.4 Discussion of Labour Market and RTW Policy Factors that May Explain Country Differences in RTW Performance

In the previous section, we discussed how the cross-country variances in RTW outcomes may be attributed to issues such as loss to follow-up and several other methodological differences between studies. We argued that such differences likely explain some difference in RTW performance between countries, precluding any direct comparisons based on precise estimates. However, we also argued that countries could be roughly categorized in terms of RTW performance. In our inter-country comparisons, Denmark and Norway—representing the social democratic welfare state—had proportionally fewer TBI patients returning to work compared to countries with a conservative welfare state (France and the Netherlands), a liberal welfare state (USA), and, in particular, a development welfare state (Brazil).

Drawing on this rough assessment, this section provides a conjectural discussion of these countries' performance in terms of the wider labour market and RTW policy factors. The likelihood that TBI patients will RTW is dependent on numerous factors, beyond the quality of medical services in the acute and post-acute phase. These factors relate to the state of the labour market, policies to encourage the supply and demand of labour among people with disabilities, and the overall institutional setting of the welfare state.

7.4.1   Welfare Models

To understand the welfare state's institutional setting, one can consider Esping-Andersen's (1990) welfare state typology. He proposes three different welfare state models that vary in their manner and extent of intervention in the wage-labour nexus (cf. Chap. 2 of this volume). The social democratic model has an underlying philosophical basis of socialism (Van Voorhis 2002). Social protection is based on equality, with little need for private/commercial involvement. In this model, labour enjoys a high degree of de-commodification, constituted by generous and universal benefits, allowing workers some degrees of freedom vis-à-vis market forces. The welfare states in Denmark and Norway approximate this model. Strong degrees of de-commodification, reflected in TBI patients having the option to receive a generous permanent disability pension, may disincentivize participating in RTW programmes, not because people lack motivation to work per se, but because the RTW trajectory may lead to vulnerable and disadvantageous positions, while also removing the option of permanent disability benefit.

The conservative model is oriented towards preserving the male bread-winner model and established occupational hierarchies (Van Voorhis

2002). Social protection is largely based on contribution, with different groups receiving different protection levels. In this model, labour has a moderate degree of de-commodification (i.e. high for insiders, low for outsiders), and labour market integration and civil rights are moderate for people with disabilities (Tschanz and Staub 2017). France and the Netherlands are examples of this model, although the latter case has also been found to exhibit social democratic traits (for another conservative case, see Chap. 3 on Germany).

The liberal state has an underlying philosophical basis of classical liberalism (Tschanz and Staub 2017). It allocates most social protection on a residual (targeted) basis, and only as a last resort. In this model, labour has a low degree of de-commodification. The liberal model is detailed in Chap. 4 of this volume, which focuses especially on the UK. In this chapter, the USA represents the liberal model.

In countries with low de-commodification, such as the USA, insufficient support might force a person with TBI into the labour market when they are not ready, driving them into low-quality and low-skilled work, with little opportunity of gradually returning to their pre-injury work. The high RTW rate in Brazil may reflect a similar lack of sufficient social protection for TBI survivors, forcing them into employment. However, conclusions should be tentative. While social protection in Brazil, being a middle-income country, is low compared to countries such as Denmark and Norway, spending on social programmes was relatively high compared to other Southern American countries, at the time covered in the Brazilian study (Tillin and Pereira 2017).

7.4.2 The Functioning of the Labour Market

To understand the functioning of a country's labour market, one needs to understand how labour markets are interwoven with the welfare state. In the Nordic countries, comprehensive state-provided welfare benefits and relatively lax regulation of employment has emerged. This combination has been a suitable option for small and open economies, characterized by small and medium export-oriented enterprises (Engelstad 1999). In its most pure form, this combination of a comprehensive welfare state and lax labour market regulation is termed the 'flexicurity model'. The model grants employers relatively high degrees of freedom in managing their workforce as needs change according to export markets and business cycles, while employees can rely on relatively generous benefits if made redundant (Berglund and Madsen 2010). It is, however, likely that this set-up hampers the RTW of people with disabilities, including TBI patients,[2] since it abandons quotas and other requirements on employers to stimulate the employment of people with disabilities.

Hence, one barrier to RTW in Denmark and Norway may be that employers are not obliged to retain workers following long-term sickness. By contrast, in the Netherlands, 70% of sick people are re-employed by their former employer (OECD 2008), perhaps because employers are required to take action, such as developing a 're-integration plan', and pay contributions to the disability benefit system, including levies on allowances granted to employees (OECD 2010c).

In Denmark, only 40% of sick people are employed by their former employer (OECD 2008), as Danish legislation facilitates the dismissal of sick employees. Instead, the welfare state (incorporated into job centres) carries the responsibility for social security and helping disabled persons to find a job. Therefore, Danish people with disabilities are generally less likely to be re-employed by their former employers. Hence, it may be easier for job centres to create a fully dependent welfare client, rather than a working person. This is important, as effective RTW interventions for people with severe TBI requires workplace involvement (Donker-Cools et al. 2015), which is impractical if the TBI survivor has no workplace.

---

[2] The flexicurity model is primarily associated with the Danish system, but a broader perspective on flexibility, considering not only degrees of employment protection but also the general regulatory system for doing business, suggests that all the Nordic countries are characterized by flexicurity. The flexicurity label is also applied to the Dutch case, but here the element of flexibility concerns the deregulation of part-time, fixed-term, and agency work, as well as the encouragement of leave schemes (Wilthagen and Tros 2004). These differences may be important, as we shall discuss later in this chapter.

7.4.3 Post-Industrial, High-Productivity Labour Markets

Another important feature is labour market productivity. People with reduced work capacities may experience more exclusion, due to difficulties of competition, in labour markets characterized by high productivity. The Nordic countries have especially high productivity (Annenkov and Madaschi 2005), and are characterized by large service sectors with many knowledge-intensive service jobs, strong digitalization, internationalization of working life, and a strong requirement for soft skills and dispositions such as flexibility, communication, and teamwork skills (Harsløf et al. 2013). Such requirements are likely to constitute barriers for people in the process of RTW following a brain injury.

7.4.4 Disability Policies

When discussing labour market disability policies, different clusters of countries may be considered, each manifesting different patterns of combining social protection, labour market integration, and civil rights. The social democratic countries tend to score highest in social protection, labour market integration, and civil rights for people with disabilities (Tschanz and Staub 2017).

In Denmark and Norway, people with health problems and disabilities are entitled to generous benefits. The Norwegian programmes are particularly generous (OECD 2006). However, these countries also have several state-funded RTW initiatives for people who are sick or disabled (Ministry of Children, Gender Equality, Integration and Social Affairs 2014). In 2007, Denmark, Norway, and the Netherlands were three of five OECD countries spending 10% more on active rehabilitation programmes than 'passive' benefits, and in the OECD index of work integration of general disability claimants, Denmark and Norway ranked highest among OECD countries (OECD 2010c). People with severe TBI require lower-skilled work, part-time work, and/or flexible work arrangements, which people with other disabilities may not require. Therefore, RTW after severe TBI is dependent on whether such jobs are available in the labour market. As mentioned earlier, Denmark and Norway are dominated by highly skilled jobs, which severe TBI survivors are less likely to occupy. There is also lack of part-time work (OECD 2010b), although there are programmes to assist the employment of people with permanent health deficits (such as the permanent 'flexjob' in Denmark).

7.5 Conclusion

This chapter has assessed several studies of RTW among severe TBI patients, and roughly grouped several countries into low, moderate, and high RTW performers. Compared to the other considered countries, Denmark and Norway have conspicuously low RTW rates, particularly given their relatively favourable overall employment situation. This may be attributable to the welfare state's institutional setting. While the strong level of de-commodification does not seem to hamper general participation in working life, it may disincentivize severe TBI patients from embarking in RTW programmes. Other reasons for low RTW may include inappropriate work opportunities—lack of part-time work and low-skilled jobs (less cognitively demanding)—and a flexicurity model that places the onus of RTW on the welfare state, as Danish employers are not required to re-employ people following injury.

We end this chapter by discussing possible strategies for improving RTW rates in the Nordic countries.

Potential Strategies to Improve RTW Outcomes for Severe TBI Survivors in Denmark and Norway
There is a discrepancy in Denmark and Norway between the RTW rate of severe TBI survivors and the employment rate of the overall disabled population. We have argued that this may partly result from the policy directives typical of a social democratic state, which transfer responsibility from employers and TBI survivors to the welfare state. It should also be noted that high RTW performance is not necessarily the ideal outcome, as it may reflect a harsh employment regime forcing TBI survivors in a poor health condition to seek paid work for lack of sufficient social protection. While changing an established system may be difficult, we

have identified inadequacies in the system and recommend several modifications to increase societal inclusiveness of people with deficits resulting from severe TBI. Suggested modifications are as follows:

- Evidence suggests that effective RTW interventions for people with severe TBI require workplace involvement, combined with skills training, education, and coaching (Donker-Cools et al. 2015), that is, involving employers in the RTW process is crucial if the aim is to make people with severe TBI return to work.
- To involve employers, the government could adopt a carrot-and-stick approach. If employers are involved and responsible for re-employment, it is likely that some lower-skilled jobs and/or part-time jobs suitable for severe TBI survivors may develop. The carrot could be offering financial incentives to companies to re-employ people with severe TBI, whereas the stick could be mandatory 're-integration plans' developed by the employers and/or mandatory contribution to the disability benefit system, as in the Netherlands (OECD 2010c).
- To adequately cater for severe TBI survivors, those assisting in RTW efforts require additional skills, capacity, and training. Such initiatives take time and planning, and may not be a priority in the current employment landscape. This should be considered and addressed by policymakers.
- In Denmark, younger age was the only significant predictor of stable RTW following severe TBI. This may indicate that the system assists the young to find work, while ignoring the needs of older people. Both younger and older people are capable of neurological recovery, so the difference observed could be a result of differential treatment between age groups, indicating employer discrimination against older people with severe TBI. Therefore, schemes to actively promote hiring older people with TBI could be implemented.

Acknowledgements This chapter reproduces, in part, material published in Odgaard, Johnsen, Pedersen, and Nielsen (2017a), Odgaard, Johnsen, Stubbs, et al. (2017b), and Odgaard, Pedersen, et al. (2018). As such, we acknowledge our earlier co-authors and thank them for their contributions to this work.

References

Access Economics. (2009). *The economic cost of spinal cord injury and traumatic brain injury in Australia*. Report by Access Economics for the Victorian Neurotrauma Initiative (p. 31). Canberra: Access Economics.

Andelic, N., Hammergren, N., Bautz-Holter, E., Sveen, U., Brunborg, C., & Røe, C. (2009). Functional outcome and health-related quality of life 10 years after moderate-to-severe traumatic brain injury. *Acta Neurologica Scandinavica, 120*(1), 16–23.

Annenkov, A., & Madaschi, C. (2005). *Labour productivity in the Nordic EU countries: A comparative overview and explanatory factors 1980–2004*. ECB occasional paper no. 39.

Arango-Lasprilla, J. C., Ketchum, J. M., Lewis, A. N., Krch, D., Gary, K. W., & Dodd, B. A., Jr. (2011). Racial and ethnic disparities in employment outcomes for persons with traumatic brain injury: A longitudinal investigation 1–5 years after injury. *PM&R: The Journal of Injury, Function, and Rehabilitation, 3*(12), 1083–1091.

Berglund, T., & Madsen, P. K. (2010). Nordic labour market and welfare systems from a flexicurity perspective. In *Labour market mobility in Nordic welfare states* (pp. 37–60). Copenhagen: Nordic Council of Ministers.

Biering, K., Hjøllund, N. H., & Lund, T. (2013). Methods in measuring return to work: A comparison of measures of return to work following treatment of coronary heart disease. *Journal of Occupational Rehabilitation, 23*(3), 400–405.

Corrigan, J. D., Harrison-Felix, C., Bogner, J., Dijkers, M., Terrill, M. S., & Whiteneck, G. (2003). Systematic bias in traumatic brain injury outcome studies because of loss to follow-up. *Archives of Physical Medicine and Rehabilitation, 84*(2), 153–160.

Corrigan, J. D., Lineberry, L. A., Komaroff, E., Langlois, J. A., Selassie, A. W., & Wood, K. D. (2007). Employment after traumatic brain injury: Differences between men and women. *Archives of Physical Medicine and Rehabilitation, 88*(11), 1400–1409.

Corrigan, J. D., Cuthbert, J. P., Whiteneck, G. G., Dijkers, M. P., Coronado, V., Heinemann, A. W., et al. (2012). Representativeness of the traumatic brain injury model systems national database. *The Journal of Head Trauma Rehabilitation, 27*(6), 391–403.

Cuthbert, J. P., Corrigan, J. D., Whiteneck, G. G., Harrison-Felix, C., Graham, J. E., Bell, J. M., & Coronado, V. G. (2012). Extension of the representativeness of the traumatic brain injury model systems national database: 2001 to 2010. *The Journal of Head Trauma Rehabilitation, 27*(6), E15–E27.

Dex, S., & McCulloch, A. (1998). The reliability of retrospective unemployment history data. *Work, Employment and Society, 12*(3), 497–509.

Diaz, A. P., Schwarzbold, M. L., Thais, M. E., Cavallazzi, G. G., Schmoeller, R., Nunes, J. C., et al. (2014). Personality changes and return to work after severe traumatic brain injury: A prospective study. *Revista Brasileira de Psiquiatria, 36*(3), 213–219.

Dillahunt-Aspillaga, C., Nakase-Richardson, R., Hart, T., Powell-Cope, G., Dreer, L. E., Eapen, B. C., et al. (2017). Predictors of employment outcomes in veterans with traumatic brain injury: A VA traumatic brain injury model systems study. *The Journal of Head Trauma Rehabilitation, 32*(4), 271–282.

Doctor, J. N., Castro, J., Temkin, N. R., Fraser, R. T., Machamer, J. E., & Dikmen, S. S. (2005). Workers' risk of unemployment after traumatic brain injury: A normed comparison. *Journal of the International Neuropsychological Society, 11*(6), 747–752.

Donker-Cools, B. H. P. M., Daams, J. G., Wind, H., & Frings-Dresen, M. H. W. (2015). Effective return-to-work interventions after acquired brain injury: A systematic review. *Brain Injury, 30*(2), 1–19.

Engelstad, F. (1999). Demokrati og makt – samfunn og bedrift [Democracy and power – Society and enterprise]. In Ø. Østerud (Ed.), *Mot en ny maktutredning* [Towards a new investigation of power in Norway] (pp. 19–42). Oslo: Gyldendal Akademisk.

Esping-Andersen, G. (1990). *The three worlds of welfare capitalism.* Cambridge: Polity Press.

Grauwmeijer, E., Heijenbrok-Kal, M. H., Haitsma, I. K., & Ribbers, G. M. (2012). A prospective study on employment outcome 3 years after moderate to severe traumatic brain injury. *Archives of Physical Medicine and Rehabilitation, 93*(6), 993–999.

Grauwmeijer, E., Heijenbrok-Kal, M. H., Haitsma, I. K., & Ribbers, G. M. (2017). Employment outcome ten years after moderate to severe traumatic brain injury: A prospective cohort study. *Journal of Neurotrauma, 34*(17), 2575–2581.

Griep, Y., Kinnunen, U., Nätti, J., De Cuyper, N., Mauno, S., Mäkikangas, A., & De Witte, H. (2016). The effects of unemployment and perceived job insecurity: A comparison of their association with psychological and somatic complaints, self-rated health and life satisfaction. *International Archives of Occupational and Environmental Health, 89*(1), 147–162.

Hankemeier, A., & Rollnik, J. D. (2015). The Early Functional Abilities (EFA) scale to assess neurological and neurosurgical early rehabilitation patients. *BMC Neurology, 15*(1), 207.

Harsløf, I., Scarpa, S., & Andersen, S. N. (2013). Changing population profiles and social risk structures in the Nordic countries. In I. Harsløf & R. Ulmestig (Eds.), *Changing social risks and social policy responses in the Nordic welfare states* (pp. 25–49). Basingstoke: Palgrave Macmillan.

Hjollund, N. H., Larsen, F. B., & Andersen, J. H. (2007). Register-based follow-up of social benefits and other transfer payments: Accuracy and degree of completeness in a Danish interdepartmental administrative database compared with a population-based survey. *Scandinavian Journal of Public Health, 35*(5), 497–502.

International Labour Organization. (2016). *Key indicators of the Labour market: Unemployment rate.* https://www.ilo.org/ilostat/. Accessed 1 July 2018.

Jourdan, C., Bosserelle, V., Azerad, S., Ghout, I., Bayen, E., Aegerter, P., et al. (2013). Predictive factors for 1-year outcome of a cohort of patients with severe traumatic brain injury (TBI): Results from the PariS-TBI study. *Brain Injury, 27*(9), 1000–1007.

Jourdan, C., Bayen, E., Bahrami, S., Ghout, I., Darnoux, E., Azerad, S., et al. (2016). Loss to follow-up and social background in an inception cohort of patients with severe traumatic brain injury: Results from the PariS-TBI study. *The Journal of Head Trauma Rehabilitation, 31*, E42.

Ketchum, J. M., Almaz Getachew, M., Krch, D., Banos, J. H., Kolakowsky-Hayner, S. A., Lequerica, A., et al. (2012). Early predictors of employment outcomes 1 year post traumatic brain injury in a population of Hispanic individuals. *NeuroRehabilitation, 30*(1), 13–22.

Ministry of Children, Gender Equality, Integration and Social Affairs. (2014). *Social security.* http://sm.dk/en/responsibilites/social-security. Accessed 15 June 2015.

Odgaard, L., Poulsen, I., Kammersgaard, L. P., Johnsen, S. P., & Nielsen, J. F. (2015). Surviving severe traumatic brain injury in Denmark: Incidence and predictors of highly specialized rehabilitation. *Clinical Epidemiology, 7*, 225–234.

Odgaard, L., Johnsen, S. P., Pedersen, A. R., & Nielsen, J. F. (2017a). Return to work after severe traumatic brain injury: A nationwide follow-up study. *The Journal of Head Trauma Rehabilitation, 32*(3), E57–E64.

Odgaard, L., Johnsen, S. P., Stubbs, P. W., Pedersen, A. R., & Nielsen, J. F. (2017b). Alternative measures reveal different but low estimates of labour market attachment after severe traumatic brain injury: A nationwide cohort study. *Brain Injury, 31*(10), 1–9.

Odgaard, L., Pedersen, A. R., Poulsen, I., Johnsen, S. P., & Nielsen, J. F. (2018). Return to work predictors after traumatic brain injury in a welfare state. *Acta Neurologica Scandinavica, 137*(1), 44–50.

OECD. (2006). *Sickness, disability and work: Breaking the barriers: Norway, Poland and Switzerland* (Vol. 1). Paris: OECD Publishing. Tables available at: https://www.oecd.org/norway/sicknessdisabilityandworkvol1norwaypolandandswitzerland.htm

OECD. (2008). *Sickness, disability and work: Breaking the barriers: Denmark, Finland, Ireland and the Netherlands* (Vol. 3). Paris: OECD Publishing. https://doi.org/10.1787/9789264049826-en.

OECD. (2010a). Executive summary and policy conclusions. In *Sickness, disability and work: Breaking the barriers: A synthesis of Findings across OECD countries*. Paris: OECD Publishing. https://doi.org/10.1787/9789264088856-en.

OECD. (2010b). Insufficient labour market integration of people with disability. In *Sickness, disability and work: Breaking the barriers: A synthesis of finding across OECD countries*. Paris: OECD Publishing. https://doi.org/10.1787/9789264088856-en.

OECD. (2010c). Sickness, disability and work: Improving social and labour-market integration of people with disability. Fact sheet based on *Sickness, Disability and Work: Breaking the Barriers*. Paris: OECD Publishing. https://www.oecd.org/els/soc/46488022.pdf

Ponsford, J. L., Downing, M. G., Olver, J., Ponsford, M., Acher, R., Carty, M., & Spitz, G. (2014). Longitudinal follow-up of patients with traumatic brain injury: Outcome at two, five, and ten years post-injury. *Journal of Neurotrauma, 31*(1), 64–77.

Sherer, M., Madison, C. F., & Hannay, H. J. (2000). A review of outcome after moderate and severe closed head injury with an introduction to life care planning. *The Journal of Head Trauma Rehabilitation, 15*(2), 767–782.

Tillin, L., & Pereira, A. W. (2017). Federalism, multi-level elections and social policy in Brazil and India. *Commonwealth & Comparative Politics, 55*(3), 328–352.

Tschanz, C., & Staub, I. (2017). Disability-policy models in European welfare regimes: Comparing the distribution of social protection, labour-market integration and civil rights. *Disability & Society, 32*(8), 1199–1215.

Van Voorhis, R. A. (2002). Different types of welfare states? A methodological deconstruction of comparative research. *Journal of Sociology & Social Welfare, 29*, 3.

Wilthagen, T., & Tros, F. (2004). The concept of 'flexicurity': A new approach to regulating employment and labour markets. *Transfer: European Review of Labour and Research, 10*(2), 166–186.

Young, A. E., Wasiak, R., Roessler, R. T., McPherson, K. M., Anema, J. R., & van Poppel, M. N. (2005). Return-to-work outcomes following work disability: Stakeholder motivations, interests and concerns. *Journal of Occupational Rehabilitation, 15*(4), 543–556.

8

Severe Brain Injury and Boundary Work

Anette Lykke Hindhede

8.1 Introduction

Today, as increasing numbers of people survive traumatic brain injury (TBI), correspondingly more are living with complex negative health effects afterwards (Danish Health Authority 2011; Juengst et al. 2015). These effects may appear as impaired physical, mental, and social functioning, and can be devastating for both the individual and their social relations (Das-Gupta and Turner-Stokes 2002). Predominantly, research on TBI survivors tends to consider this group as homogeneous in terms of how they experience their disability (Lefebvre et al. 2008). However, lifestyles in general negotiate between the objective structures of a society and the subjective practices possible within it. Thus, TBI is an example of a condition that individuals of diverse socioeconomic statuses bear across various previous life standards, practices, or 'modes of existence' (Bourdieu 1984, p. 741). One of the implications of this is that

A. L. Hindhede (✉)
Department of Learning and Philosophy, Aalborg University Copenhagen,
Copenhagen, Denmark
e-mail: alh@learning.aau.dk

© The Author(s) 2019   **171**
I. Harsløf et al. (eds.), *New Dynamics of Disability and Rehabilitation*,
https://doi.org/10.1007/978-981-13-7346-6_8

the changing of one's social status may challenge TBI survivors differently, as they carry with them from their pre-injury life various amounts of, for example, embodied forms of capital in the form of long-lasting dispositions of the mind and the body.

In his work examining the relationship between class and status or *stand*, the German sociologist Max Weber (1864–1920) captured the rational and cognitive dimensions of this issue through the following quote: 'Status honour is normally expressed by the fact that above all else a specific *style of life* can be expected from those who wish to belong to the circle' (Weber 1946/1991, p. 187; emphasis in original). There is little research that focuses on the way in which TBI survivors themselves might make distinctions in order to categorize people, themselves, practices, attitudes, and manners post injury in their 'wish to belong to the circle'. Bourdieu (1984, p. 4) uses the notion of 'taste' to explain the individual's culturally and socially based patterns of choice and preferences. According to him, individuals constantly choose between what they find 'aesthetic' and what they consider 'vulgar'. Whilst many scholars have considered the exclusionary impact of differenced lifestyles in general, the present study seeks to investigate empirically the various repertoires of valuation that TBI survivors draw upon to demarcate themselves symbolically from others, and how this approach relates to them as a group that is being categorized by society.

8.2   Systems of Classification and Boundaries in Relation to TBI

Social scientific studies on the role of systems of classification and boundaries have traditionally proposed that these systems serve to construct and maintain social and personal orders. Within such research, 'social order' refers to the distinctions provided by classifications to construct, reconstruct, and sustain cultural–organizational structures, while 'personal order' refers to the way in which symbolic classifications and distinctions act to shape subjectivity and self-management in everyday life. While not all symbolic distinctions matter equally with respect to their effect on power relations, constructions of 'difference' have historically been used to stratify groups in society based on, for example, gender, religious orientation, and race. Such symbolic distinctions have also contributed to the stratification of people according to mental and/or physical disabilities. As reviewed in Chap. 1 of this book, a reorganizing of welfare services and provisions throughout the 1990s in Northern Europe has reinforced an active and work-oriented approach that mobilizes marginal labour power. Thus, the ability to emphasize TBI rehabilitation as a form of inequality is based on the use of social boundaries (i.e., structures of thought) by those in power when, for example, macro and political–economic forces categorize TBI patients as a group of benefit recipients that needs 'activation' (see Chap. 1).

The sociologist Thomas Gieryn (1983) originally proposed the concept of 'boundary work' as a process central to the constitution of the self. He used it in the context of scientific knowledge production, arguing that science has no fixed set of characteristics but, rather, is the result of scientists' discursive positioning of what they do as special, as distinct from what others do. Gieryn (1995, p. 406) defined boundary work as 'rhetorical games of inclusion and exclusion' that are a step 'toward a cultural interpretation of historically changing allocations of power, authority, control, credibility, expertise, prestige, and material resources among groups and occupations'.

In line with this definition, Epstein (1992, p. 232) argued that symbolic boundaries are 'the lines that include and define some people, groups, and things while excluding others'. According to Lamont (1992), boundaries can be divided into two: social and symbolic. Social boundaries are 'objectified forms of social difference'; thus, widely agreed-upon boundaries between people. Symbolic boundaries, on the other hand, are 'conceptual distinctions made by social actors to categorize objects, people, practices, and even time and space' (Lamont and Molnár 2002, p. 168). Thus, symbolic boundaries are cognitive distinctions that operate as invisible and often taken-for-granted mechanisms through which people try to 'concentrate themselves, separate themselves from others' (Lamont and Fournier 1992, p. 1, citing Marcel Mauss 1929/1969) as well as ways in which this is done for and to them by those in power. At the micro level, individuals use symbolic distinctions to define who they are and to situate themselves in relation to others in society. At the meso and macro levels, symbolic boundaries reinforce general organizing practices such as collective norms, social codes, and behaviours (Lamont 1992).

As boundary work is related to delimiting who is 'in' and who is 'out', it directly refers to culture understood as 'the institutionalized repertoires that have as powerful an effect on the structuration of everyday life as do economic forces' (Lamont and Fournier 1992, p. 7). Thus, the cultural is structural and is shaped and maintained through interactions with network members. It involves both valuation practices (i.e., what is giving worth) and evaluation practices (i.e., assessing how an entity attains a certain type of worth) (Lamont 2012, p. 205). Thus, the judgement of what is good or preferable above other things is exchanged within individuals and social groups, whereby it promotes sociability by allowing people to make connections and find commonalities with one another. Swidler (1986) stated that culture is more important during unsettled times because it makes possible new strategies of action for creating new versions of the self and new social relations (see also DiMaggio 1987). When TBI survivors learn new ways of organizing individual and collective actions, practising unfamiliar habits until they become familiar, then, according to Swidler, it is existing ideologies and available cultural repertoires that directly shape their action (Swidler 1986, p. 278) and are mobilized in boundary work. Unlike Bourdieu, Swidler does not include reference to how forms of capital, objective structures, and living conditions may also shape action.

8.3   Methods

The remainder of the chapter is structured as follows: first, I present the study's context and methods. This is followed by the analysis, wherein I consider three TBI survivors in their 20s: Fanny, Simon, and Louis. They represent various cases of the complexity of the world as they understand it at a time in their life during which plans for the future, in terms of choice of further education, has been disrupted by a TBI (see Table 8.1). Common among these respondents is how they belong to the category of

Table 8.1 Age and educational or professional statuses of the study's TBI survivor participants

Participant	Fanny	Simon	Louis	Linda	Peter
Age	27	26	27	42	41
Post-injury status	Sabbatical leave after high school	Bachelor's degree student at university	Carpenter	Sales assistant	Scaffolder
Present status	Just accomplished technical college degree	Accomplished master's degree at university	Student at bachelor's degree level, university	In work ability testing	Disability pensioner

'real fighters' leading to what they have accomplished 'despite' all odds—consequently, this analytical grip helps in addressing incongruities between symbolic and social boundaries.

This analysis is followed by an evaluation of two further cases of TBI survivors, Peter and Linda, who both had undergone several years of working life experiences before their accident. Their cases demonstrate the way that some TBI survivors do not have the dispositions or networks with which to deal with the Danish rehabilitation system as successfully as others might, and use alternative types of symbolic boundaries to normalize social boundaries. I finish the chapter by discussing how respondents' social identities are given value and meaning through comparison; they create, reproduce, and change hierarchies between groups of people, such as TBI survivors, and thus partly determine the trajectory of individuals in society through allocation of resources.

8.3.1 Context and Setting

Denmark has 5.6 million inhabitants and a tax-financed healthcare system. The organization of hospital services and rehabilitation following a TBI is set by the Danish Health Authority, and includes free access to acute care, neurosurgery, and rehabilitation.

The present study is part of a larger one for which I have drawn upon the Danish Head Trauma Database for data collection. This database was established in 2004 and includes patients with the most severe head traumas—approximately 100 patients per year—who are admitted to one of the two national hospitals that offer highly specialized rehabilitation after severe TBI. All patients registered on the database who were aged 18 years or older and had survived a severe TBI between 2010 and 2012 (approximately 170 individuals) were contacted. One third of them agreed to participate in the study, which included both a survey and qualitative interviews.

The survey was designed to explore everyday and leisure activities, as well as how structural and social aspects of friendships were distributed. It reconstructed cultural capital, economic capital, health capital, and social capital. Because survey data do not fully allow us to understand how symbolic boundaries are used in everyday assessments of others to develop and maintain friendships, I complemented a quantitative analysis of the surveys as a social network analysis (Hindhede and Aagaard-Hansen 2017; Scott 2017) through directed, in-depth qualitative interviews with 20 respondents. For the present study, I referred to the results of the qualitative interviews with five respondents. These respondents represent various ways of enacting boundaries, in terms of definitions of values and attitudes that TBI survivors consider essential in separating themselves from everyone else—and how this was also being done for or to them by those in power.

Each interview was conducted directly with the TBI survivor—in some cases, together with a relative/significant other of the interviewee's own choice. Here, the focus was on co-constructed stories of both supportive elements and tensions. Common among the respondents was the experience of a recent unsettled period of their lives, in terms of social network disruption and identity transformation. There was slight variance in their cognitive and physical limitations. In the analysis, in my construction of themes, I followed the suggestion from Lamont (2012, p. 205) to consider both valuation practices and evaluative practices. I also considered the mechanisms that are associated with activation, maintenance, and the transposition of boundaries, along with where boundaries are disputed or may be dissolved (Lamont and Molnár 2002, p. 187).

Approval of the project from the Danish Data Protection Agency was obtained (journal No 2015-57-001). Informed consent was obtained prior to the interviews taking place, and participants were assured that anonymity in connection to publication would be respected. Accordingly, individuals have been anonymized and the identification of locations has been disguised.

8.4   Findings

In general, relational difficulties were informed by respondents' desires to disassociate themselves from negative associations with being brain injured. Therefore, many of the respondents did not want to associate with people who show signs of TBI, even though TBI persons most often were the group of people they met during their rehabilitation process. Thus, on the one hand, they find friendships with non-brain-injured individuals necessary and desirable, but, on the other hand, they find it difficult to make new ones, as this reminds them of their lack of capabilities in this regard. The following three cases represent this finding in various ways.

8.4.1 'Bad Taste' at the College Level and Displacement

Fanny is 27 years old and has just completed a year-long course at technical college. Six years ago, Fanny was involved in a traffic accident on a Sunday morning; she was the driver, and she lost control of her car and severely injured her head. At that time, she was still living at home with her parents and her younger sister. She had finished high school at a private institution and had plans to enrol in higher education. At the time of our interview, Fanny showed no visible signs of sequelae after the accident. Her mother was present during the interview, and explained that she had decided to quit her job after Fanny's accident to support her daughter full time in the rehabilitation process. The mother also described how Fanny is sharp, and that she had just finished her education with very high grades, even though everyone in the rehabilitation system had said that Fanny was not ever going to complete any kind of education:

> FANNY'S MOTHER: Fanny has hit the frontal lobe. She has lost it, so to speak. So, regarding feelings and all that, Fanny does not have much left of this capability.
> FANNY: And I hate being brain injured. I hate my life after the accident, I hate it! … One activity [at the neurorehabilitation centre] was to go shopping along with the staff to the supermarket. It was not very funny, but you had to do it … because I'm not very old, and everybody knows that I've hit my head, when I come with the staff. … Lynton is a small town … so, if you come with one of those with the Lynton Rehab logo on their uniforms, then you are sure to be one of them [the brain injured].

Fanny undertakes boundary work when thinking back to her experiences at the highly specialized rehabilitation centre, disassociating herself age wise from the other patients. She finds her new life and position miserable, as what she has accomplished does not reflect her own ideals of the 'style of life' she had hoped for. She had plans for pursuing further education, and disputes the social boundaries that categorize her as the kind of person who will never be able to complete education at that level. However, only with very strong efforts has she been able to disconnect to this category by completing a one-year-long technical college-level education programme. When reflecting on this, she distances herself from her fellow students, only to realize, when she encounters real life, that her capabilities are not in accordance with her tastes and distastes (Bourdieu 1984, p. 61):

> FANNY: There were some completely different types of people than I have ever known in my life, because I'm very targeted; I'm very like 'This is what I'm going to do', and 'This study I will complete', and 'I can do this', and 'I want this' … there, it was the kind of people who just sit on their butt and want everyone else to do everything for them. Of course, they were not all like that, but there were many of these types … it [the brain damage] has not affected my memory. I almost remember as [well as] an elephant. … In the brain injury centre, I was one of the best. I was good at all tasks. And then I started at school and realized, 'What the fuck; I've been cheated!', 'I'm miserable, I'm really lousy'. I could not do anything at all.

As can be seen, Fanny constructs symbolic boundaries based on elusive social class differences. She draws on a hierarchy of cultural practices when evaluating her fellow students and ranks her own practice as higher than theirs. In doing so, she represents the case of a TBI survivor who produces stereotypes of TBI patients in order to differentiate herself from others in this category. However, although she does better than many of the other patients and distances herself from the classmates at college, she realizes that this distinction does not work well for her as she has difficulties in keeping up with the demands to her brain, and therefore, in practice, she does not belong anywhere any longer.

8.4.2   Cultural Incompatibility at University and Displacement

Simon is the study's second case who had his accident six years ago. At the time of the interview, he was 26 years old and in the final year of his master's degree programme of study. Since late adolescence, he has been an elite swimmer. Five years ago, Simon was a first-year bachelor's degree student at a university in Copenhagen. One day, while out on a bike ride with his friend, he was hit by a motorist and severely injured his head. Present at the interview was also Simon's father, who explained how, after the accident, he moved into the highly specialized hospital and stayed with his son 24/7. The father became close friends with the hospital staff and learned 'what to do so as not to have my son end up completely retarded'. Currently, Simon has clear scars on the face and scalp, but otherwise no apparent sequelae. He has lived with his girlfriend for six years in an apartment in the Copenhagen area. In the following quote, Simon is reflecting on the time between the accident and when he went back to his studies, and thinking about that university time does not bring any positive memories:

> In retrospect, it would probably have been better to wait another year [to continue university studies] … it did not have anything to do with me not being able to read or concentrate, but there were so many people around me—all those new impressions—and what did they think of me? Could I do the same as before the accident? Was I the same person as before? … I'm pretty sure I would have had better relationships if I had waited another year. Because then I would have been more confident about myself, I guess.

Simon distances himself culturally from the group of TBI patients who have difficulties concentrating or memorizing. He also distances himself from fellow students, and does not have a sense of shared belonging as he worries if he might seem weird to them compared to how he was before the accident. In this way, Simon describes a dialectic interplay of processes of both internal and external definitions, wherein his internal identification—according to his perception of the interplay—does not seem to be recognized by his fellow students. Therefore, he withdraws from the group. Equally, Simon seems to bridge boundaries to the category of TBI survivors when relating this to frontal lobe damage as an argument for his behaviour. However, he eventually generates differentiation by categorizing himself in the group of 'normal' people with quite a temper:

> I have always been temperamental, and we come from a family where, in general, there is quite a lot of temper in the house and we say things a lot like they are. But it was just pointed out by people around me that it had just gotten an extra touch [worse] for me after the accident. But I'm happy that I have temperament, because, if you don't have a temper, you're indifferent. Well, of course, it should not be that people around me are adversely affected by it.

Simon experiences discrete entities when saying that 'we' have tempers in 'our family'. This presupposes a perception of some boundaries surrounding them, and defines his mental entities he comes to experience as 'us' and 'them'. According to Zerubavel (1993, p. 14), these boundaries 'constitute the basis of our sense of identity and determine much of the scope of our social relations'. Moreover, Simon reproduces moral symbolic boundaries that prescribe certain attitudes and govern behaviour for university students when he explains how he felt he ought to go back to studying, thereby constructing a group of individuals who one would expect to act like this:

> SIMON: There are many who never come back from such an accident, and many people spend at least five years on rehabilitation before they are ready. I think it has been a combination of, firstly, having the family I have; secondly, I'm used to pushing myself and exercising a lot.

As with Fanny, Simon's boundary-making strategy is to define himself as distinct from other TBI survivors, emphasizing that, despite the boundaries at the structural level they are confronted with as rehabilitation clients, they valorize the struggler and hard worker who is able to challenge the predictions of the health professionals.

8.4.3   Mould Breaking, Academic Competences, and Displacement

The study's third case of young TBI survivors in their 20s is Louis. He represents the struggles of young TBI survivors who have been diagnosed with severe frontal lobe injury. For them, the diagnosis relates to constructions of what normality is, which in turn can impact healthcare professionals' advice and judgements. Thus, symbolic boundaries regarding what can be expected from severe TBI survivors seem to have been incorporated into the social consciousness. At the time of the interview, Louis was 26 years old and at bachelor-degree level at a university in the eastern part of Denmark, where he lives alone in a flat. Louis was involved in a car accident five years ago in which he was the driver and 'survived against all odds'. At that time, he worked as a carpenter and lived with a girlfriend. Due to having a lot of disputes and disagreements with his girlfriend and with his mother and father in the time after the accident, he cut off all contact, and, a year ago, he chose to move to another part of the country 'to start a new life'. During the interview, Louis explained about all the struggles he had had in convincing healthcare workers that he was indeed capable of completing higher education. After taking a course in philosophy, through which he was introduced to the work of the cognitive psychologist Howard Gardner, Louis felt that he understood himself much better:

> LOUIS: I will also constantly argue that my intersocial intelligence has also been hit.
> INTERVIEWER: How does this show?
> LOUIS: In the past, I was able to get along with people; I'm not like that today. Everything is going completely wrong, and I cannot figure out how to be with my friends and I say some stupid things. I push things too hard, I do not know when enough is enough, I just continue. People become annoyed or furious at me before I figure out what is happening.
> INTERVIEWER: You do not even have a sense of what is going on?
> LOUIS: None!
> INTERVIEWER: So who corrects you?

Louis: No one! That's why I've always wanted someone to explain to me what the hell is going on. … In the past, I could just run the noble style and then just do things without thinking about them. Now I analyse everything. I analyse my weight, my fat percentage, my daily rhythm, my food, my exercise. All of it! People [too]: 'What did she say to him?', 'What did he say to her?', 'Why does she change the tone of voice when she tells him this?', [and] how he gets sad but she does not understand it.

Louis distances himself from the way he was before the accident; he creates a boundary to his new and more reflexive self. However, he also evaluates himself according to standard symptoms of front lobe brain damage and how he offends other people by not having appropriate social skills. He distances himself from physical labour (i.e., his life as a carpenter before the accident) but not from investing in doing hard work; thus, post injury, he is applying acquired classical virtues from physical labour to mental labour when constructing a post-injury self.

Louis reflected further on his struggles through the rehabilitation system. An example of this concerned Denmark's political–economic decision to entitle persons with TBI to receive social security benefits, which often conflicted with respondents' ideas about the chronological age at which retirement should begin. In Louis' case, social workers were surprised that he was not pleased by the fact that he qualified for a disability pension. For Louis, though, a disability pension was not his goal. Rather, he preferred to use his energy to navigate through rules and regulations, and emphasized how he—compared to 'ordinary people'—was particularly skilled in seeing through it all. In this way, he creates a categorization of ordinary TBI survivors and himself as not ordinary:

Ordinary people cannot manage the [rehabilitation] system. It's crazy. My strategy has been to enrol in specific courses, finalize them, and then I decide that I need to continue. What my neuropsychologist did not want to tell me, that's what I could just read in a book. What everybody else could not tell me about life and society, philosophy could. And why the hell is there not one single responsible person in that messy public system to say such basic things?. … I do not know what to use [higher education] for, because I have a different focus than my classmates … to me, it is still part of the disease, part of the rehabilitation. I'm just doing it for myself because I think the system is not up to the task.

As shown, during his rehabilitation process, Louis has had to deal with institutions such as the educational system, which, according to him, create inequality and impose boundaries when dividing TBI survivors into those who are suited for certain types of education and those who are not. These types of respondents may also be 'the product of a moral passage; that is, of an informed decision taken after considering options' (Lamont and Fournier 1992, p. 13).

8.4.4 Working Identity and Displacement

Many TBI survivors have a reduced work capacity and are therefore unable to retain their pre-injury job or employment status (Odgaard et al. 2017; van Velzen et al. 2009). In Denmark, despite there being a welfare system in place that purports to provide equal opportunities to all citizens, returning to work after a severe TBI is predicted by several pre-injury socioeconomic factors such as being of a younger age, having higher levels of education, and not receiving benefits (Odgaard et al. 2018).

These forms of social boundaries were also revealed in the present study's interviews, when respondents compared themselves with their previous identity through which they had had attachment to the labour market. The prevailing ideology in the Western world and in Scandinavia in particular urges people, even those recovering from a serious injury, to avoid unemployment or at least to continue as many aspects of working life as possible. This ideological tenet was reflected in the interviews too, in that many of the respondents explained how they had initially tried to go back to their old job, only little by little realizing that this was not realistic. In the following extract from her interview, Linda exemplifies this process. She is in her early 40s and, at the time of the interview, in work ability testing. She had formerly been employed as a sales assistant in a large furniture company. Linda was injured in a traffic accident, wherein she was on a motorcycle at a traffic light and collided with a passenger car. Linda lost half a foot and now wears foot prosthesis when she walks outside of the house. She lives in a residential neighbourhood with her cohabitant, who is a bricklayer. They have a daughter 22 years of age and a grandson who is 1 year old. Linda here explains about going back to her old job six months after the accident:

> It turned out that actually you spend much more time at work than you thought you did. And, therefore, your job is your identity, right? So, I found it so depressing when I finally realized that I could not work full time … there were many things I no longer could do. Later, I've been told that maybe it was not such a good idea to return to what you did before, because you will always be able to compare yourself with before [the accident]. But, I thought it would be an advantage that I knew everything already. But I couldn't. I was reminded all the time. It was not just remembering things, it was also physical tasks that you were no longer able to perform. It was absolutely terrible.

Linda constructs symbolic boundaries when making distinctions between working full time and part time, wherein worth for her is working full time as she used to do. She also constructs symbolic boundaries of time and space when reflecting on how she previously had not thought about how much time she used to spend on work compared to now. The boundaries are tools by which she struggles over and agrees upon her definition of reality. They reflect her way of classifying right from wrong and good from bad. They separate her from other kinds of people and include her into a group of people with only a few resources. However, they are not *social* boundaries, as 'only when symbolic boundaries are widely agreed upon can they take on a constraining character and pattern social interaction in important ways' (Lamont and Molnár 2002, p. 169).

Linda also constructs boundaries between herself and other groups of people. This boundary work does not seem to be in relation to her brain damage, though. She explains it like this:

> I have always been a very happy, optimistic, and positive type, so, when my husband or daughter complained about stuff, I always replied, 'It's going to be all right' and 'We can do it' or 'We'll figure it out'. Now, I very often fall into a deep hole and can't see the positive side of things. … I divide people

into real people and those who just pretend they are real people, such as my mother-in-law and father-in-law; they are not real people. It's like, if you are having them for dinner, in their opinion, you need to behave like this and the table should look like that and so on. ... And there are so many of these types. That's why I like David [the social worker] so much, and I have said to him several times, 'If it had not been for you, David-dear, I would have gone all the way down the drain'. David is the type of guy who expresses his opinions and what he says comes straight from the heart.

For Linda, having a social worker who can support her in her struggles to be a part of working life again has kept her from taking her own life. Other respondents had given up going back to a real job but still related themselves to and distanced themselves from the stereotyped nature of the collective identity of people with intellectual challenges. This led the respondents to adopt a range of equalization strategies in response to the stigmatization that they felt. However, contrary to the findings of prior literature on oppositional groups, in general, this group were less likely to want to equalize and gain cultural membership. Rather than being concerned with maintaining group boundaries with which to maintain economic advantage in respect to an unskilled labour market, they seemed more preoccupied by the politics of recognition as a collective good in and of itself. Peter is an example of this. He is 41 years old, single, a scaffolder, and now a disability pensioner. He fell from a scaffolding site six years ago, and now has poor eyesight in both eyes and walks with a limp. He is living alone in an apartment in the Copenhagen area, where he is from, and has two adult children. In the following extract, Peter illustrates an example of the type of boundary work that individuals perform in relation to their own past and present selves:

PETER (*regarding the first time after the accident, where he fell down from a scaffolding structure*): At first, I could not go, so I had to ride a wheelchair, and I thought, 'What the hell? Is that my life?' ... I just didn't want to live anymore, because my brain did not work very well. And my leg—I could not walk by myself and I thought, 'Okay, will I end up a vegetable?' I didn't want this—because I've always been in good shape, right? Maybe it's something else if you were born handicapped, right?

But, when you're well and ... I just couldn't handle it. ... I have difficulties in contacting people now.

INTERVIEWER: Why is that?

PETER: Because—I do not know—I have ... an inner dislike of myself. Because I do not feel that I'm good enough anymore.

INTERVIEWER: Why are you not good enough anymore?

PETER: Because I'm handicapped ... I walk a little skewed sometimes, right? So sometimes people may—I do not know if they do—they may think that I am drunk or crooked. And my speech is not so good, either. But, if I bring with me a blindfold, then everybody is much more friendly.

Being labelled as 'brain injured' creates challenges for friendships among peers who are not brain damaged. Impersonal pronouns such as 'they' or 'these people' are used to distinguish between peer groups and often related to perceived or real negative associations of being brain damaged. Thus, Peter classifies himself as handicapped, as opposed to those individuals who are not. He also puts himself in the category of those who are not 'good enough'. Institutional categories become the material for his individual boundary work. The moral distinctions that Peter draws on not only delimit his own social spaces and expectations, but also serve as a way to maintain collective representation about who is 'one of us' and 'one of them' (Lamont and Fournier 1992).

I also talked to Peter about his experiences of being part of a rehabilitation system:

INTERVIEWER: What did they suggest you do? Did you get any advice?

PETER: No, no, no. And I think that was very bizarre, not being helped in any way. So, I tried: 'What should I do? I have not been handicapped before.' And it may be that they are not trained to help me. But there has always been handicapped people, that's not something new. I do not know if it's new to the job centre but talk to the handicapped or talk to some people who know something. In my opinion, they did not do anything like that ... when you survive an accident and are not used to being disabled, then you should get some kind of advice or help, like 'There you can go' or 'There you can get help'. And I just felt that I was all by myself in the world, right? I had become a 'spaz' and I could not do anything about it. Well, it was difficult. Of course, I have a strong psyche, right? But that should not be what counts. I had to fight to get information.

Peter feels that he is met by an indifferent welfare system, and so he himself tried to engage in life and at one time applied for courses in cooking, English, and computer training. This was, however, too demanding, and eventually Peter dropped out:

> PETER: It was a bit weird because, um ... they seemed like ordinary people, right? They may have been mentally ill or something but you could not see or hear anything extraordinary, right? And then I just felt like a little cookie, right? ... But I'm comfortable with my old friends. They do not treat me as handicapped at all. They treat me like before [the accident]. They speak as ugly to me as they did before. Maybe they do not ask me to get the beer or the food, but they do not behave like if I'm spurned. Not at all. And it's actually very nice. It's very liberating sometimes.

According to Bourdieu (1984), practices cohere symbolically to form a whole (a 'style of life'). These practices serve to constitute social collectivities by establishing symbolic boundaries between individuals occupying different locations in social space, like when Peter stresses how he has a sense of belonging with his old friends. Cultural tastes including preferences and experiences are used in identity shaping and presentation, and allow individuals like Peter to symbolically represent his place in the world. He has to adjust the activities he can engage in due to bodily limitations, particularly his partial blindness. Thus, TBI is enacted not only through social bodies but also at the level of the individual body where it can lead to particular distinctions.

8.5   Discussion

With his work *Distinction*, Bourdieu (1984) focused on the French bourgeoisie, its tastes and preferences, and provided an insightful understanding of cultural consumption. However, its theoretical framework has been criticized for failing to capture the processes that transformed the cultural domain by the end of the twentieth century, in that cultural boundaries are now so blurred that 'his account has become obsolete' (Warde 2008, p. 327). Lamont's (1992) theoretical framework on boundary work offers a different approach to taste and preferences. She focuses on the variations in the strategic uses of taste and distaste between cultures and between groups within the same culture. This allows for a more nuanced understanding of the relations among social structures, cultural tastes, and symbolic boundaries. To her, symbolic boundaries relate to patterns of inequality, in that groups use symbolic differences to justify and maintain their status, monopolize resources, and minimize threats to their structural positions.

In the present study, the participants constructed nuanced symbolic distinctions that related to their pre-injury socioeconomic positions, tastes, and distastes. Independently of dispositions, though, they all evaluated themselves as belonging to a marginalized group and conveyed an experience of a devalued status. However, they had differing strategies with which to deal with the categorization. For Fanny and Simon, their mindset as 'fighters', along with the support of dedicated parents, had been the capital needed to navigate through the system. Louis has a working-class background, and he drew on his 'new' mindset as constantly curious and never accepting the status quo to help him through his struggles with the system. Peter, on the other hand, who also had a working-class background, but was in a different phase of his life when his accident happened, did not have family or close friends supporting him (for further discussion on the role of the family, see Chap. 9), and his position was to wait for the system to tell him what to do. In this light, it is important to understand how the enactment of boundary work in daily practice influences both status and exclusion. This process varies within the category of TBI and its context. This finding is particularly relevant because it demonstrates that, for TBI survivors, social locations and their power differentials are not uniformly experienced.

According to Lamont and Molnár (2002, p. 168), social boundaries are 'manifested in unequal access to and unequal distribution of resources (material and nonmaterial) and social opportunities'. Moreover, symbolic and social boundaries should be viewed as equally real. In this study, the former exists at the intersubjective level whereas the latter can be seen as groupings of individuals with TBIs.

The TBI patients in my study came from various regions of Denmark and had different experiences with how government policies were implemented at the municipal level. These differences influenced the provision of and access to rehabilitation services, which meant that moving from one municipality to a neighbouring one had huge impacts on what was provided with regard to rehabilitation services.

Lacking sufficient endowment of the embodied type of cultural capital is the deficit that induces the most symbolic violence, as it is difficult to acquire. Therefore, individuals like Peter and Linda, who had less embodied cultural capital than the other respondents, such as social skills and the ability to navigate through the Danish rehabilitation system, are faced with a double articulation of symbolic violence, as they do not comply with the demand for normalized collective identities ('if only you had asked for the help'), thus leaving them at the margins of the Scandinavian welfare state.

The older respondents like Peter and Linda reinforced collective norms of the typical brain-injured individual, thus manifesting strong symbolic boundaries at the level of both the individual and the collective identity. The younger respondents, such as Louis, Simon, and Fanny, however, who had more at stake, sought to affect the predominant stereotypes, such as not being able to work, and to transform their collective identity by expressing equalization strategies. They had various levels of success, due to strong social boundaries manifesting themselves through unequal patterns of access to work (primarily owing to health and social workers' lack of knowledge and stereotypical classifications of TBI survivors) affecting their life chances.

As shown, the advantages and disadvantages of being categorized as having endured a severe TBI are not experienced uniformly within any given category because these categories overlap in complex ways. The respondents challenge collective norms of the typical brain-injured individual, thus manifesting strong symbolic boundaries at the level of both individual and collective identity. As argued by Hofstede (2001), these collective norms contain a component of national culture and vary among nations. In my study, TBI survivors engaged in identity work and group distinction between themselves and others based on their assessment of one another's behaviour—sometimes as perceived as 'abnormal'.

Additionally, political and economic discourse shaped boundaries and power differentials between them as a group and in comparison to their peers in the wider society.

8.6   Conclusion

This chapter has considered TBI survivors' discursive repertoires of valuation and evaluation in order to explore the relationship between social boundaries and symbolic boundaries—and, thus, class and status. Insight into these relations may improve our understanding of the cultural and social mechanisms that shape TBI survivors' boundary work.

I explored boundary work at the level of the daily lives of five TBI survivors across age, gender, and residential arrangements in Denmark. I was concerned with how boundary work is accomplished—that is, with what kinds of typification systems or inferences concerning similarities and differences individuals diagnosed with TBI mobilize to define who they are.

I found that, in their narratives, respondents identified the social categories they perceive as either complying with or violating their own norms. Their social identity is given value and meaning through comparison. They create, reproduce, and change hierarchies between groups of people, such as TBI survivors, and thus partly determine the trajectory of individuals in society through the allocation of resources. The study's findings suggest two diverse age-related constructions of boundary work. The older respondents reinforced collective norms of the 'typical' brain-injured individual, thus manifesting strong symbolic boundaries at the level of both individual and collective identity. The younger respondents, however, who arguably had more at stake, sought to affect the predominant stereotypes, such as not being able to work, and thus to transform their collective identity.

Boundary work for people having survived a severe TBI is a continuous process, even many years after their accident, as they negotiate the official categories into which they are placed along with the types of discourse that sustain them even while they are relatively well rehabilitated. However, these boundaries are culturally constructed and hence arbitrary and changeable. This is an important insight, especially as it pertains to the formation or implementation of general rehabilitative, social, health, and welfare policies.

References

Bourdieu, P. (1984). *Distinction*. Cambridge, MA: Harvard University Press.

Danish Health Authority. (2011). *Hjerneskaderehabilitering – en medicinsk teknologivurdering* [Brain injury rehabilitation – A health technology assessment]. www.sst.dk/~/media/CB8CCFE77832456C8B1BABF2F558A661.ashx. Accessed 26 Jan 2019.

Das-Gupta, R., & Turner-Stokes, L. (2002). Traumatic brain injury. *Disability & Rehabilitation, 24*(13), 654–665.

DiMaggio, P. (1987). Classification in art. *American Sociological Review, 52*(4), 440–455.

Epstein, C. F. (1992). Tinkerbells and pinups: The construction and reconstruction of gender boundaries at work. In M. Lamont & M. Fournier (Eds.), *Cultivating differences: Symbolic boundaries and the making of inequality* (pp. 232–256). Chicago: University of Chicago Press.

Gieryn, T. F. (1983). Boundary-work and the demarcation of science from nonscience: Strains and interests in professional ideologies of scientists. *American Sociological Review, 48*(6), 781–795.

Gieryn, T. F. (1995). Boundaries of science. In S. Jasanoff, G. Markle, J. Petersen, & T. Pinch (Eds.), *Handbook of science and technology studies* (pp. 393–443). Thousand Oaks: SAGE.

Hindhede, A. L., & Aagaard-Hansen, J. (2017). Using social network analysis as a method to assess and strengthen participation in health promotion programs in vulnerable areas. *Health Promotion Practice, 18*(2), 175–183.

Hofstede, G. (2001). *Culture's consequences: Comparing values, behaviors, institutions, and organizations across nations* (2nd ed.). Thousand Oaks: SAGE.

Juengst, S. B., Adams, L. M., Bogner, J. A., Arenth, P. M., O'Neil-Pirozzi, T. M., Dreer, L., et al. (2015). Trajectories of life satisfaction after traumatic brain injury: Influence of life roles, age, cognitive disability, and depressive symptoms. *Rehabilitation Psychology, 60*(4), 353–364.

Lamont, M. (1992). *Money, morals, and manners: The culture of the French and American upper-middle class*. Chicago: University of Chicago Press.

Lamont, M. (2012). Toward a comparative sociology of valuation and evaluation. *Annual Review of Sociology, 38*(1), 201–221.

Lamont, M., & Fournier, M. (Eds.). (1992). *Cultivating differences: Symbolic boundaries and the making of inequality*. Chicago: University of Chicago Press.

Lamont, M., & Molnár, V. (2002). The study of boundaries in the social sciences. *Annual Review of Sociology, 28*, 167–195.

Lefebvre, H., Cloutier, G., & Levert, M. J. (2008). Perspectives of survivors of traumatic brain injury and their caregivers on long- term social integration. *Brain Injury, 22*(7–8), 535–543.

Mauss, M. (1929/1969). *Les civilisations. Éléments et formes. Exposé présenté à la Première Semaine Internationale de Synthèse, Civilisation. Le mot et l'idée, La Renaissance du livre* (pp. 81–106). Paris, 1930. Texte reproduit in Marcel Mauss, Oeuvres. 2. *Représentations collectives et diversité des civilisations* (pp. 456–479). Paris: Les Éditions de Minuit, 1969.

Odgaard, L., Johnsen, S. P., Stubbs, P. W., Pedersen, A. R., & Nielsen, J. F. (2017). Alternative measures reveal different but low estimates of labour market attachment after severe traumatic brain injury: A nationwide cohort study. *Brain Injury, 31*(10), 1298–1306.

Odgaard, L., Pedersen, A. R., Poulsen, I., Johnsen, S. P., & Nielsen, J. F. (2018). Return to work predictors after traumatic brain injury in a welfare state. *Acta Neurologica Scandinavica, 137*(1), 44–50.

Scott, J. (2017). *Social network analysis*. London: SAGE.

Swidler, A. (1986). Culture in action: Symbols and strategies. *American Sociological Review, 51*(2), 273–286.

van Velzen, J. M., van Bennekom, C. A. M., Edelaar, M. J. A., Sluiter, J. K., & Frings-Dresen, M. H. W. (2009). How many people return to work after acquired brain injury? A systematic review. *Brain Injury, 23*(6), 473–488.

Warde, A. (2008). Dimensions of a social theory of taste. *Journal of Cultural Economy, 1*(3), 321–336.

Weber, M. (1991). *From Max Weber: Essays in sociology*. New York: Routledge. (Original English-language translation published 1946).

Zerubavel, E. (1993). *The fine line: Making distinctions in everyday life*. Chicago: University of Chicago Press.

9

Conversion of Social Capital in the Rehabilitation Process of Adolescents Following an Acquired Brain Injury

Mette Ryssel Bystrup and Anette Lykke Hindhede

9.1 Introduction

The Danish welfare state is often considered to be a prototypical social democratic, universal welfare system (Esping-Andersen 1990). This is true for the allocation of health services, including treatment and rehabilitation, which are free of charge for all, regardless of income (Ministry of Health 2016). However, health inequalities in Denmark among different socioeconomic groups are large and growing (Diderichsen et al.

M. R. Bystrup (✉)
Department of Learning and Philosophy, Aalborg University Copenhagen, Copenhagen, Denmark

Hammel Neurorehabilitation and Research Centre and University Research Clinic, RM, University of Aarhus, Hammel, Denmark
e-mail: mrb@learning.aau.dk

A. L. Hindhede
Department of Learning and Philosophy, Aalborg University Copenhagen, Copenhagen, Denmark
e-mail: alh@learning.aau.dk

© The Author(s) 2019
I. Harsløf et al. (eds.), *New Dynamics of Disability and Rehabilitation*,
https://doi.org/10.1007/978-981-13-7346-6_9

2011). These inequalities concern not only the uneven distribution of illness but also socioeconomic differences in the outcome of treatment/ rehabilitation in terms of survival, dependence on care, and quality of life (Andersen et al. 2014; Geckler and Hansen 2014).

This unevenness of outcomes regarding treatment and rehabilitation also seems to be closely related to the patient's family, despite Scandinavian healthcare services in theory being largely independent of interventions by relatives (Geckler and Hansen 2014; National Board of Health 2011). On the other hand, it is becoming an increasing political priority to involve relatives in the decision-making and rehabilitation processes within the Danish healthcare system, with one of the arguments for this change being the reduction of inequality (Ministry of Health and Prevention 2014). The supposition is that, if socioeconomically advantaged patients and relatives have the tools and framework to be more active and take on more responsibility, healthcare resources can be allocated to patients with more need. Generally, prior studies have shown that the involvement of relatives is connected to better rehabilitation outcomes for individuals with a traumatic brain injury (Foster et al. 2012), and that severe brain injury strongly increases the patient's dependence on others (Doser et al. 2018). Yet, to date, little attention has been paid to the rehabilitation courses of those with the most severe brain injuries (National Board of Health 2011).

Adolescents—already a potentially vulnerable group because of the many life changes and challenging situations they encounter over a short period of time—may suffer increased damage to their emotional and social lives, as well as their physical and cognitive abilities, when they acquire a severe brain injury (Doser et al. 2018). Support from family for children and young people may therefore be particularly significant in terms of a successful rehabilitation and return to their lives thereafter (Gan et al. 2006; Sander et al. 2002). However, 'family' is not a fixed entity, and varies in size, constitution, quality, and the way its resources can be converted into rehabilitative assets (Guldager et al. 2018; Norup 2012). In other words, the levels of resources that families possess and are able to mobilize are valued differently among health professionals within the rehabilitation system. Despite our knowledge of the existing inequalities in the Danish healthcare sector, we know little about how to approach and handle diagnosis, treatment, and rehabilitation for different social groups (Kamper-Jørgensen and Rasmussen 2008). In addition, most previous research on relatives concerns spouses;

there is less focus on parents, and even less still on siblings (National Board of Health 2011). Thus, there is a dearth of studies that seek to comprehend the capitalization and cultivation of assets among families alongside the variations in the outcomes of rehabilitation processes, and thus on the role that these assets play in health inequality.

In this chapter, we investigate how intangible, non-material assets in the form of the family connections of the relatives of young people with an acquired brain injury are invested and converted to services and 'goods' during the process of rehabilitation. We show that some families understand the health system better than others and therefore reap greater benefits through their networks in terms of advantage, preferential treatment, or additional rehabilitation services from the welfare state. The set of resources that accrue to the families through their social relationships is a form of social capital that facilitates the attainment of goals. Moreover, social relations only turn into capital when that so-called 'social capital' is valued. According to Portes (1998), these unequal possibilities of conversion help to explain some of the asymmetries in benefits gained by two actors in a relationship. Our study therefore contributes to the establishment of a theoretical context for the empirical investigation and explanation of the impact of social capital by asking: How are forms of social capital invested and converted by the relatives of young people with a severe acquired brain injury during the rehabilitation process?

9.2 Social Class and Social Capital in the Context of Neurorehabilitation

Although the origins of the notion of social capital lie in the nineteenth-century classics of sociology, the most influential contemporary manifestations of the concept seem to be Bourdieu (1986), Coleman (1988), and Putnam (1993). In his renowned paper on the origin and application of social capital in modern sociology, Portes (1998) drew parallels with Bourdieu and Coleman's earlier conceptualizations and theories. He argued that social capital can be considered (a) a source of social control generated in closed networks, where the potential for social control is highest; (b) a source of family-mediated resources; and (c) a source of resources mediated by non-familial networks. According to Portes, the first of these aspects follows on from Coleman's usage of the term 'closure', the second partly intersects with what Bourdieu considers 'cultural capital', and the third aspect comes close to Bourdieu's understanding of social capital. We consider these three sources to be productive in the investigation of social capital in the context of neurorehabilitation.

Bourdieu and Coleman's theories were developed more or less at the same time, and both focus on the existence of several forms of capital and on the transformation and outcome of both economic and non-economic resources. However, they also differ in several ways. Bourdieu's conceptualization of social capital is part of his broader theory of fields, which also addresses power and structural inequalities. Capital, according to Bourdieu, is a resource that solely exists and functions in relation to specific fields, and these fields operate according to their own internal logics and dynamics (Bourdieu and Wacquant 1992). For Bourdieu, social capital is the sum of the resources that accrue to an individual (or a group) by virtue of being enmeshed in 'a durable network of more or less institutionalized relationships of tacit acquaintance and recognition—or, in other words, to membership in a group' (Bourdieu 1986, p. 248). Bourdieu's interest in (social) capital primarily concerns the constant struggle for domination existing among the positions in a field. Hence, the accumulation of social capital can be considered a strategy of investment in order to strengthen one's position:

> The volume of the social capital possessed by a given agent thus depends on the size of the network he can effectively *mobilize* and on the volume of the capital (economic, cultural, or symbolic) possessed in his own right by each of those to whom he is connected. (Bourdieu 1986, p. 249; our emphasis)

Each field can be understood to have a specific doxa in the understanding of its own logic and common beliefs, its own forms of social control, its own structures of opportunity, and specific types of resources. In this study, the field we relate to is the Scandinavian field of (neuro)rehabilitation, which is considered a multidisciplinary subfield, though it is dominated by the medical field, in alliance with the political field (Carlhed 2007; Feiring and Solvang 2013; Sandholm Larsen and Larsen 2008).

Cultural capital exists in three forms: embodied (dispositions), objectified (cultural goods), and institutionalized (educational qualifications)

(Bourdieu 1986). For Bourdieu, the social capital of the family also encompasses cultural capital in the form of involvement in cultural practices and possession of cultural goods, as these may facilitate children's access to, for example, education. However, Bourdieu's concept of social capital 'does not lend itself either to a precise definition or a close empirical assessment' (Hindhede 2016, p. 539), nor does he explicitly discuss forms of social capital. Following Bourdieu, we stress the importance of considering social capital as both an actual and a potential resource. By 'actual', we mean that the resources are capitalizable or interchangeable in the here and now. 'Potential' social capital, on the other hand, reflects long-term strategies that include the cultivation of networks that might be useful in an unforeseen situation. As Bourdieu (1980, p. 2; our translation) explained, what characterizes groups of individuals that possess social capital is that they 'are not only endowed with common properties (likely to be perceived by the observer, by others, or by themselves), but are also united by permanent and useful relationships'.

Meanwhile, Coleman's theory of social capital combines rational choice theory and structuralism. He defines social capital as consisting of any social and structural features that are useful to individuals for specific actions. A central difference between Bourdieu and Coleman is the latter's focus on 'closure' in social relations, constituted by the relations between parents and children or other close members of the family (Coleman 1988). When families are more connected to one another, trust, norms, and effective sanctions from parents are more likely, and parents can therefore more effectively enforce their interests. The strength of the relation between these family members is a measure of the strength of social capital. This delimitation of the outside world is necessary in order for the relation to constitute social capital. Coleman (1988) claimed that social capital in the family can create human capital, such as when the parents are involved in the lives of their children. Portes's (2000) testing of social capital, in his study on the educational attainment of immigrant children, stressed that such factors as both biological parents being present, parental involvement, network closure, and socioeconomic status were criteria for estimating social capital effects. Norms, trust, authority, and so on also constitute solidifying forces of social capital that facilitate certain actions while constraining others (Coleman 1988). As Coleman (1990, p. 243) stated, 'a norm concerning a specific action exists when the socially defined right to control the action is held not by the actor but by others'. In everyday life, the right of control is informal and diffuse; it extends to almost everyone considered to be a competent social actor. However, Coleman disregarded the structural elements of social capital. Moreover, his framework obscures the relations among the formation, distribution, and operation of social capital as both an action and a process, while, as set forth by Portes (1998, p. 5), 'equating social capital with the resources acquired through it can easily lead to tautological statements.'

A network approach to researching social capital, such as 'social network analysis', aims to overcome the limitations of both Coleman and Bourdieu by examining in more detail the actors in a network and the ties between them. Social network analysis has its focus in the structure, function, and composition of the network ties surrounding the individual. The current chapter is inspired by this theoretical and methodological thinking, in order to better understand the kinds of network connections families draw upon in rehabilitation processes. According to Borgatti et al. (2013, p. 7), network theorizing is based on a view of ties as 'conduits through which things flow – material goods, ideas, instructions, diseases, and so on'. Thus, social network analysis is based on the assumption that the behaviours, attitudes, and values of individuals are shaped through contact and interaction with others. Interpersonal ties most often come in three versions: strong, weak, and absent ties (Granovetter 1973). Strong ties typically are among individuals characterized by emotional intimacy, intensity, and trust; weak ties are non-frequent and transitory relations; and absent ties are instances when you might expect a tie but it does not exist, such as in a group of friends in which two members are still distant from each another (Montgomery 1994).

Social networks are typically illustrated as graphs with two sets of data: (1) actors and (2) the ties connecting the actors. We are interested in the structure, function and composition of personal network ties which is called the egocentric network. This type of network consists of all the alters around the ego(s) who can be considered as providing resources (family and other relatives, friends, healthcare professionals, social workers, etc.). Our focus is on the nature of the ties connecting the egos and the alters, as well as the characteristics of the alters (Borgatti et al. 2013, p. 262). Taken together, these approaches contribute to answering our research question.

9.3 Methods

The relatives of eight young people (aged 15–30) with a severe acquired brain injury[1] represent the focal point of this study. In order to empirically investigate how relatives invest their social capital and convert it into rehabilitative goods, a triangular and longitudinal study design was adopted, comprising direct observations of hospital discharge meetings, focus group interviews with relatives six months after discharge, questionnaires answered by each of the closest relatives, and medical records from the rehabilitation hospital where the young people were treated. The principal eight cases were supplemented with interviews with an additional six families of young people (also between 15 and 30 years old) with an acquired brain injury of a different severity. These additional families were interviewed at various times after hospitalization (in contrast to the eight original interviews, which all took place six months after the hospital stay), varying from six months to two and a half years after hospitalization. Altogether, the families of eight young boys and six young girls are represented in this study. The gender mix, with a predominance of males, approximates with general patterns in the study population (Corrigan et al. 2010). Twelve of the participants were ethnic Danes and two had a different ethnic background. All of the young people were recruited at one of the two specialized rehabilitation hospitals for patients with severe brain injuries in Denmark.

The data were analysed using a deductive approach revolving around the theoretical frameworks of Bourdieu and Coleman. We used NVivo (version 11; QSR International) qualitative data analysis software to assist in obtaining an overview and coding the data. The families were given

---

[1] In neurorehabilitation, an acquired brain injury is often classified into one of three categories: mild, moderate, or severe. One set of criteria is that of the National Board of Health's (2011) categorization, which is based on the number of days of hospitalization, wherein more than 28 days is considered 'severe'.

both verbal and written information regarding the study before we obtained their informed consent for participation. The identities of the families have been anonymized and pseudonyms used in the reported findings. The study received approval from the Danish Data Protection Agency and the data were handled according to its requirements.

9.3.1   Observations

The discharge meeting at the rehabilitation hospital is considered a crucial juncture during the rehabilitation process because important decisions are made concerning the rehabilitation course after hospitalization and through life thereafter. At the discharge meeting, many actors (including various professionals from the rehabilitation hospital, the municipality, and, in some cases, a residential rehabilitation institution, as well as relatives and sometimes the patient themselves) are brought together. In six out of the eight cases in our study, a discharge meeting was held and observed. The meetings were offered to patients living in a specific Danish region, or when the patient was under the age of 18. In two cases, the meetings were conducted via video conferencing, with the municipality representatives participating online. The number of participants varied from 10 to 16. Nonparticipant observation was adopted by the first author (MRB), with acceptance from the participants of the meeting. Theory-based observational field notes were written on the basis of a constructed observational guide, with a focus on the positioning of the relatives, their adopted roles, and negotiable topics. The meetings were recorded digitally and transcribed verbatim.

9.3.2   Interviews

Focus group interviews with the eight principal families and four additional families were conducted by MRB (in total, 33 relatives; 25 plus an additional eight relatives). The relatives were parents (or step-parents) and, in most cases, siblings; the young people themselves were not present. The families (primarily, the parents) themselves decided who would be defined as the closest relatives and participate in the interviews. The families were all interviewed in their own homes, in an attempt to minimize the asymmetry of power as well as to use their physical framing as an empirical observation. The interviews were digitally recorded and transcribed verbatim. A semi-structured interview guide was constructed, based on Bourdieu's concepts of capital (1980, 1986), to explore the families' experience of the rehabilitation process and their life situation, in order to reveal resources and strategies.

9.3.3 Questionnaires

We used a questionnaire constructed with inspiration from Fischer (1982) and Alexander (2009) to map the families' personal network. The questionnaire was answered by the relatives during the in-depth interview session. The questionnaire included questions on income, education, occupation, and co-habitation. Using this information we classified each family according to Olsen et al.'s (2012) social classes in the Denmark categorization scheme. This categorization contains a five-factor social class index, as follows: 'upper class' (1% of the Danish population), 'upper-middle class' (9%), 'middle class' (24%), 'working class' (47%), and 'underclass' (20%). Our study featured two families representing the middle class, three families belonging to the working class, and three families identified as underclass. In addition, the questionnaires contained questions to generate egocentric networks of the relatives corresponding to both before and after the young person's injury (Bidart and Charbonneau 2011). From this questionnaire, we analysed the different attributes of the relationships between ego and the various alters. We looked at the *quality* of the relationship, that is, how often they are in touch (as indicated in the diagrams by the thickness of the arrow), *reciprocity* of the relationship between the egos (indicated by the arrows being one or two way), as well as its *nature* in terms of being family, friend, boy-/girlfriend, partner, or involving a welfare professional as alter (e.g., a social worker), and so on (as indicated by different colours of the circles). The ego (the relative who has answered the questionnaire) is placed in a square-like figure in contrast to the alters placed in circles).

The green contours are placed in order to show who constitute the family core estimated on the professionals' (medical) journals as well as interviews with the families.

9.3.4 Medical Records

Medical records from the rehabilitation hospital for each of the young persons constituted supplementary empirical material pertaining to the description and timeline of the rehabilitation process.

9.4 Findings

9.4.1 Network Structures and Resources in the Rehabilitation Process

Among the families of the young people, three structures were identified, which involved various levels of closure: (1) a split family structure; (2) a strong, closed family structure; and (3) a small and weak family structure. These family structures were related to the family's social positioning in society.

9.4.1.1 A Split Family Structure

This family structure is considered to feature only a little cohesion, as its members are not well connected because there are few to no single ties between family members, and, in some cases, there is conflict in the relations between some of the closest family members (e.g., between the biological parents), or because there is a wide opening up of the non-familial network that thereby has precluded it being a strong, closed (family) unit. This lack of cohesion hinders both trustworthiness and trust building, which, according to Coleman (1988, p. 101), is crucial for a family's ability to mobilize social capital: 'A group within which there is extensive trustworthiness and extensive trust is able to accomplish much more than a comparable group without that trustworthiness and trust'.

In our study, the case of 'Agnes' is an example of a working-class family that is in conflict. Agnes is a woman in her late 20s who acquired a severe traumatic brain injury in a vehicle accident involving her boyfriend, after which she experienced strong interactional limitations. The internal conflicts among Agnes's family members hinders family closure and prevents them from mobilizing social capital to use as leverage towards a better rehabilitation process. Agnes's mother, stepfather, maternal aunt, and the husband of the maternal aunt attended the discharge meeting. The maternal aunt had, for a period of time before the injury, served as the official contact person for Agnes, and thus was positioned close to her. Half a year later, when Agnes's mother, stepfather, and siblings were interviewed, it was revealed that the family was in conflict with the maternal aunt, and they were suing each other due to conflicts concerning guardianship and choice of rehabilitation institution among other issues:

> SIBLING: We do not really talk to her [maternal aunt] because she wants parental jurisdiction over Agnes – or … what is it called? That's litigation you are in process with, aren't you?
> MOTHER'S HUSBAND: No, she wants guardianship.
> MOTHER: She [the maternal aunt] got angry at the time when I got guardianship of Agnes.
> INTERVIEWER: Because …? Why did she get angry about it?
> MOTHER'S HUSBAND: Because the problem was that it became a [nursing home].
> MOTHER: Because I chose she was at [nursing home], and my sibling became very angry and said it was the worst place I could place my [child]

In addition, the family was in a custody battle with the father of one of Agnes's children. Network analysis established that the family was split both before and after the injury. Notably, Agnes was not mentioned by any of the family members as a relation during the answering of the questionnaires, either before or after the injury. This could be an oversight or explained by the severity of the brain injury leaving Agnes with very limited interactional possibilities, which might be why she is not considered a relation, but it could also be an indication of the family not being close. They have a significant geographical distance between them (the mother moved several hours' drive away from her children because of her new husband). Medical records also indicate that the mother disapproves of Agnes's boyfriend, and therefore the tie between them was already weak before the incident. Through the in-depth interview, we found that the relationship between the mother and her injured child was reduced to a visit once a month, while the siblings had only seen her a couple of times at the care home. One of the siblings participating in the interview declined to answer the questionnaire. In addition, the younger sibling left the interview in tears before its completion and therefore did not answer the questionnaire either. No one followed her, but the mother asked the brother's new girlfriend (who had no relationship with the younger sibling) if she would go and console her. The younger sibling lives several hours away from her mother and close to an hour's drive from her siblings, and was not mentioned as a relation by any of them either. Neither the mother nor the stepfather mentioned any of the children as a relation. The relation between the mother and the stepfather exists, according to the questionnaires (see the network mapping in Fig. 9.1); however, the in-depth interview suggests that the emotional relationship and support provided by the stepfather is limited. For example, he commented, 'It is, at any rate, a daily challenge that she [mother] feels so bound by [Agnes and her situation] and cannot let go of it', and showed a lack of understanding of the mother's need to keep her hopes up and stay near the phone in case of an urgent call from the nursing home. Agnes ended up in a discontinued rehabilitation process (e.g., in-between periods with no rehabilitation, and uncertainty regarding the next step in the process) and at a care home with elderly residents that offered no expertise in neurorehabilitation, despite the possible rehabilitation possibilities expressed by hospital professionals at the discharge meeting.

9.4.1.2   A Strong, Closed Family Structure

This family structure was identified in various sizes, and it is characterized by a strong and relatively closed core, consisting, at the very least, of both biological parents, both before the injury and six months following the

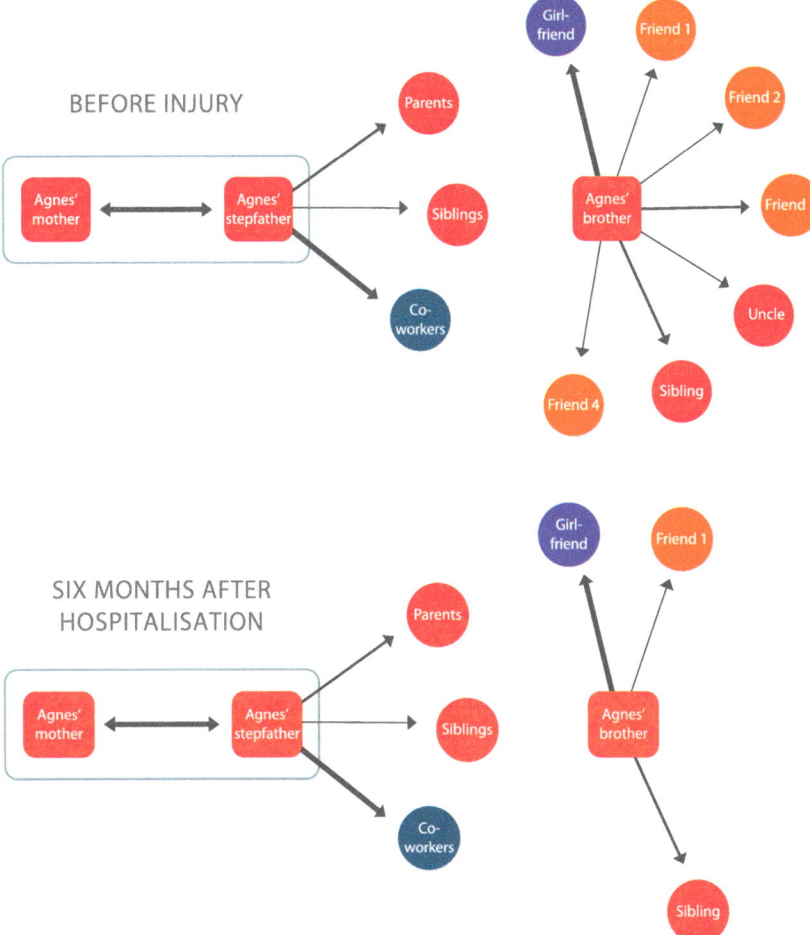

Fig. 9.1 Network maps of a split family structure, exemplified by the relatives of 'Agnes' before the injury and six months after her discharge from the rehabilitation hospital. The 'family core' is marked with a green contour

individual's discharge from the rehabilitation hospital. These families had strong, supportive involvement in each other's lives and in the rehabilitation process of the young patient, and formed strong connections to the professionals that worked with their children. Notably, these families mentioned the injured family member as a relation regardless of the severity of the brain injury. This might be a sign of a preserved family closeness including the young injured person despite the brain injury as well as the complex life situation this has entailed for the family.

An example of this family structure is the case of 'Smilla', who comes from a middle-class family. She is younger than 20 and acquired her brain injury in a vehicle accident also involving another close family member. During the interview, the family mentioned in various ways that the four of them are closely connected, and also that, prior to the accident, family closeness was always highly prioritized and appreciated. These expressions were supported by the findings from the network analysis, which demonstrates that, while the families' networks are reduced, the family core and closeness remain intact (see Fig. 9.2). Smilla's mother expresses in this regard the need they felt for family closure when the crisis struck them:

> SMILLA'S MOTHER: You are so much in a crisis and you do not have the need to communicate anything to anyone. It might sound crazy, but the care from others is completely indifferent, because you close yourself up in a closed unit [comprising the four family members], where you only focus on what is essential – it's your child's life.

This is despite the fact that, as Smilla's sibling explains, the family closure is challenged by the many professionals constantly surrounding the family:

> SMILLA'S SIBLING: Now, there are all kinds of people around us all the time. I think that it's problematic. I don't need to be anything for you or any of them at [residential rehabilitation institution], but, on the other hand, I should. It is not like being the three of us [living at home] or together with Smilla.

Despite the challenges to family closure, they remain a strong unit, meaning they have advantages with regard to the rehabilitation process, such as an extended period with compensation for loss of earnings and psychotherapeutic treatment granted for the whole family, as well as other benefits mentioned in the following sections.

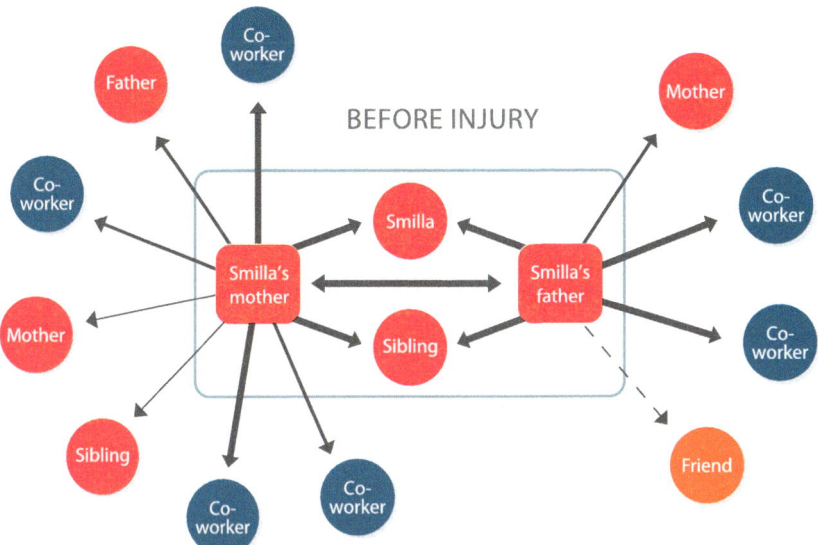

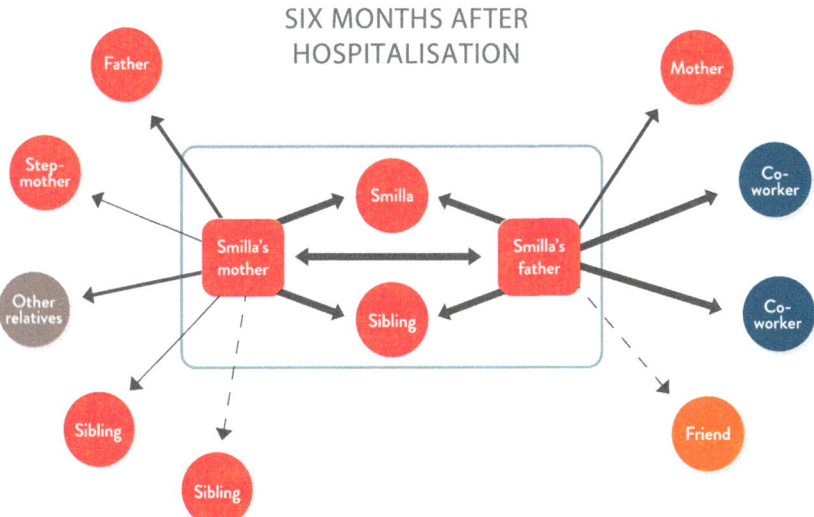

Fig. 9.2 Network maps of a strong, closed family structure, exemplified by the relatives of 'Smilla' before the injury and six months after the rehabilitation hospital. The 'family core' is marked using a green contour

9.4.1.3   A Small and Weak Family Structure

This family structure was found to consist of only a few relations close to the young person, and involved persons who were in relatively vulnerable life situations themselves (e.g., because of their own illness, few socioeconomic resources, ethnicity, living in deprived areas, few close relatives). This family structure is the one least involved in the rehabilitation process of the young person (e.g., few visits, little familiarity between the family and the professionals), and is characterized by frustrated, powerless, passive, and/or despairing family members not making demands for rehabilitation services.

An illustration of this structure is the case of 'Rasmus', a young man who, in his late 20s, acquired a severe traumatic brain injury through a vehicle accident. He stayed at a rehabilitation hospital and, at the time of inclusion in this study, was being considered for rehospitalization almost three years after the injury because he had shown signs of development at the care home in which he was institutionalized. Rasmus comes from an underclass family. He has an older sibling with renewable disability. In other words, his parents have been in a vulnerable situation far longer than the parents of the other young people included in the study. This fact may help explain their limited numbers of social relations, as sustaining friendships takes effort and work. This already vulnerable situation may also be part of the explanation for why their conception of their network (as inferred through the questionnaires) was exactly the same before as it was after the injury. Notably, they did not mention each other as relations, thus reflecting a structure of only weak or almost absent ties (see Fig. 9.3). This could be an oversight, since they live together, visit Rasmus together, and so on. On the other hand, it could also be the case that the parents do not consider each other as a relation worthy of mentioning, as the interview was characterized by a defeated and strained atmosphere and an attitude of blame between them. The mother also expressed that she didn't share her innermost emotions:

> MOTHER: It is not all we let out to each other. No, it is not ... issues that come very close. It isn't all you're told [*directed to her husband*]. You should not believe that.

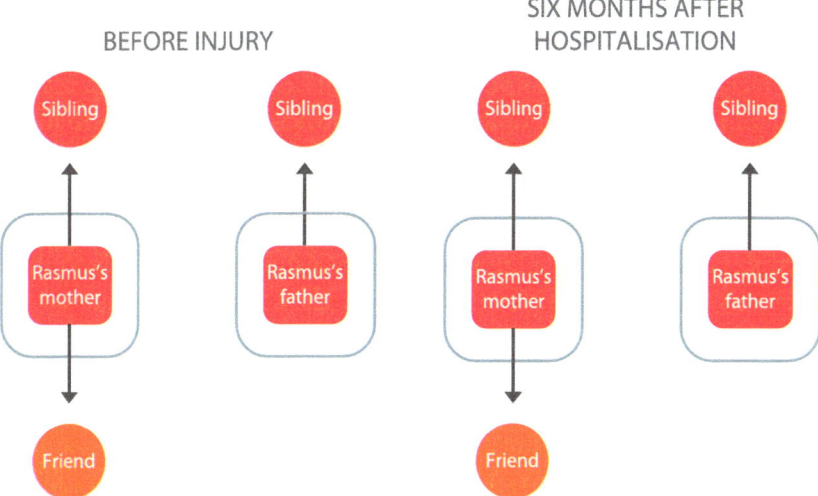

Fig. 9.3 Network maps of a small and weak family structure, exemplified by the relatives of 'Rasmus' before the injury and six months after the rehabilitation hospital. The 'family cores' are marked with green contours

These family structures are characterized by making no or few demands on rehabilitation services and tacitly accepting what they were offered—for example, regarding where the young family member was placed. This was even the case when one of the young persons was evicted from a residential rehabilitation institution and was returned home without any rehabilitation.

9.4.2   Sources of Family-Mediated Resources

Family-mediated resources are, according to Portes (2000), in line with Bourdieu's concept of cultural capital, in that a family facilitates their children's access to, for example, education and transmits a set of values and outlooks, variously classified as 'low-' to 'high-brow' culture. Here, we draw on Bourdieu's ideas of cultural capital in the form of involvement in cultural practices and the possession of cultural goods. In the case of rehabilitation, the 'goods' strived for are scarce healthcare services, such as longer stays at the rehabilitation hospital and residential rehabilitation institutions, stays at specific, preferable residential rehabilitation institutions, compensation for loss of earnings, psychotherapeutic treatment, and facilities/devices to improve the patient's everyday life (e.g., a large iPad for improving communication, reconstruction in the home to make space for a wheelchair, etc.). In the empirical material, different strategies to invest in the cultural capital of families in order to enhance their situation have been identified, which shows how the relatives in various ways (and to various extents) understood the doxa and used it actively in their strategies (Bourdieu and Wacquant 1992). These strategies include a willingness to cooperate, showing the rehabilitation potential of the injured individual, mobilizing various forms of power to use as threats, and confronting professionals with their mistakes.

An example of using threats is seen in the case of 'William', who is in his early 20s and acquired a brain injury because of a work accident. William is from a working-class family. His mother was dissatisfied with the rehabilitation services and therefore wanted to put pressure on the municipality to induce them to provide better services. She used knowledge gained from her work with another vulnerable group of people, as well as her understanding of how to use the media (attained through a contact of another relative, who, in cooperation with a TV station, was producing a documentary film), to bring attention to this issue:

> MOTHER: I also know what [the municipality] like and what they dislike. If I take it one step further, for example, to the city councillor, or if I tell [the municipal coordinator of brain injuries] that 'this is not a threat, but the next step will be contacting the media' ... [William] only gets one chance... So, I know [because of her work] which buttons to press ...
> INTERVIEWER: Do you have any contacts with the media, or which strategy do you choose?
> MOTHER: You have probably read about [name of female], her from [a television programme about a person acquiring a brain injury and his wife and the subsequent life implications] ... I correspond quite a lot with her on Facebook in closed messages ... and she says, 'You shouldn't doubt, you call [TV channel] and then they'll tell your story'.

As shown here, the mother uses her knowledge as a strategy with which to obtain better rehabilitation services, by threatening to go to the city councillor or contacting the media.

In the case of Smilla, the parents' involvement in the rehabilitation process seems to be an advantage because it has taught them the 'game', consisting of a special preoccupation with the physical body in the process of rehabilitation, a shortage of professional time and 'hands', and the necessity to show rehabilitation readiness and improvement and respond to this by showing willingness to invest their own time, energy, and acquired knowledge. This is demonstrated in the quote below, expressed by the mother during the discharge meeting:

> SMILLA'S MOTHER: We [parents] take part in all this work with Smilla. She is very confident with us doing the things and we know Smilla's body just as well as [the physiotherapist] … and do things the same way. And we keep a close eye on what the professionals do … to be able to do as much as possible, because we know that there are only limited resources to work with Smilla, and therefore it is very important that someone can take over when the professionals let go. And this is still the case when Smilla is at [residential rehabilitation institution]. So, the time we spend with Smilla will be used with the focus on training in our being together, and we will continue doing so, because she benefits a lot from that.

9.4.3 Sources Related to Non-familial Network

According to Portes (2000), social capital viewed as a non-familial network constitutes what Bourdieu conceptualizes as social capital—that is, a *potential* resource in which a family may or may not invest. The magnitude of the possible network to become an object of investment varies among the families. However, due to the service-intensive Danish welfare state, family members will always have at least an external network of professional support. In the empirical cases, three primary forms of non-familial network were identified and activated by the families: (1) a network of known relations (friends, family, neighbours, and colleagues),

(2) a professional network, and (3) a network of tacit and peripheral acquaintances. These will be explained in more detail below.

9.4.3.1   A Network of Known Relations

The data show that the networks vary with regard to the types of relations prompted, the kind of support they contribute, and in which situations and stages of the rehabilitation process the network is valued and becomes an object of investment. The largest and most immediate provided network was that of 'Christian', a young man (less than 20 years old) living in a small village with a large group of friends. Immediately after the vehicle accident that inflicted the brain injury, many of his friends made the long drive to the hospital to offer their compassion and support. Furthermore, the entire group of friends offered their help to the family. During the interview with the family, Christian's older sibling noted, 'When the accident happened, they [Christian's friends] all dropped everything and drove to the hospital [several hours' drive from home], and suddenly 20 people show up.' A year after the accident, the group of friends were still supportive of the whole family, and were helping to prepare for Christian's return home after a stay at a residential rehabilitation institution. The whole year, they had offered practical and emotional support, and, to some extent, also financial and counselling support to the family. An example of this support is when the group of friends took over the housework in the family home while the parents were at the hospital, including taking responsibility for the younger sibling (cooking, sleeping over, preparing packed lunches, bringing her to school, driving her to leisure activities, etc.). The year when Christian was being rehabilitated several hours away from their home, they visited him once a week and contributed by picking him up and returning him for the weekends. Also, they contributed with emotional support to the family. As the older sibling confirmed:

> CHRISTIAN'S SIBLING: Well, I can say that I couldn't have done it without [the support]. Without the boys. Without his friends. I couldn't have in any way. They helped with the little [sibling] every day, they helped with

the food; well, they were just there for me, whether it was a hug or to go for a drive or whatever the hell was needed.

9.4.3.2 A Professional Network

When a person acquires a brain injury and is hospitalized, the Danish welfare state allocates more or less automatically and free of charge the services of professionals. Nonetheless, despite ideals of equal access, our observations during the discharge meetings revealed that families' familiarity with the professionals varies, as does the extent of professional services as a source of information and resources provided. The number of resources and professionals are limited, meaning that some families profit more than others. This inequality in gaining benefits is captured by Portes (1998, p. 15) in the observation that 'the same strong ties that bring benefits to members of a group commonly enable them to bar others from access'. Our empirical findings show that it is predominantly the families with a strong, closed family structure that draw on the professional network as a resource to the greatest extent.

An example of a professional source of social capital provided by the state can be seen in the case of Smilla, who was hospitalized for ten months with her mother co-hospitalized with her during the week and her father on weekends. This situation contributed to the strong ties between the family and the professionals at the rehabilitation hospital. In addition, they had a certain amount of familiarity with one of the representatives from the municipality over a long period (approximately four years), due to their child's mental illness. This familiarity, and hence the provision of as well as appreciation for the professional network as a resource, was apparent at the discharge meeting in several ways. The father expressed, with humour, 'Unfortunately, we have for quite some years known how good you are.' A reciprocal appreciation was also expressed by the professionals from the residential rehabilitation institution and the rehabilitation hospital—for example, while talking about Smilla's transfer to the new institution: 'There is no doubt that this [the parents] is also a resource for us, that somebody comes who knows her that well.' Likewise, the physiotherapist (at the rehabilitation hospital) added, 'It is a HUGE help.' The familiarity was expressed by the mother, contributing with small details during the description of the treatment and revealing that she has been closely involved in Smilla's everyday rehabilitation and has almost served as a colleague. It was also apparent that the mother had consulted the municipality, the professionals at the residential rehabilitation institution, and the chairman of the discharge meeting ahead of the meeting, regarding topics to be discussed. This was revealed, for example, when the chairman at the end of the meeting said, 'I believe this was pretty much what we had been talking about ... [*directed at mother*]?' This familiarity and appreciative relationship between the family and professionals was reflected in a good atmosphere at the discharge meeting, where everyone present showed a willingness to sacrifice a little extra to provide the best for Smilla, including extra professional resources, for example, in the transition from the rehabilitation hospital to the residential rehabilitation institution:

> MEDICAL SOCIAL WORKER: Then we can hear from the residential rehabilitation institution what they think about that task [rehabilitation of Smilla].
> HEAD OF DEPARTMENT, RESIDENTIAL REHABILITATION INSTITUTION: We have been attentive on the sideline and had your [family] visit; unfortunately, I was not working that day, but, when I consider the things you're talking about, we can easily continue that. But, we really want to send two of our employees to meet [Smilla] here [at the rehabilitation hospital] at the beginning of September.

Taken together, these efforts create both tangible and intangible advantages, such as smoothness in the rehabilitation process, where the next step of the rehabilitation process is planned ahead of time because the agreements have been made and the institutions and professionals are well prepared. Another example of this extra willingness is evident in the following further extract:

> SOCIAL WORKER, MUNICIPALITY: As a rule, full lost earnings wouldn't be granted to the mother when the child is being placed or when a young person is being placed, but this is a special situation [because of Smilla's

mental illness], so what [the management group] actually decided is a month to one and a half months, where you [mother] have a period of time to accompany Smilla [starting up at the residential rehabilitation institution].

9.4.3.3   A Network of Tacit and Peripheral Acquaintances

Portes (1998, p. 7) stated that, 'To possess social capital, a person must be related to others, and it is those others, not himself, who are the actual source of his or her advantage.' He argued that, in general, immigrant families compensate for the absence of the form of resource embedded in outside networks and instead capitalize on the second source of social capital: familial support. The case of 'Ahmad', who is a young man (less than 20 years old), offers an example of an immigrant family comprising a network with sources of capital only for a limited time and a form of capital that is not convertible to rehabilitation services. Ahmad lives with his chronically ill mother on social welfare, with an absent father living abroad. The two of them live in a deprived area with a significant number of people on welfare. He has two older siblings living in different regions of the country, where they are occupied with work and education. The family is categorized as belonging to the underclass. The network map of the mother shows a small network outside the four of them: the mother has only two friends, and, apart from them, has experienced social isolation since the return of her child, as she described in the interview:

AHMAD'S MOTHER: When Ahmad came home, I didn't dare to go out. I took care of him the whole time. That is a natural thing that a mother should ... my son has been in an accident and is at home the whole time, and not going out. What should I do if I go outside, if something suddenly happens?

The reduced physical network in their daily life is, however, compensated for by a huge network provided virtually. The sibling explains how, in the religious milieu of which they are a part, people are there for one another in case of emergency. The sharing of Ahmad's situation on social media provided a huge number of network members, compensating for the vulnerability of the family:

> AHMAD'S SIBLING: Of course we are there for each other, also at the hospital. There were more than 100 people visiting us. That was cool. Yes, and it was all the time he was there, there were people there all the time, and people brought food to my mom and clothes and everything.
> INTERVIEWER: And was it your [friends] or friends of the family?
> AHMAD'S MOTHER: It was friends of the family.
> AHMAD'S SIBLING: There were all sorts of people who we do not know at all, who have seen it on Facebook, it was my friends who went there instead of me because I couldn't be there until the day after because of a storm, and it was my mother's friends, it was his friends, it was all kinds of people. I actually cried because I was so grateful that we had so much support in the beginning.

As indicated in the quote, this source of network relations was an important support for the family in the beginning of the rehabilitation process, but, overall, seems to have played a rather peripheral role in relation to the rehabilitation process, by 'only' supporting the family with their presence and material goods during a limited period of time; they did not act as promoters for allocating rehabilitation services.

9.4.4   Family Structure and Social Class

In the family cases constructed in this study, the *split* family structure is represented by the working-class families (those of Agnes, Christian, and William); the *small and weak* family structure is represented by the underclass families (Rasmus and Ahmad); and, finally, the *strong, closed* family is primarily represented by middle-class families (Smilla, and also 'Maria', whose family's case is not detailed above), but also by the working class ('Caroline', whose case, like Maria's, is not discussed in detail in the current text). The same representation was found when exploring the cases of the additional six young people and their families (see Table 9.1). The latter cases also contained families from the upper-middle class (those of 'Harriet' and 'Christine'), which also presented the strong, closed family structure.

Table 9.1 Family structures connected to social class

Class[a]	Small and weak family structure	Split family structure	Strong, closed family structure
Upper class			
Upper-middle class			(Harriet), (Christine)
Middle class			Maria, Smilla
Working class		Agnes, Christian, William	Caroline, (Harry)
Underclass	(Wassim), Ahmad, Rasmus, (Jens), (Marcus)		

Notes: The families of the study's principal eight young persons were interviewed six months after hospitalization. The names of the additional six young persons whose families were interviewed as part of the study are presented in parentheses
[a]Social class designations based on Olsen et al. (2012)

It is notable that, in this analysis, the families with ethnic backgrounds other than Danish belong to the underclass of Danish society and are characterized as having a small and weak family structure. This family structure may be the result of family members not living in the country, and the family members surrounding the injured person already being burdened (e.g., psychologically, physically, financially, socially) before the injury because of the situation that brought them to Denmark. According to statistical studies, there exist ethnic disparities in the risk of traumatic brain injury (Corrigan et al. 2010). The strong representation of the lower social classes in this study is in line with epidemiological studies showing socioeconomic status as a predictor of increased risk of acquiring a traumatic brain injury (Corrigan et al. 2010; Feigin et al. 2010).

9.5 Conclusion

Our approach, following that of Portes, of splitting the phenomenon of social capital into different aspects contributes to a nuanced understanding of how and what kind of a social network can be transformed into the most beneficial assets in a rehabilitation process for young people with an acquired brain injury. Social capital is, in this situation, more potent than economic capital, because money is not the strongest commodity in government-funded rehabilitation. In applying this approach, we have gained an understanding of the inequality that occurs in the rehabilitation process, despite the extended welfare state.

To sum up, we found that the structure and mediated resources of the family, as well as the ability to make use of networks based on ethnicity, are important for the rehabilitation process. Families with a strong, closed family structure were found to be the most successful at transforming their resources in the rehabilitation process—for example, due to the ability to draw on a professional network. This family structure was characterized by resources being concentrated in close, cooperating family members and that subsequently transformed into cultural capital in the rehabilitation process. The identified benefits included both tangible advantages and, to a larger extent, smoothness and continuity in the rehabilitation process. Thus, this type of structure demonstrates the so-called 'Matthew effect' of accumulated advantage (Gladwell 2008), in that credit will be given to those already relatively rich on capital. The small and weak family structure, together with the split family structure, on the other hand, were the least beneficial in the rehabilitation processes of the young persons. These network structures were associated with a low degree of negotiation and cooperation between the family and service professionals, and entailed discontinued and interrupted rehabilitation processes, leaving the families with little influence on the rehabilitation process and their own life situation—a situation that left them relying only on hope.

References

Alexander, M. (2009). Qualitative social network research for relational sociology. In S. Lockie (Ed.), *The annual conference of the Australian Sociological Association: The future of sociology* (pp. 1–15). Canberra: Australian Sociological Association. https://tasa.org.au/wp-content/uploads/2015/03/Alexander-Malcolm-paper-1.pdf. Accessed 10 Oct 2018.

Andersen, K., Dalton, S., Steding-Jessen, M., & Olsen, T. (2014). Socioeconomic position and survival after stroke in Denmark, 2003 to 2012: A nationwide hospital-based study. *Stroke, 45*, 3556–3560.

Bidart, C., & Charbonneau, J. (2011). How to generate personal networks: Issues and tools for a sociological perspective. *Field Methods, 23*(3), 266–286.

Borgatti, S. P., Everett, M. G., & Johnson, J. C. (2013). *Analyzing social networks*. Thousand Oaks: SAGE.

Bourdieu, P. (1980). Le capital social. Notes provisoires. *Actes de la recherche en sciences sociales, 31*, 2–3.

Bourdieu, P. (1986). The forms of capital. In J. Richardson (Ed.), *Handbook of theory and research for the sociology of education* (pp. 241–258). New York: Greenwood Press.

Bourdieu, P., & Wacquant, L. J. D. (1992). *An invitation to reflexive sociology*. Chicago: University of Chicago Press.

Carlhed, C. (2007). *Medicinens lyskraft och skuggor – om trosföreställningar och symbolisk makt i habiliteringen, 1960–1980* [The glow and shadows of the medicine: Doxa and symbolic power in the area of services to young children with disabilities, 1960–1980]. Doctoral dissertation, Uppsala University, Studies in Education 116.

Coleman, J. S. (1988). Social capital in creation of human capital. *American Journal of Sociology, 94*, S95–S120.

Coleman, J. S. (1990). *Foundations of social theory*. Cambridge, MA: Belknap Press of Harvard University Press.

Corrigan, J. D., Selassie, A. W., & Orman, J. A. (2010). The epidemiology of traumatic brain injury. *The Journal of Head Trauma Rehabilitation, 25*(2), 72–80.

Diderichsen, F., Andersen, I., & Manuel, C. (2011). *Ulighed i sundhed – årsager og indsatser* [Inequality in health – Reasons and initiatives]. Copenhagen: National Board of Health. https://www.sst.dk/da/udgivelser/2011/ulighed-i-sundhed-aarsager-og-indsatser. Accessed 27 Aug 2018.

Doser, K., Poulsen, I., Wuensch, A., & Norup, A. (2018). Psychological outcome after severe traumatic brain injury in adolescents and young adults: The chronic phase. *Brain Injury, 32*(1), 64–71.

Esping-Andersen, G. (1990). Three worlds of welfare state capitalism. In C. Pierson, F. G. Castles, & I. K. Naumann (Eds.), *The welfare state reader* (pp. 160–174). Cambridge: Polity Press.

Feigin, V. L., Barker-Collo, S., Krishnamurthi, R., Theadom, A., & Starkey, N. (2010). Epidemiology of ischaemic stroke and traumatic brain injury. *Best Practice & Research Clinical Anaesthesiology, 24*(4), 485–494.

Feiring, M., & Solvang, K. (2013). Rehabilitering mellom medisin og samfunnsfag – en feltanalytisk skisse [Rehabilitation between medicine and social science – A field analytical outline]. *Praktiske Grunde, 1–2*, 73–84. http://praktiskegrunde.dk/2013/praktiskegrunde(2013-1+2h)feiring-solvang.pdf. Accessed 24 Aug 2018.

Fischer, C. S. (1982). *To dwell among friends: Personal networks in town and city.* Chicago: University of Chicago Press.

Foster, A. M., Armstrong, J., Buckley, A., Sherry, J., Young, T., Foliaki, S., et al. (2012). Encouraging family engagement in the rehabilitation process: A rehabilitation provider's development of support strategies for family members of people with traumatic brain injury. *Disability and Rehabilitation, 34*(22), 1855–1862.

Gan, C., Campbell, K. A., Gemeinhardt, M., & McFadden, G. T. (2006). Predictors of family system functioning after brain injury. *Brain Injury, 20*(6), 587–600.

Geckler, S., & Hansen, H. (2014). *Afdækning af uligheder i behandling* [Uncovering inequalities in treatment]. Copenhagen: Centre for Alternative Social Analysis. https://casa-analyse.dk/wp-content/uploads/2016/08/2014-Afd%C3%A6kning-af-uligheder-i-behandling.pdf. Accessed 10 Apr 2015.

Gladwell, M. (2008). *Outliers: The story of success.* Boston: Little, Brown and Company.

Granovetter, M. S. (1973). The strength of weak ties. *American Journal of Sociology, 78*(6), 1360–1380.

Guldager, R., Poulsen, I., Egerod, I., Lundback Mathiesen, L., & Larsen, K. (2018). Rehabilitation capital: A new form of capital to understand rehabilitation in a Nordic welfare state. *Health Sociology Review, 27*(2), 199–213. https://doi.org/10.1080/14461242.2018.1434808.

Hindhede, A. L. (2016). Neighbourhood renewal, participation, and social capital in deprived areas: Unintended consequences in a Nordic context. *European Societies, 18*(5), 535–559.

Kamper-Jørgensen, F., & Rasmussen, J. G. (2008). Ulighed i behandling [Inequality in healthcare]. In F. Diderichsen, J. G. Rasmussen, & N. Döllner (Eds.), *Den tunge ende: sandheden om ulighederne og uretfærdighederne i den danske sundhed: debatbog* (pp. 27–45). Copenhagen: Dagens Medicin Bøger.

Ministry of Health. (2016). *Announcement of health legislation.* https://www. retsinformation.dk/forms/r0710.aspx?id=183932#idf6ac9508-afcf-4580-b7e0-18102ee7352c. Accessed 3 Oct 2017.

Ministry of Health and Prevention. (2014). *Dialogpapir om øget inddragelse af patienter og pårørende* [Dialogue paper on increased involvement of patients and relatives]. https://www.sum.dk/Aktuelt/Publikationer/Dialogpapir-om-oeget-inddragelse-af-patienter-og-paaroerende.aspx. Accessed 16 Aug 2018.

Montgomery, J. D. (1994). Weak ties, employment, and inequality: An equilibrium analysis. *American Journal of Sociology, 99*(5), 1212–1236.

National Board of Health. (2011). *Hjerneskaderehabilitering – en medicinsk teknologivurdering: hovedrapport* [Brain injury – A health technology assessment]. Copenhagen: National Board of Health, Danish Centre of Health Technology Assessment (DACEHTA). https://www.sst.dk/da/udgivelser/2011/hjerneskaderehabilitering. Accessed 20 July 2018.

Norup, A. (2012). *Severe brain injury: Impact on family members in the early phases of rehabilitation.* Doctoral dissertation, Copenhagen University Hospital, Glostrup. http://www.neuropsykologi.dk/Neuropsykologi/Upload/Anne%20Norup.pdf. Accessed 24 Aug 2018.

Olsen, L., Plough, N., Andersen, L., & Juul, J. S. (2012). *Det danske klassesamfund – Et socialt Danmarksportræt* [The Danish class society – A social portrayal of Denmark]. Copenhagen: Gyldendal.

Portes, A. (1998). Social capital: Its origins and applications in modern sociology. *Annual Review of Sociology, 24*(1), 1–24. https://doi.org/10.1146/annurev.soc.24.1.1.

Portes, A. (2000). The two meanings of social capital. *Sociological Forum, 15*(1), 1–12.

Putnam, R. D. (1993). The prosperous community: Social capital and public life. *The American Prospect, 4*(13), 35–42.

Sander, A. M., Caroselli, J. S., High, W. M., Becker, C., Neese, L., & Scheibel, R. (2002). Relationship of family functioning to progress in a post-acute rehabilitation programme following traumatic brain injury. *Brain Injury, 16*(8), 649–657.

Sandholm Larsen, N., & Larsen, K. (2008). Rehabilitering og 'motion på recept' – sociologiske perspektiver [Rehabilitation and 'exercise by prescription' – Sociological perspectives]. In K. Jensen, J. N. Rosendahl, M. Nørholm, & U. Brinkkjær (Eds.), *Studier af pædagogisk praksis: eksempler på brug af teori, metode og empiri* [Studies of pedagogic practices: Examples of the use of theory, methods and empirical knowledge] (pp. 35–56). Copenhagen: Danish School of Education.

10

Complex Problems in Need of Inter-organizational Coordination: The Importance of Connective and Collaborative Professionalism Within an Organizational Field of Rehabilitation

Tone Alm Andreassen

10.1 Introduction

Rehabilitation processes of working-age citizens comprise various health and welfare services and professions and involve several organizations and disciplines, requiring inter-organizational and inter-professional coordination and collaboration (Wade and de Jong 2000). How to organize

This analysis is based on the project 'Transitions in rehabilitation: Biographical reconstruction, experiential knowledge, and professional expertise' (Norwegian Research Council, grant no. 229082). I would like to thank the project group for valuable discussions, and am especially grateful to Mirela Slomic and Ole Kristian Håvold, who have undertaken large parts of the data collection, as well as Bjørg Christiansen, Per Koren Solvang, and Ivan Harsløf, who, like me, have also contributed in this task.

T. A. Andreassen (✉)
Centre for the Study of Professions, Oslo Metropolitan University, Oslo, Norway
e-mail: toaa@oslomet.no

© The Author(s) 2019
I. Harsløf et al. (eds.), *New Dynamics of Disability and Rehabilitation*,
https://doi.org/10.1007/978-981-13-7346-6_10

225

provision of coordinated services to citizens with chronic conditions or complex problems crossing professional, organizational, and sectoral boundaries has been a major issue in European welfare policy (Gröne and Garcia-Barbero 2001; Nolte et al. 2008), as this means integration between different levels of healthcare system and also integrated care across health and social care (Antunes and Moreira 2011; Mur-Veeman et al. 2008). This chapter derives presumptions from institutional perspectives on organizations and professions to contribute to the understanding of conditions that facilitate or impede coordinated services.

From the perspective of institutional theories of organizations and professions, professionals who provide rehabilitation services are institutionally embedded. Their values, interests, and practices are partially determined by the institutional logics that structure the organizations in which they work (Garrow and Grusky 2012; Thornton and Ocasio 2008; Thornton et al. 2012). Organizational fields are presumed to be significant sources of pressure for institutional conformity (DiMaggio and Powell 1983). Hence, inter-organizational coordination and collaboration will take place more easily between organizations *within* an organizational field than between organizations situated in separate fields. The first presumption thus is that, if healthcare and social welfare services, including employment services, resemble a joint organizational 'field of rehabilitation', accomplishing coordinated services will be easier than if these services belong to separate organizational fields.

Furthermore, in organizations populated by professionals, not only will institutional logics of organizations guide the actions taken but also logics of professionalism (Freidson 2001). However, professionalism and organizational logics intertwine in diverse ways and subsequently professionalism can take on different forms (Evetts 2003; Muzio and Kirkpatrick 2011; Noordegraaf 2011). The second presumption thus is that the forms of professionalism in operation, and the extent that professionalism includes organizing and connective capacities, will impact on inter-organizational coordination and collaboration. Hence, the existence of boundary-spanning tasks and workers (Aldrich and Herker 1977; Williams 2002) will facilitate inter-professional and inter-organizational cooperation and collaboration.

I explore these presumptions with empirical data, and previous analyses of these data, from three types of services involved in rehabilitation processes in Norway: (1) hospital-based rehabilitation programmes, (2) community-based rehabilitation services in the municipalities, and (3) the frontline offices of the Norwegian Labour and Welfare Service (NAV) providing employment assistance to citizens in the margins of the labour market.

10.2   Theoretical Perspectives

A core assumption in institutional theories of organizations is that the interests, identities, values, and assumptions of individuals and organizations are embedded within prevailing institutional logics (Friedland and Alford 1991; Garrow and Grusky 2012; Thornton and Ocasio 2008; Thornton et al. 2012). The concepts of embedded actors and embedded action turn attention to the influence of institutions on actors' behaviour, and to how the means and ends of individuals' and organizations' interests and agency are both enabled and constrained by prevailing institutional logics (Battilana and D'Aunno 2009; Phillips et al. 2000). The postulation is that institutional logics shape individual preferences and organizational interests as well as the repertoire of behaviours by which they may attain them (Friedland and Alford 1991). However, the institutional logics themselves have to be maintained and can be disrupted and transformed by institutional work (Lawrence and Suddaby 2006; Lawrence et al. 2009). Through processes of de-institutionalization and institutional change—among others, through the work of professionals (Greenwood et al. 2002)—patterns of action and interaction can be transformed.

Institutional logics operate at the level of organizations, as well as on the level of the organizational field. An organizational field (or 'institutional field') consists of organizations with different but related functions that, in the aggregate, constitute a recognized area of institutional life (DiMaggio and Powell 1983). Key features are interaction among organizations in the field, inter-organizational structures of domination and patterns of coalition, an information load with which organizations in a field must contend, and a mutual awareness among participants in a set of organizations that they are involved in a common enterprise (DiMaggio and Powell 1983).

Collaborative processes are more complex when they involve interaction of multiple sets of institutional rules and standards that may be in conflict with one another. A critical factor affecting the dynamics of collaboration involves the range of institutional fields in which participants are located (Phillips et al. 2000). Coordination and collaboration are presumed less complex within an organizational field than across fields because organizational fields are characterized by increasing homogenization instigated through processes of 'isomorphism' (DiMaggio and Powell 1983).

Professions can be important sources of isomorphism; in particular, professionals can contribute to what DiMaggio and Powell (1983) term 'normative isomorphism'. This is due to the legitimacy of formal education and a cognitive base produced by university specialists, as well as to professional networks that span organizations. Professional networks across organizations contribute to rapid diffusion of normative rules about organizational and professional behaviour. Recruitment of professionals who possess comparable orientations and dispositions to occupy almost similar positions across a range of organizations contributes to similar practices in a range of organizations.

Institutional theories of organizations emphasize professions as important agents in processes of creation, maintenance, or disruption of institutions (Muzio et al. 2013; Scott 2008). Professionals are institutional carriers or facilitators of institutional change, and organizations are sites and vehicles for professional action (Muzio et al. 2013).

Professionalism, in the 'pure' sense (Noordegraaf 2007), means exclusive ownership of an area of expertise (jurisdiction), jurisdictional autonomy and discretion in work practices, collegial control and accountability to one's peers, grounded in expertise based on abstract, theoretical knowledge and practical skills applied in diagnosing, reasoning and taking action in individual cases (Abbott 1988; Freidson 2001). The assumption is that when jurisdictional autonomy is achieved, professionals will protect their core task domains, and resist inter-professional and inter-organizational collaboration if this challenges their jurisdictions

(Kellogg 2014). Professionals' boundary maintenance will be a barrier to collaboration across disciplines and organizations (Lindsay and Dutton 2012).

In contrast to such 'pure' professionalism, new notions of the concept aim to grasp the increasing importance of organizations to professional work and of professionals' orientation to the work of the organizations in which they are employed. Notions of reconfigured, hybrid, or collaborative professionalism (Adler et al. 2008; Carvalho 2014; Noordegraaf 2007, 2013) point to forms of it in which professionals take up tasks and develop knowledge and skills outside their core activities.

This means that the traditional concept of professionalism becomes reconfigured (Noordegraaf 2013). Reconfiguration occurs through reorganization due to new circumstances that call for coordinated services and interdisciplinary approaches. 'Organized professionalism' denotes 'professional practices that embody organizational logics' (Noordegraaf 2011, p. 1351). Professionals take up organizing roles and professionals develop organizational capacities in order to face changing work circumstances. Professionalism becomes increasingly 'connective', linked to other professionals and to the outside world. In the context of the present study, this professionalism includes the crossing of specialist boundaries and organizational borders in order to support chronic patients effectively, and involves professionals who apply not only skills within their own specialized field of expertise but also connective capacities, communication, cooperative, and learning skills.

The concept of 'collaborative professionalism' indicates a professionalism taking place in network communities characterized by constructive diversity rather than unity, and by transdisciplinary forms of working (Adler et al. 2008). According to Adler et al. (2008), when professionals learn to work in heterogeneous teams and learn to see other professionals as sources of learning and support, assumedly also professional self-identities are transformed.

Hence, when reconfigured forms of professionalism are present in service-providing organizations, inter-professional or inter-organizational activities and collaboration across organizational boundaries will be supported. In particular, this will take place if professionals take up 'boundary-spanning roles' that link between an organization and important outside organizations (Aldrich and Herker 1977). By understanding how issues are differently defined, influenced by the involved organizations' different values and interests, competent boundary spanners can facilitate inter-organizational cooperation (Lindsay and Dutton 2012; Williams 2002). By buffering between different professions, 'brokerage professions' can facilitate cooperation across professional and organizational boundaries (Kellogg 2014).

Based on these perspectives, I will investigate whether hospital-based rehabilitation services, community rehabilitation services, and employment services constitute a joint organizational 'field of rehabilitation', because, if not, identification of a common ground for collaboration would be more difficult. Indicators of the field status of rehabilitation services are inter-organizational structures of domination and coalition that delineate divisions of labour and responsibilities and ascribe mandates in the rehabilitation process, an infrastructure of coordination and collaboration, and an awareness among the participants that they are involved in a common rehabilitation enterprise. Furthermore, the analysis will look for signs of professionals being carriers of homogenization processes, such as similarities in the ways that the healthcare and the employment services respectively approach persons with traumatic injuries.

Second, acknowledging that the professionals' actions will be influenced by their professional identity and the forms of professionalism that guide their perception of the problems in need of rehabilitation and their approach to easing these problems, the analysis will examine indicators of 'pure' professionalism focused on diagnosing, reasoning, and taking action in the individual cases, and on relationships to a collegium of peers. The analysis will also look for indicators of more collaborative, communicative, and cooperative forms of professionalism, which may include boundary-spanning tasks, and for the existence of brokerage professions crossing professional and organizational boundaries.

10.3   Field of Study, Empirical Material, and Analytical Approach

10.3.1   Field of Study: Services Involved in Trauma Rehabilitation in Norway

This analysis studies the rehabilitation processes of people experiencing multi-trauma with or without traumatic brain injury (TBI). Rehabilitation processes of TBI/multi-trauma patients are exemplary cases for in-depth investigation of the organizational and professional dynamics enabling or hindering coordinated services. These disabling conditions affect many different aspects of everyday life, including social and vocational participation (Andelic et al. 2009). This causes rehabilitation processes of long duration involving many different healthcare and social welfare services, and, according to the injured persons themselves, several unmet needs (Andelic et al. 2014).

An advantage in centring the study on a specific patient group, rather than coordination in general, is the opportunity to investigate approaches towards specific problems and situations instead of generalized presentations of overarching procedures and intentions. The Transitions in Rehabilitation project aimed to grasp conditions surrounding two critical transitions in the rehabilitation processes of individuals: (1) between hospital-based specialized rehabilitation and community-based rehabilitation (within municipal healthcare), and (2) between healthcare services and employment services.

In Norway, specialized hospital-based rehabilitation is the responsibility of the state and the Ministry of Health and Care Services via four regional health authorities. In this research, hospital-based rehabilitation includes two inpatient clinics and one outpatient clinic. One of the inpatient clinics serves patients in a subacute phase; the other—like the outpatient clinic—serves patients later in their rehabilitation process, with a specific rehabilitation programme oriented towards patients who have been living at home for a while. From these services, patients are discharged to community-based rehabilitation services and/or employment offices.

Community-based rehabilitation services are the responsibility of Norway's politically autonomous municipalities. Legal regulations set some standards that the local governments have to fulfil, but, due to their autonomy and the variations among the municipalities in size, geography, and centrality, the services vary in organization, volume, and character.

Employment services for citizens in the margins of the labour market are provided by the frontline offices of NAV, a responsibility of the Ministry of Labour and Social Affairs. Besides employment service provided by the frontline offices, NAV also administers national insurance benefits to all citizens in Norway and social welfare to those in need but not entitled to national insurance benefits, as well as assistive technology to compensate for impairments. Thus, for citizens as well as professionals from other services, NAV is associated with more than just employment services.

10.3.2 Empirical Basis of the Analysis

The empirical material from hospital-based rehabilitation was collected through observation of team meetings and subsequent interviews with some of the participating professionals. The sample comprised three different inter-professional teams from three rehabilitation programmes, allowing for interviews with 16 professionals and observation of an additional 25 professionals—in total, 41 professionals. Eight one-hour inter-professional meetings were observed.

The empirical material from the community-based rehabilitation and from the employment services was collected through group interviews. The interviews in relation to employment services involved eight frontline offices and, in total, 27 professionals. The interviews conducted with representatives of community-based rehabilitation services involved eight municipalities and, in all, 34 professionals. Table 10.1 presents the educational backgrounds of all the professionals interviewed.

The community-based rehabilitation services and the employment offices were selected from a list, prepared by the hospitals, of municipalities that, during the previous year, had had patients discharged from the hospital. This was done to increase the likelihood that the frontline

Table 10.1 Educational backgrounds of the interviewed professionals

	Health sciences[a]	Social work/ social education	Pedagogy/ social sciences	Other
Hospital-based rehabilitation (n = 16)	11	3	1	1
Community-based rehabilitation (n = 34)	27	4	–	3
Employment service (n = 27)	4 (+ 1)[b]	7	9	7[c]

[a]Primarily nursing, occupational therapy, or physiotherapy, but, for the hospital-based rehabilitation professionals, also psychology and medicine
[b]One social worker was also a psychologist
[c]Primarily internal training from the former National Insurance Administration merged into NAV, but also education in law

professionals will have had experience with traumatic injuries. The sample comprises small and large municipalities in both central and peripheral areas.

While hospital-based rehabilitation is specialized in relation to specific target groups (here, trauma patients), frontline services in municipalities are generalists, in the sense that their services in principle cover every kind of illness, injury, or impairment. Therefore, studying trauma patients in hospital-based rehabilitation meant observations and interviews about the daily life of the professionals. In generalist-oriented frontline services, the case of trauma patients had to be introduced by a vignette describing a trauma patient at discharge from hospital-based rehabilitation, similar to a discharge summary in the kind of information given. The vignette was developed by two researchers with background as a physician and as a trauma patient respectively, and discussed with clinicians in hospital-based rehabilitation and with a panel of citizens with personal injury experience.

The patient/client in the vignette is a 34-year-old male carpenter with a wife and two small children. He is diagnosed with traumatic brain injuries, cerebral haemorrhage, and temporary paralysis in the left extremities due to an accident. The focus groups were introduced to his situation 12 months after injury, the point at which a patient stops receiving sickness absence benefits and approaches the crossroads of either permanent disability benefit or a process aimed at returning to work supported by a temporary benefit. At that time, the study's patient is still suffering from reduced muscular strength, some problems in daily activities due to a lack of fine motor skills in his hands, balance problems, memory loss, strong headaches, light to moderate depression (for which he receives psychological treatment), and a loss of energy. Further training is recommended by the hospital. The wife has 50% unpaid leave from her job to be his carer at home. He considers his wife to be of very valuable support, and he himself would like to have more energy to play with his children. His motivation for employment is low, and his general practitioner (GP) has declared him 100% disabled for the time being. Although the vignette case was not a typical case for the frontline services, in all interviews, at least some of the participants stated that they have had similar cases, which they also referred to during the discussion.

Data were collected during autumn 2014 and spring 2015. Two PhD students[1] have previously analysed parts of the empirical material. The current analysis draws on the findings from their analyses. Their publications are referred to within the analysis below.

10.3.3   Analytical Approach

The analysis is theoretically informed, guided by perspectives from institutional theories of organizations and drawing on organizational discourse analysis (Phillips and Oswick 2012) to examine the social construction of the institutions that characterize a particular empirical case. Organizational discourse analysis sees organizations as linguistically shaped and studies how language, broadly defined, constructs social phenomena, and how language in use is an expression of the social context in which they occur. This suggests that the talk and actions of the interviewed professionals should be treated as expressions of institutionalized perceptions of the organizational context of their work, of their role as professionals, and of the problems of the injured individuals.

---

[1] Mirela Slomic and Ole Kristian Håvold.

In the analysis, not only the utterances are important but also how the professionals relate to one another in group interviews and team meetings. Accordingly, both the observed team meeting in the hospitals and the group interviews were instances of observation. Moreover, the focus is not just on the topical content of the talk but also on the ways of talking, and on the interaction among the participants, such as signs of consensus or disagreement.

In contrast to the observed meetings at the hospitals, which are instances of actual work performance, in the group interviews in community-based rehabilitation and in the employment service, the professionals talk about what they *would* do or should have done, but do not necessarily do—omissions to which they sometimes admit, as do the hospital professionals in the interviews. One example is a professional who, in the interview, speaks about several kinds of consequences of the traumatic injuries that regularly are discussed in team meetings, yet the related observation demonstrates that none of these consequences have been explicitly discussed.

The analysis involved the following steps: first, a case description of each team, office, or service was developed; second, a comparison across the cases of each service was performed, in order to understand if it made sense to describe them as unified services; and, third, a comparison between the three services was undertaken, in order to shed light on (a) whether the services could be seen as part of a common organizational field, and (b) the extent that the professionalism expressed by the professionals included organizational tasks and boundary-spanning roles.

In the analysis below, the professionals of the three services appear as a collectivity or community—as a unified 'they'. This is in accordance with the informants' own talk. In the interviews, they often spoke of a 'we' taking action in a patient's or client's case. During the analysis, I have carefully noted to whom a 'we' refers, and whether any significant divergence or disagreement appears in the group discussions. Their use of 'we' underlines the professionals as organizational members, but is also in keeping with the fact that they were invited to be interviewed as members of the organizations that employ them.

10.4   Analysis

Considering the field status of the services involved in rehabilitation, the fact that the sectors of healthcare and of employment services belong to different bureaucratic hierarchies, and are regulated by different laws, indicates that dissimilarities between the sectors are significant. Furthermore, the sectors are given different political mandates (cure, care, and rehabilitation versus activation towards labour market participation and self-support). On the other hand, healthcare services and employment services are both part of a politically governed welfare state (in a small country of around five million people). Furthermore, many citizens are users in both sectors; healthcare and social service professionals share a common aim and professional ethics of providing help to people in need; and, to some extent, the same occupations populate both sectors. This is illustrated by the educational backgrounds of the interviewed professionals (see Table 10.1). Furthermore, during their work careers, several of the interviewed professionals had moved between services. Hence, from a broader perspective, the services could be seen as belonging to the same organizational field.

10.4.1   Inter-organizational Structures of Divisions of Labour and Responsibilities

Across the sectors of healthcare and labour and welfare services, inter-organizational structures exist that delineate divisions of labour and responsibilities and ascribe mandates to the different services involved in the rehabilitation process. This appears both in the professionals' interpretation of their organizations' mandates and in their understanding of and relationships to the other services involved.

The hospital-based rehabilitation teams are constructed to treat multi-problem cases holistically. They operate according to a common goal of providing interdisciplinary interventions to rehabilitate patients in relation to all areas of life. To the professionals, employment is one such area of a patient's life. Social workers or occupational therapists could therefore communicate with the employment service and/or with the patient's employer.

The hospital-based rehabilitation teams and their organizations are set up to perform the task of rehabilitating an injured patient sufficiently to discharge the patient from hospital, and to produce clinical information and recommendations to the frontline services. The end of the treatment period instigates a conclusion about possible needs for further rehabilitation, summed up in a report prepared for the frontline services; in particular, a discharge summary sent to the patient's GP. In the present study, the professionals in the community rehabilitation services and the employment offices, for their part, seemed well aware of the kind of services provided by the hospitals.

Likewise, across the frontline offices of the employment service, a shared understanding of the mandate—return to work and income security during this process—seemed present. In all offices, the professionals appeared internally coherent, and, across offices, locations, and sizes, consistency in the approach towards the clients was widespread. The professionals described many of the same kinds of measures and procedures to be applied in the vignette case, and they presented a shared understanding and evaluation of his problems (Håvold 2019). According to the employment professionals, their environment seemed to hold the same conception of their mandate—except for a lack of knowledge about the opportunities offered by the employment service.

The community-based rehabilitation services differed. In some municipalities, the professionals presented well-established procedures for needs assessment, as well as programmes for rehabilitation and other forms of service provision to the person in the vignette case. In others, the professionals revealed uncertainty, and apparently approached this kind of situation on an ad hoc basis. In several municipalities, the professionals talked about a lack of adequate services.

The professionals searched for opportunities in the services offered by the municipality (Slomic et al. 2017). Some stated that they could provide an adequate rehabilitation programme to an injured young man. Others concluded that neither their resources nor their expertise sufficiently covered his need for long-term, specialized rehabilitation. Correspondingly, compared to the hospitals and the employment services, community rehabilitation services seemed more diffuse.

The employment offices described 'work' as their mission, and work was a question in hospital-based rehabilitation (in particular, in late-phase rehabilitation programmes), but, in community-based rehabilitation, work was mostly out of the scope of the professionals. To them, the frontline offices of NAV were associated with benefits and irrelevant as collaborators in rehabilitation.

10.4.2   Traces of Normative Isomorphism

Despite the differences above, the analysis revealed a similarity in the ways that the healthcare and the employment services respectively addressed individuals with multi-traumatic injuries—how they understood the problem and how they approached the situation. In hospital-based rehabilitation, the professionals stated that they are holistically oriented towards the whole person, attentive to the patients' individual goals, and adjust their services to each individual situation. As one said, 'In the end, it is their goals that define the focus of our work'. They meet patients whose lives have been dramatically transformed, but, for a patient to realize the need for a radical reorganization of their life, the professionals have to apply a gradual and soft approach.

In community-based rehabilitation, the professionals' approach to the vignette case was to stimulate motivation of the person—'to implant in him a confidence that the situation will improve' and 'help him realize that, with such an injury, one year is not very long'. They wanted to approach lack of motivation 'from every possible angle', and 'take the backdoor' if necessary. In doing so, they will search for the patient's personal goals, and start there. They considered the vignette patient's recovery process to be of a long duration and emphasized that a long-term perspective would be necessary. Hence, despite municipal variation in the range of services available to injured people, the professionals' approach to injured patients was strikingly similar.

In the employment offices, the professionals' approach was also to stimulate motivation (Håvold 2018). They described their focus as being on 'opportunities despite health problems'. Their job is to try out any possible route that may lead to a return to work. Relating to the vignette case, the professionals considered individuals with brain injuries to be complicated cases, and they assumed a long-term perspective regarding his return to work process. It was important to stimulate a move in the right direction—towards hope and a future. They talked about 'being careful, not too pushy' and about having to consider when to introduce the question of job and employment.

Across the different services, the professionals' approach was quite similar. In all services, the professionals stated that their point of departure is a person's individual situation, wishes, and goals, and that these are their basis for enhancing motivation. They will listen to a person's opinions and wishes, but not fully accept wishes that contradict what they perceive to be in the person's best interest. Rather, they will motivate for stepwise changes, which during the process could initiate motivation and goals that are more 'constructive' from the professionals' point of view.

Despite different sectors, organizations, and ownership (municipalities and ministries), policies and professional knowledge seem to travel across organizational boundaries, and contribute to shared approaches to the problems that the services deal with. The similarities in professional approaches across a range of organizations in the healthcare services and the frontline employment offices show traces of normative isomorphism. They indicate that processes of homogenization have taken place through professionals who possess similar orientations and understanding of the problems of injured individuals.

10.4.3   An Infrastructure of Interaction and Awareness of a Common Enterprise

Across the different service organizations, an infrastructure of interaction, coordination, and sharing of information seemed to be in operation. In this infrastructure, the GPs seemed to hold a key position in terms of their receiving discharge summaries from hospitals. While both the community rehabilitation services and the employment offices stated that differences between GPs existed, in general, the GPs often appeared distant and difficult to involve in collaboration.

In community-based rehabilitation, the GPs seemed seldom involved in interdisciplinary assessments of an injured individual's needs. The responsibilities and tasks linked to GPs concerned medication and referrals to specialist healthcare, such as psychologists. When in doubt about assessment of a patient, the municipal medical officer could be consulted.

In employment services, the professionals depend on medical declarations, but they make their own judgements about job requirements and aspects of the employer that will affect the opportunities for returning to work. In the vignette case, they did not take on face value the GP's statement that the client is 100% incapacitated (Håvold et al. 2017). According to the professionals, the employment service has many measures and programmes that can enable an individual to return to work, and, for a young man like the one in the vignette case, only after every opportunity is tried out will permanent disability benefit be the conclusion. If in doubt, the workers will consult NAV's own medical or neuropsychological expertise.

To both frontline services, the hospitals seemed more important than the GPs as providers of specialized diagnostic information about an injured person as in the vignette case. A shared understanding across the interviewed services was that, in the infrastructure of interaction, the hospitals have a position as providers of specialized services, and the community-based rehabilitation and the employment services, for their part, are in the position of receivers of patients, information, and advice.

In some municipalities, the professionals were certain that they would receive a discharge report from the hospitals; in others, they stated that they would not know about the existence of an injured young man unless his GP or the employment office reported a need for further rehabilitation. From the point of view of the municipal rehabilitation services, the hospitals' recommendations for further rehabilitation and assistance were given without sufficient insight into the available services in the municipalities (Slomic et al. 2017). Therefore, from this perspective, hospital recommendations were challenging.

In relation to community-based rehabilitation, the hospital professionals described efforts to recommend a patient's need for follow up. They tried to write 'explicit instructions', such as 'the patient needs …' an occupational therapist, or a support person to motivate towards an activity, or contact with a psychiatric nurse or a psychologist for help with coping with their life. Hospital professionals framed the needs of the patients as needs for specific professionals, rather than as descriptions of injury implications, prognosis, or functional ability. Apparently, they acted as if the discharge summary sufficiently provided this kind of information. Nothing in the hospital professionals' discussions pointed to the knowledge needs of the frontline services. The professionals named the kind of professionals that the patients needed, but not the kind of problems for which professional help was required. In line with their expressed patient centeredness, their focus was primarily on the patient's needs, not on the frontline services' needs for sufficient information to serve the patient after discharge from hospital. When municipal services lacked the professionals named, the hospital recommendations did not help the frontline professionals to identify alternative ways to meet that patient's needs.

In relation to the employment service, the hospital professionals considered it within their mandate to give an accurate picture of a patient's situation, including a judgement on whether the patient at discharge was ready for a (gradual) return to work or whether a workable everyday life was the only achievable goal. In the employment offices, assessing a client's work capability is important in judgements about opportunities for returning to work. The professionals reported that they received medical declarations from the GPs, or discharge summaries from hospitals, and sometimes hospital professionals made direct contact. They relied on medical expertise about the health conditions and on recommendations for further treatment ('presumably, the specialists know what they are talking about'), but they found the vignette's discharge summary too focused on injuries and impairments. They complained about medical declarations regularly lacking useable information about a client's functional ability and prognosis (Håvold et al. 2017).

The analysis of hospital-based rehabilitation to some degree confirmed the opinion of employment professionals that healthcare professionals' primarily pay attention to problems and deficits, which is understandable given their mandate of rehabilitating impairments. Still, it is worth noting that, in the hospital teams' discussions about discharging patients' opportunities for returning to work, the professionals (ostensibly experts on the implications of injuries) seldom made judgements about how the impairments their tests revealed affected a patient's ability to match the requirements of their job. Rather, they discussed work capacity and work stress in general.

The analysis of employment services to some extent confirmed the hospital professionals' opinion that employment professionals lack sufficient knowledge about the implications of traumatic injuries, which is understandable given their generalist character of serving clients with all kinds of health conditions or social problems. Hospital professionals reported that some of their patients found collaboration with the employment service difficult. However, they also emphasized that, when they explained the health problems of an individual to the employment service, the professionals understood and accepted these explanations.

This analysis points to an inter-organizational structure of domination and dependencies, in which the hospitals, as providers of specialized services, are in position to set premises for the work of the frontline services—in deciding the point of time for discharge and in holding the professional expertise on the traumatic injuries. The frontline services—as receivers of patients, information, and advice—although they can ask for further information and advice, seem not to be in a position to require of the hospitals that their knowledge transfer answers to the needs of frontline professionals.

Although the professionals pointed to several insufficiencies and missing links that impeded a well-functioning collaboration (Slomic et al. 2017), and despite relationships of dominance in the infrastructure of interaction, all three services seemed to hold an awareness of being part of a common enterprise of contributing to the rehabilitation of injured people. This indicates a shared organizational field across the sectoral divide between healthcare services and the labour and welfare services.

10.4.4   Professionalism and Boundary-Spanning

The forms of professionalism guiding the professionals' work appear in their discussions about their work, but must be understood in light of the organizational structures in which they work.

The hospital-based rehabilitation services are organized in inter-professional teams with working relationships on a daily basis. The professionals talked about their inter-professional teams as 'we' and 'us' understood as units of professionals connected by common goals and shared knowledge (Slomic et al. 2017). In team meetings, this was demonstrated through frequent confirming with a 'yes' or nodding. The professionalism of the hospital professionals seemed extensively linked to the team's organizational task of providing specialized rehabilitation services. Furthermore, their inter-professional collaboration was facilitated by brokerage professionals—team coordinators who are mostly passive in the inter-professional discussions, but who are the 'oil in the machinery' and arrange for the teams and their external responsibilities to function. Here, the classic 'pure' professionalism is transformed, underpinned by dedicated brokerage professionals. Subsequently, reconfigured patterns of action and interaction can take place.

The employment offices are organized in teams, units, or departments. The interviews identified an organizational structure in which clients are assigned to one professional, and, although the professionals are organized in teams, they most often assess and follow up clients on their own. Still, close collegial relationships based on being members of the same organizations seemed prevalent. During the interviews, the professionals added to or even concluded one another's statements, or they confirmed each other's accounts by nodding. They used the terms 'we' and 'us' with reference to the organization. Their professionalism related to the mandate of the organization.

The community-based rehabilitation services are organized in a purchaser–provider-like model in which one unit assesses the patients' needs, whilst other units provide the services granted to the patients. In addition, physiotherapy and occupational therapy services are often organizationally separated from nursing homes and homebased care. This organizational divide was manifested as a sort of fragmentation. While the professionals knew or knew of each other, they did not operate or talk as unified teams (as in the hospitals) or colleagues in working relationships (as in the employment service). They worked in parallel, each professional individually, rather than together (Slomic et al. 2017). Their professionalism related mainly to their respective occupations, as did the 'we' in their statements. While the professionals would perform an interdisciplinary assessment of the vignette case, the actual rehabilitation measures would be autonomously undertaken by each professional or service.

The professionals in the hospitals and in the employment service seemed to operate with a professionalism linked to the mandate of the organizations in which they worked, resembling a form of 'organized professionalism'. In contrast, in community-based rehabilitation, the professionalism seemed linked to occupational groups, rather than to a municipal responsibility of providing rehabilitation services, and thus was more aligned to a 'pure' professionalism. Rather than this being an effort to protect their professional domain against challenges from inter-professional or inter-organizational collaboration, it appeared to be a withdrawal into a collegium of peers, which was possibly due to the fragmented organizational structure in the municipalities, and, in several of the municipalities, no coordination stimuli from the management.

The hospital-based rehabilitation teams and the employment offices both included professionals who took up boundary-spanning tasks of establishing links from their organization to relevant actors in the outside world. In hospitals, social workers and occupational therapists performed boundary-spanning tasks in conveying to the patients' employers and the employment service any adjustment requirements in respect of a reduced work capacity, opportunities for self-support, and needs for public income security. In the employment service, seemingly, all professionals could take up the boundary-spanning tasks of collecting information from the healthcare services and of involving employers in discussions of opportunities for the patient to return to work. Through such information processing, these professionals enacted a form of 'connective' professionalism aimed at influencing their environment.

In contrast, the boundary-spanning task of coordinating an individual care plan (to which citizens with complex problems have a legal right) seemed often avoided by the professionals in community-based rehabilitation. While the professionals considered such a plan to be beneficial with respect to the vignette case, they were reluctant to initiate a joint plan process. They regarded the coordination task burdensome, and seemed to apply an approach of 'self-targeting', leaving the initiative to the patients or the families (Harsløf et al. 2019). No brokerage professionals existed to assist with coordination tasks. Apparently, 'connective' professionalism was absent, which might be due to a lack of organizational incentives to take up organizing tasks.

10.5   Conclusion

This analysis has demonstrated that, across the sectors of healthcare and labour and welfare services, inter-organizational structures exist that delineate divisions of labour and responsibilities and ascribe mandates to the organizations involved in rehabilitation processes. Between these organizations, differences exist in political 'owners' (ministries and municipalities), organizational mandates, and professional focuses. However, there are also significant similarities in professional approaches across organizations and sectors, specifically regarding how the professionals understood traumatic injury and how they would support the injured person's rehabilitation process. These similarities can be understood as traces of normative isomorphism. The organizations seemed incorporated in an infrastructure of interaction, coordination, and sharing of information, and the professionals appeared to have an awareness of being part of a common rehabilitation enterprise. These are all manifestations of a joint organizational field of rehabilitation, which, according to the introductory presumption derived from institutional perspectives on organizations, should support collaboration and coordinated services.

Furthermore, the analysis has revealed deficits in the infrastructure of coordination and collaboration, such as the key position but lack of involvement of GPs, knowledge transfer from hospitals that does not answer to the needs of frontline professionals, who, on their part, are not in a position to place requirements on the hospitals.

However, not only infrastructure deficits impede coordination and collaboration. Knowledge sharing and joint action seem also hindered by the lack of a professionalism anchored in the mandate of the organization and including boundary-spanning tasks. A 'pure' professionalism focused on diagnosing, reasoning, and taking action in the individual case seems insufficient to meet complex, sector-crossing problems. Connective and collaborative professionalism including boundary-spanning tasks seems necessary to ensure smooth transitions, undisrupted pathways, and coordinated services being provided for injured individuals. Ostensibly, such professionalism involves professionals acting as members of an organization, understanding professional work as part of a totality of services, and seeing rehabilitation services not merely as a contribution of their own discipline but also as the contribution of the organization and the organizational field of rehabilitation. Puzzlingly perhaps, this means a professionalism that pays attention not merely to the needs of the injured individuals, but that also, in order to ensure coordinated services, meets the needs of the services that serve these individuals.

References

Abbott, A. (1988). *The system of professions: An essay on the division of expert labor.* Chicago: University of Chicago Press.

Adler, P. S., Kwon, S.-W., & Heckscher, C. (2008). Perspective–professional work: The emergence of collaborative community. *Organization Science, 19*(2), 359–376.

Aldrich, H., & Herker, D. (1977). Boundary spanning roles and organizational structure. *Academy of Management Review, 2*(2), 217–230.

Andelic, N., Hammergren, N., Bautz-Holter, E., Sveen, U., Brunborg, C., & Røe, C. (2009). Functional outcome and health-related quality of life 10 years after moderate to severe traumatic brain injury. *Acta Neurologica Scandinavica, 120*(1), 16–23. https://doi.org/10.1111/j.1600-0404.2008.01116.x.

Andelic, N., Soberg, H. L., Berntsen, S., Sigurdardottir, S., & Roe, C. (2014). Self-perceived health care needs and delivery of health care services 5 years after moderate-to-severe traumatic brain injury. *PM&R, 6*(11), 1013–1021.

Antunes, V., & Moreira, J. P. (2011). Approaches to developing integrated care in Europe: A systematic literature review. *Journal of Management & Marketing in Healthcare, 4*(2), 129–135. https://doi.org/10.1179/1753303 11X13016677137743.

Battilana, J., & D'Aunno, T. (2009). Institutional work and the paradox of embedded agency. In T. B. Lawrence, R. Suddaby, & B. Leca (Eds.), *Institutional work: Actors and agency in institutional studies of organizations* (pp. 31–58). Cambridge, UK: Cambridge University Press.

Carvalho, T. (2014). Changing connections between professionalism and managerialism: A case study of nursing in Portugal. *Journal of Professions and Organization, 1*(2), 176–190.

DiMaggio, P. J., & Powell, W. W. (1983). The iron cage revisited: Institutional isomorphism and collective rationality in organizational fields. *American Sociological Review, 48*(2), 147–160.

Evetts, J. (2003). The sociological analysis of professionalism: Occupational change in the modern world. *International Sociology, 18*(2), 395–415. https://doi.org/10.1177/0268580903018002005.

Freidson, E. (2001). *Professionalism: The third logic*. London: Polity Press.

Friedland, R., & Alford, R. R. (1991). Bringing society back in: Symbols, practices, and institutional contradictions. In W. W. Powell & P. J. DiMaggio (Eds.), *The new institutionalism in organizational analysis* (pp. 232–263). Chicago: University of Chicago Press.

Garrow, E. E., & Grusky, O. (2012). Institutional logic and street-level discretion: The case of HIV test counseling. *Journal of Public Administration Research and Theory, 23*(1), 103–131.

Greenwood, R., Suddaby, R., & Hinings, C. R. (2002). Theorizing change: The role of professional associations in the transformation of institutionalized fields. *Academy of Management Journal, 45*(1), 58–80. https://doi.org/10.2307/3069285.

Gröne, O., & Garcia-Barbero, M. (2001). Integrated care: A position paper of the WHO European office for integrated health care services. *International Journal of Integrated Care, 1*(2), e21.

Harsløf, I., Håvold, O. K., & Slomic, M. (2019). Establishing individual care plans for rehabilitation patients: Traces of self-targeting in the Norwegian, universal welfare state. *Nordic Journal of Social Research 10*(1).

Håvold, O. K. (2018). Opportunity talk, work talk and identity talk: Motivating strategies used by the Norwegian labour and welfare offices. *Nordic Social Work Research, 8*(2), 158–170. https://doi.org/10.1080/2156857X.2017. 1405836.

Håvold, O. K. (2019). All roads lead to Rome: Discretionary reasoning on medically objective injuries at the Norwegian Labour and Welfare Offices. *Professions & Professionalism, 9*(1). http://doi.org/10.7577/p2283.

Håvold, O. K., Harsløf, I., & Alm Andreassen, T. (2017). Externalizing an 'asset model' of activation: Creative institutional work by frontline workers in the Norwegian Labour and Welfare Service. *Social Policy and Administration, 52*(1), 178–196.

Kellogg, K. C. (2014). Brokerage professions and implementing reform in an age of experts. *American Sociological Review, 79*(5), 912–941. https://doi. org/10.1177/0003122414544734.

Lawrence, T. B., & Suddaby, R. (2006). Institutions and institutional work. In S. R. Clegg, C. Hardy, T. B. Lawrence, & W. R. Nord (Eds.), *The SAGE handbook of organization studies* (2nd ed., pp. 215–254). London: SAGE.

Lawrence, T. B., Suddaby, R., & Leca, B. (2009). *Institutional work: Actors and agency in institutional studies of organizations.* Cambridge, UK: Cambridge University Press.

Lindsay, C., & Dutton, M. (2012). Promoting healthy routes back to work? Boundary spanning health professionals and employability programmes in Great Britain. *Social Policy & Administration, 46*(5), 509–525.

Mur-Veeman, I., van Raak, A., & Paulus, A. (2008). Comparing integrated care policy in Europe: Does policy matter? *Health Policy, 85*(2), 172–183. https:// doi.org/10.1016/j.healthpol.2007.07.008.

Muzio, D., & Kirkpatrick, I. (2011). Introduction: Professions and organizations – A conceptual framework. *Current Sociology, 59*(4), 389–405.

Muzio, D., Brock, D. M., & Suddaby, R. (2013). Professions and institutional change: Towards an institutionalist sociology of the professions. *Journal of Management Studies, 50*(5), 699–721. https://doi.org/10.1111/joms.12030.

Nolte, E., Knai, C., & McKee, M. (Eds.). (2008). *Managing chronic conditions: Experience in eight countries.* Brussels/Copenhagen: European Observatory on Health Systems and Policies/World Health Organization.

Noordegraaf, M. (2007). From 'pure' to 'hybrid' professionalism: Present-day professionalism in ambiguous public domains. *Administration and Society, 39*(6), 761–785. https://doi.org/10.1177/0095399707304434.

Noordegraaf, M. (2011). Risky business: How professionals and professional fields (must) deal with organizational issues. *Organization Studies, 32*(10), 1349–1371. https://doi.org/10.1177/0170840611416748.

Noordegraaf, M. (2013). Reconfiguring professional work: Changing forms of professionalism in public services. *Administration and Society, 48*(7), 783–810. https://doi.org/10.1177/0095399713509242.

Phillips, N., & Oswick, C. (2012). Organizational discourse: Domains, debates, and directions. *Academy of Management Annals, 6*(1), 435–481.

Phillips, N., Lawrence, T. B., & Hardy, C. (2000). Inter-organizational collaboration and the dynamics of institutional fields. *Journal of Management Studies, 37*(1). https://doi.org/10.1111/1467-6486.00171.

Scott, W. R. (2008). Lords of the dance: Professionals as institutional agents. *Organization Studies, 29*(2), 219–238.

Slomic, M., Soberg, H. L., Sveen, U., & Christiansen, B. (2017). Transitions of patients with traumatic brain injury and multiple trauma between specialized and municipal rehabilitation services – Professionals' perspectives. *Cogent Medicine, 4*(1). https://doi.org/10.1080/2331205X.2017.1320849.

Thornton, P., & Ocasio, W. (2008). Institutional logics. In R. Greenwood, C. Oliver, R. Suddaby, & K. Sahlin (Eds.), *The SAGE handbook of organizational institutionalism* (pp. 99–129). Los Angeles: SAGE.

Thornton, P., Ocasio, W., & Lounsbury, M. (2012). *The institutional logics perspective: A new approach to culture, structure and process*. Oxford: Oxford University Press.

Wade, D. T., & de Jong, B. A. (2000). Recent advances in rehabilitation. *British Medical Journal, 320*(7246), 1385–1388. https://doi.org/10.1136/bmj.320.7246.1385.

Williams, P. (2002). The competent boundary spanner. *Public Administration, 80*(1), 103–124.

11

Transfer Practices During Acquired Brain Injury Rehabilitation: A Descent in the Medical Hierarchy

Karin Højbjerg, Ingrid Egerod, and Ingrid Poulsen

11.1 Introduction

Inequality in treatment and rehabilitation in general is well documented in Western countries (Devaux and de Looper 2012; Eikemo et al. 2008; Willis et al. 2016). Although most health expenses are paid through taxes in the Nordic welfare states, and therefore cost is not a barrier for accessing healthcare services, inequality in health still exists (Kamper-Jørgensen

K. Højbjerg (✉)
Department of Learning and Philosophy, Aalborg University Copenhagen, Copenhagen, Denmark
e-mail: kah@learning.aau.dk

I. Egerod
Intensive Care Unit, Rigshospitalet, University of Copenhagen, Copenhagen, Denmark
e-mail: ingrid.egerod@regionh.dk

I. Poulsen
Department of Neurorehabilitation, Rigshospitalet, University of Copenhagen, Copenhagen, Denmark
e-mail: Ingrid.Poulsen@regionh.dk

© The Author(s) 2019
I. Harsløf et al. (eds.), *New Dynamics of Disability and Rehabilitation*,
https://doi.org/10.1007/978-981-13-7346-6_11

and Rasmussen 2008; Bambra 2012; Larsen et al. 2013; Mackenbach et al. 2008). Socioeconomic variables such as education, income, housing, and family situation among patients are commonly used to examine the success of rehabilitation in Denmark (Andersen et al. 2014; Guldager 2018). In this study, though, we have chosen a different approach by exploring the role of healthcare organizations and healthcare professionals (HCPs) in relation to inequality in health outcomes. By empirically focusing on transfer practices during the rehabilitation of patients with severe acquired brain injury (sABI), our ambition is to gain knowledge about how inequality may also be generated among HCPs in organizations. This chapter presents an empirical study of the trajectories of patients with sABIs, including severe traumatic and non-traumatic brain injury (e.g., stroke and subarachnoid haemorrhage from acute to long-term rehabilitation), to investigate how HCPs at different levels influence transfer practices. The analysis is based on Pierre Bourdieu's theory of practice and key concepts of Andrew Abbott's theory of profession.

11.2 Rehabilitation of Patients with Acute Brain Injury

Rehabilitation after acute brain injury has developed in recent years from nonspecialized practice with limited expertise and access to highly specialized interdisciplinary neurorehabilitation units in many Western countries (Engberg et al. 2006). Specialization and centralization of neurorehabilitation has resulted in better patient outcomes (Anke et al. 2015; Engberg et al. 2006). The typical trajectory for the most severely injured patients is acute hospital admission via the trauma centre and neurointensive care unit, followed by transfer to in-house specialized rehabilitation and finally rehabilitation in primary care (National Board of Health 2011). The length of stay at hospitals has been reduced dramatically in recent years (Husted et al. 2012) and, consequently, HCPs must ensure that patients are transferred to the 'right' department for the 'right' treatment and care at the 'right' time. The constant focus on cost and effectiveness also sets standards for streamlining the HCPs' work. Incentive structures have been introduced to direct professional practices (e.g., rates according to the 'diagnose related groups' system) (Bossen et al. 2016). Efficient transfer has traditionally been driven by physicians, as they represent the group of professionals with authority to make decisions on diagnoses and treatment. However, because of the involvement of interdisciplinary staff working in more specialized healthcare institutions, we assume that decision-making in this context is no longer solely a medical issue. We regard organizational and professional values and standards as an integrated part of clinical decision-making when it comes to transferring patients in a highly specialized healthcare sector.

11.3   Design and Methods

The study featured a prospective qualitative design using ethnographic fieldwork and in situ interviews at three institutions in the Capital Region of Denmark. We strategically selected the sites and settings according to their levels and areas of specialization. The institutions represented three stages in the rehabilitation trajectory: the acute stage (institution A), including acute hospital admission and intensive care; the subacute stage (institution B), including highly specialized intensive neurorehabilitation; and the stable stage (institution C), including long-term outpatient rehabilitation at the municipal level.

The intention with the ethnographic fieldwork was to focus on observations of interdisciplinary meetings in which we assumed that decisions were made about patient transfer to the 'next' institution/ department according to each patient's specific rehabilitation needs. It was discovered, however, that transfer decisions were not necessarily made at the regular meetings. The procedures at the acute and stable stage institutions were more ad hoc, emerging during the everyday work, whereas formal discharge meetings were held at the subacute institution.

We emphasize that the empirical material reflects the differences in transfer-related decisions. Our data consist of field notes and interview transcripts from institutions A, B, and C. The three institutions were each visited for three days as an introduction to fieldwork to get a feel for the work and organization of patient transfer. At institutions A and C, fieldwork was conducted as nonparticipatory observation for five days at each site, focusing on the ad hoc situations wherein transfer was negotiated. At institution B, where specific transfer meetings were organized, we observed ten meetings and supplemented our notes from these with debriefings and interviews.

At institution A, the physicians were the primary objects of observation because they were formally in charge of the transfer procedure. Coordinating nurses and a physiotherapist were also observed to describe their roles in the decision process. We interviewed the head physician, the coordinating nurse, and three other physicians at the site.

At institution B, we observed interdisciplinary meetings with potential patient and family participation. During the days of introduction, a physician, a nurse, and an occupational therapist were observed in their everyday work with severely brain-injured patients. Ten interdisciplinary meetings were observed, focusing on the dominant argument bringing the patient further in the rehabilitation process. The HCPs had to determine whether the patient should stay in specialized rehabilitation or transfer to the next stage of rehabilitation as an outpatient. Eight of the ten interdisciplinary meetings were recorded and transcribed by a student with assistance from the researcher present at the meetings. The number of participants at the interdisciplinary meetings ranged from 8 to 12 persons including the relatives. In situ interviews were conducted after the meetings with participants with or without influence on the decisions. The idea was to explore the decisional nuances and what might be at stake for the HCPs.

The main focus of fieldwork at institution C was the licensed practical nurses, also known as 'social and healthcare assistants'[1] (SHAs), since they were the active professionals with the responsibility of getting the patients further towards discharge from the institution. Other HCPs were interviewed, such as an occupational therapist, the leader of a volunteer group, and the leader and deputy of the institution. Although our data

---

[1] Licensed practical nurses—or, directly translated, 'social and healthcare assistants'—complete two years, nine months, and three weeks of education, admitting students with a secondary school diploma. In comparison, registered nurses are admitted with a high school diploma and complete a three-year, six-month baccalaureate education.

are heterogeneous, we argue with the ethnographic tradition that a 'desk design' of our study must adapt to real-life practices and not the other way around (Hammersley and Atkinson 2007; Walford 2009).

We adhered to the ethical principles of the Declaration of Helsinki (World Medical Association 2018). Managers and staff at the three institutions were informed of the aim of the study, as well as the planned observations and interviews. The HCPs and relatives who were observed and interviewed provided their informed consent to participate. The HCPs involved were advised that participation was voluntary and that they could withdraw their consent at any time.

11.4   Analytical Framework and Operationalization

The theoretical approach is mainly based on Pierre Bourdieu's theory of practice or praxeology (Bourdieu 1990, 1994, 1997), while Andrew Abbott's concept of 'jurisdiction' is used to highlight the professional aspects of practice (Abbott 1988, 2005).

When focusing on the HCPs' practices, we rely on Bourdieu's relational and dispositional approach (Bourdieu 1997, 2002). Relations become real out of the tension emerging from the result of something being ascribed and acknowledged as having more value than something else, and the assumption that the distribution of who has the valuable 'capital' becomes bodily knowledge to the professionals and orients but does not determine their practices. This perspective gives voice to the HCPs' subjective experiences and preferences (Bourdieu 2000a; Bourdieu and Passeron 2000). However, this subjectivity must, according to Bourdieu, be contextualized by objectifying or constructing the platform on which the professionals speak and act. The introduction of the present chapter is meant to illustrate the contours of the objective conditions as a platform for practising transfer, and also the following 'descriptive analysis' of the different organizations should function as such. In this description, the material aspects and architectural conditions are included to show how

nurses, due to the high level of specialization. All patient rooms are placed on the side of the ward facing the windows. There is a front office with ward secretaries and nurses working on computers and observing patient monitors. For an outsider, the technical equipment is overwhelming. All patients' vital organs are monitored and maintained continuously. The daily cost for a patient at this unit runs at approximately EUR 3500.

Transfer Practices Maintaining Acquired Highly Prestigious Position and Managing Hyper-Specialization of Healthcare

The physicians at the neurointensive care unit are mostly neuro-anaesthesiologists. Day shifts start with an 8 a.m. conference in a room away from the unit. About 10–12 physicians and 1 coordinating nurse are present. The doctor in charge from the night shift leads the meeting, during which the most urgent patient problems are presented and discussed. All issues focus on whether the patient should stay or be transferred to another ward or hospital.

Around 9 a.m., the physicians and the coordinating nurse meet again. In the meantime, they have seen some of their patients, checked up on their computers, or participated in an academic '15-minute meeting'. The 'nine o'clock-meeting' is conducted in a different conference room within the ward. Here, more specific plans are made for the patients. Following the logic of the patient rooms, all diagnoses, treatments, and patient responses are presented by the doctor in charge of each patient. The final topic of discussion is whether the patient should stay or transfer out of the unit.

At noon, anaesthesiologists and neurosurgeons meet to discuss whether patients are fully treated from a neurosurgical perspective. If treatment has finished and the patient is free of the mechanical ventilator, the anaesthesiologists are responsible for finding a bed for the patient after transfer. If the patient has not fully responded to treatment, the physicians conclude: 'Not going anywhere'.

The neurosurgical department must at all times be triple-prepared to provide anaesthesia during (a) acute thrombectomy (blood clot removal), (b) acute magnetic resonance imaging (MRI) scans (if anaesthesia is needed), and (c) neurosurgery. These procedures provide legitimate access to the ward regardless of a patient's age. These structural conditions challenged the survival statistics as older people who have suffered strokes are given the same access to acute treatment. The ward manager and physicians experience constant pressure to admit patients and to transfer patients out of the unit. In addition to the meetings in which 'stay-or-go' decisions are a central part of the agenda, the neurosurgeons and anaesthesiologists must keep abreast of which patients might be ready for transfer. Although the neurosurgeons might consider the patient fully treated, the anaesthesiologists have the final say regarding patient transfer.

After neurointensive care, the 'next-step institution' is the subacute rehabilitation department located at a different hospital site. If a patient requiring close observation is not ready for subacute rehabilitation and a new patient is being admitted, the physicians are responsible for finding an appropriate placement for the patient transferring out of the unit.

Considered from Abbott's perspective, according to which the physician's medical specialty is seen as a jurisdiction, it might be assumed that the anaesthesiologists would try to keep compromised patients in the unit in order to control the boundaries of their jurisdiction until the patients are stable. In this way, the jurisdiction could be maintained and the anaesthesiologists could exercise their particular skills. But, this was not the case in our study. Seen as a strategy, we found that the physicians incorporate the structural conditions (i.e., all patients with severe brain trauma and compromised vital functions must be received in this ward). With Bourdieu's concept of capital, the explanation for the transfer practice seems to offer more nuances. Possessing the exceptional skills of saving lives and mastering health problems related to the vital organs represents high stakes within the medical field. When negotiating over the phone with other anaesthesiologists regarding whether or not to transfer a patient to another intensive care unit, they are also confirming each other in their exclusive positions.

Transferring to temporarily stay in another hospital is an inconvenience to the patient and their family. It represents a 'detour' in the trajectory towards the 'right place' (i.e., the neurorehabilitation department). As one physician explained:

Of course, we think that it was even better if the patient was fully treated at the intensive care unit at [hospital A], which means that he was off the ventilator and sent directly to rehabilitation unit (hospital B) where he belongs. Of course, that is the ideal ... even though [hospital A] has expanded the number of beds, it seems that there is never enough space.

Equally, an anaesthesiologist from a 'detour hospital', who received a 'detour patient', experienced the transfer procedure as 'exemplary', explaining:

Well, I think it has something to do with ... of course, besides that, we are good people and we want to help each other ... that we know each other very, very well within the intensive care units. ... It's a small specialty; often, I would know somebody's name. And we all know the problem of overcrowding; the next day, I might be in the same situation. It's not like we are talking about a random admission ... I mean, a neat and equal distribution of patients among the available beds at all hospital at all times ... You have to take the patients to where the empty beds are ...

The physicians are probably aware of the structural constraints and lack of vacant beds, and they have not completely naturalized the conditions—one anaesthesiologist referred to the transfer practice as a 'logistic hell'. At first glance, the physicians act pragmatically, but, applying the theories of Bourdieu and Abbott, it becomes apparent that the specialist physicians confirm their exclusive position while they transfer the patient. The negotiation of vacant beds at the receiving unit serves as an act of consolidating joint jurisdiction. According to Bourdieu's argument, we see a maintenance of an exclusive position strengthened by a strong network among the peer privileged.

Challenges to the Boundaries of Jurisdiction at Institution A

Following the boundaries of the jurisdiction, the structural conditions (i.e., triple-preparedness to provide anaesthesia) disturb the jurisdiction and challenge the a priori privilege of physicians to autonomously admit and discharge patients.

The physicians use an implicit algorithm for patient transfer between units and hospitals. Treating medical problems in multiple organ failure means that a dominant organ has to be defined in order to place the patient at the 'correct' ward. It is negotiable whether a patient can be accepted as a 'detour patient', but other limitations are non-negotiable: if the main diagnosis is not treated at the 'detour hospital' (i.e., intensive care needs in addition to urology, and abdominal surgery) and the specific medical specialty is not backed up at the hospital, the anaesthesiologists do not even ask for a 'detour bed'. As formulated by a 'detour anaesthesiologist' (doctor receiving a patient from hospital A, neuro-anaesthesiological ward):

> We don't want patients out here with urological problems, since we do not have an urologist at our hospital. If urology is the main problem, it is only hospital x, y, or z [regional hospitals]. We have to cooperate in this way, right? Of course, it is an advantage that we know how the region has distributed its medical specialties, but we know that, of course.

The 'necessity' of hyper-specialism of modern-day hospitals seems to be incorporated and naturalized in an uncompromised way. Exercising a medical specialty can only persist if the physicians are able to call other specialists. If the boundaries of a particular jurisdiction are blurred, though, it is hard to distinguish between specialties. In this way, transfer practices serve to maintain a specific medical specialty and to support its distinctiveness. In addition to the distinct knowledge of a prestigious medical specialty, it appears that the physicians have acquired a specific competence by knowing which hospital or ward to contact for a patient transfer. Furthermore, the physicians are aware that this knowledge is crucial and provides access to the administrative domain that often challenges their own dominant medical capital.

11.4.1.2 Institution B: The Subacute Stage

At this neurorehabilitation institution, patients are accepted when they are no longer ventilator dependent, although they still might need some breathing support. At this stage of rehabilitation, a virtue is made of the need for interdisciplinary healthcare services. All the clinical staff from the dayshift meet at 8 a.m. in the morning for a so-called safety debriefing. About 25 people sit in a large staff room. Nobody drinks coffee here. A senior physician leads the meeting, all subdepartments (divided according to patient beds) have their own rounds, and the HCPs have a chance to present specific problems, such as, 'We need to discuss patient x more'; a meeting is planned through a request from the physiotherapists; a patient coughs during physical training and it is discussed whether the timing of exercise could be rescheduled; the senior physician speaks about a report from the central working environment council; some technical equipment is re-located, and so on.

The HCPs wear uniforms in different colours: turquoise or white. Apparently, there is no particular colour code for the professions. Physicians and therapists wear T-shirts and trousers, both wear turquoise T-shirts; nurses prefer white, but wear turquoise as well. The traditional white lab coats worn by physicians over street clothes are banned, but some physicians still use them. The daily cost for a patient at this unit runs at approximately EUR 2000.

Transfer Practices as Interdisciplinary Joint Practices

Transfer decisions are made during 'treatment meetings' or 'team meetings'. Treatment meetings, held every two weeks, are used to plan ongoing rehabilitation, whereas in team meetings, held every six weeks, decisions are made regarding whether to transfer or discharge a patient or to continue rehabilitation for another six weeks.

Physicians, neuropsychologists, physiotherapists, occupational therapists, nurses, and occasionally SHAs and social workers participate in both treatment meetings and team meetings. At the latter, where transfer is the main issue on the agenda, the physician leads the meeting. When the physician for some reason has to leave the meeting early, the next in line to lead the meeting is the neuropsychologist, who also holds an academic degree. The physician gives all the HCPs a chance to speak and they each describe the positive or negative progress of the patient in question. When the round of updates is over, the physician decides whether the patient should be offered another six weeks of rehabilitation. Representatives from municipal outpatient care join the meeting at this time. Up to three different coordinators participate: the municipal coordinator, a brain injury coordinator, and a triage manager. The purpose is to find the best place to meet the needs of the patient while adhering to the municipal regulations for treatment costs. When the patient leaves the hospital, payment is transferred from the region to the municipality.

Challenges to the Boundaries of Jurisdiction at Institution B

At the subacute institution, transfer practices are organized collectively, and transfer decisions are shared among HCPs. This flatter organizational structure is a contrast to the paternalism observed in the acute organization. What can threaten the legitimacy of the ward is, as we saw at institution A, conditions preventing HCPs from exercising their specialty.

During observation, a male patient exhibited highly agitated behaviour probably due to brain damage. His uncooperative behaviour and hostility towards the staff were so extreme that it was discussed whether a psychiatric diagnosis was dominant. The physicians at institution B pushed towards transfer to the psychiatric ward, whereas the psychiatric personnel did not support this proposal. Although the meeting was led by the physician, transfer decisions were ideally based on equality among the HCPs present. The physician made the initial decision on patient transfer (stay or go), but the decision could be changed if other HCPs had a stronger argument. Relatives also had a voice and, for example, could argue for an extension of six more weeks in rehabilitation. In two of the ten observed meetings, the relatively underprivileged relatives managed to change the HCPs' (specifically, the physician's) decision. In one case, a Filipino airport housekeeper and mother in a family with strong caring values became emotional and almost begged the physician to grant the patient another six weeks of rehabilitation. Another mother, herself disabled and in a wheelchair, from a low-income family succeeded in changing the decision by using strong language. As the physician explained, 'We are not ironbound, we are open for new impressions'. Strong emotions, personalities, and family ties together with a flatter hierarchy and the opinions of additional actors, yet still with the physician as the final decision-maker, can apparently succeed in influencing an administrative and medical decision.

By being an exceptional, specialist unit (only one other institution has the same status in Denmark), the unit becomes attractive to the patients and their relatives. It also seems to be commonly acknowledged that, once the patient has moved on to the next step—either another local community institution or back to their own home—the rehabilitation is less intensive.

11.4.1.3   Institution C: The Stable Stage

The local municipality has the responsibility of organizing rehabilitation for patients in the stable stage after severe brain injury. Institution C is run as a self-governed institution managing rehabilitation tasks on behalf of the municipality. This institution is the last step before discharge to home or a permanent care institution. Patients—or 'residents', as they are called when they leave the hospital—are rehabilitated for complex reasons, but the overall criterion for admission to municipal rehabilitation is an inability to take care of oneself. The specialty of institution C is social complexity, and one of the three floors at the institution is dedicated to residents with severe alcoholic abuse issues, although residents with other problems might also have problems with alcohol abuse. Residents with acquired brain injury are located on the two other floors, mixed with residents suffering multiple health problems as well as socioeconomic issues. As the institution leader explained, 'Our main focus is to speak up for those who are unable to speak up for themselves'. The leader adheres to the principles of 'taking the side of the resident', 'being a watchdog', and 'acknowledging professional indignation'. The leader also emphasizes user participation and user involvement as institutional values. The cafeteria in the institution is open to the public but is primarily used by former residents with close relations to other residents and the institution. The staff team consists of professionals, former residents, and volunteers. The two institution leaders are equipped with degrees in sociology and psychology, whereas the 'street-level' staff are unlicensed nurses or SHAs. There are no nurses or doctors employed at the institution. The residents, like the general population, have their own municipal general practitioner (GP), who can be called by the SHA if needed. SHAs are in charge in the wards, and also in charge of the decision to transfer a patient home. The daily cost for a resident at this institution runs at approximately EUR 220.

Transfer Practices as Pulling and Pushing Tardy Structures

The institution leaders and SHAs experience the GPs as reluctant to show up when they are needed, causing major problems. One day during our study's fieldwork, the SHAs discovered an unresponsive patient/resident. The patient had multiple diagnoses, including diabetes, liver disease, and complications following a brain injury. The SHAs conferred with one another and decided that the patient's level of consciousness had changed markedly. An SHA called the GP several times, and, the next day, the GP called for an ambulance that brought the resident to the hospital. The resident was later diagnosed with pneumonia and remained at the hospital for intensive observation. The SHA said, 'His own doctor doesn't really want to have anything to do with him'.

In comparison to the acute and subacute stages of rehabilitation, where, as has been described, a patient's physical function and brain damage are the central focuses, the focal point at institution C is the wider social complexity of the situation. The following exchange observed between two SHAs demonstrates this:

INTERVIEWER: What happened to this resident? Why is he [the resident] here?

SHA1 (*rehabilitation assistant grabs the chart and starts to read*): 'A 60-year-old man admitted to the trauma centre. Patient found unconscious in his home by the janitor'...

INTERVIEWER: Oh, the janitor was there too...

SHA1: He was evicted from his apartment, I guess...

SHA2: It looks like he didn't pay the rent. He couldn't manage staying in his own apartment. They say the apartment was in a terrible condition. (*Also reading now*) 'On arrival, the patient had nomoterm'... I don't know what that means. (*Reads again*) 'The patient is probably suffering from alcohol abuse. Not further information on arrival.'

SHA1: '... showing a big subdural haematoma' ... (*mumbling ... reading to herself*)
INTERVIEWER: Could you read it aloud?
SHA1: He has had something after he fell, right?
INTERVIEWER: Yes, when was that?
SHA1: August 26th (*it is now September 18th*).
INTERVIEWER: So, that was just before he came here?
SHA1: I guess it was. That's what it says happened ...
INTERVIEWER: So ... he was at the trauma centre at [institution A]?
SHA1: I think he was ... it doesn't really say where he was, it just says 'neurosurgical clinic'...
INTERVIEWER: It's most likely [institution A].
SHA1: Then it says something about 'GCS 7 with slowly reacting pupils' ... I don't know what that means.

The complexity of a resident's needs is not limited to the body, as we had observed at the acute stage institution. Here, a body was a body regardless of age, due to the new regulations. Moreover, in addition to physical problems, the patients have severe psychosocial issues. Their housing situation, finances, social networks, and work relations (if any) are taken into consideration during negotiations regarding the final housing for a resident. Often, the brain damage was caused by risky behaviour combined with drug or alcohol abuse, and, in these circumstances, it is unclear whether a patient's behaviour is a result of brain damage or chemical abuse. Another major issue the staff had to deal with as part of the transfer practice was that the resident was illiterate in respect of the modern digitalized world, including the management of various credit cards and codes and communicating with authorities (bank, computerized information systems, etc.). Accordingly, the SHAs had to escort the residents to the bank or municipal office to acquire new cards and codes, if they for some reason had lost their cards or forgotten their codes. They organized regular visits with the residents to renew these cards and codes, and, for each individual, they had to decide how to integrate the ethics and the practicalities around these issues.

On top of this, the SHAs struggled with slow service at the municipal office that managed the housing situation as a precondition to get residents transferred to a permanent housing and healthcare situation. SHAs were continually pushing the municipal office to speed up progress regarding a resident's housing situation in the system. One SHA called several times and left messages, all in vain, while she waited for an official answer to a request for a specific apartment. She began to describe her experiences in a calm voice, but had trouble keeping her anger down:

> SHA1: So you know, Steen [resident] should have received a letter within two weeks ... And this is the problem! I tell Bob [the social worker in charge], 'Steen is suffering from amnesia, he forgets stuff, he can't do things'. Then Bob says, 'But I have sent it! Maybe I have sent it electronically?' So I think to myself, 'What is this idiot thinking? Steen has been evicted. He has no credit card. He gets a new credit card every week because he forgets where he puts it. He hasn't got a health insurance card, he has nothing ... He wouldn't even open his mail ... And then they send an e-mail?' I say, 'Very clever' ... really ... he doesn't even have a wallet.' He [the social worker] works with this kind of residents, and I think, 'Can't he even put two and two together?' I get pretty upset by these cases ...

11.5   Discussion

11.5.1   Organizationally Produced Inequalities in Transfer Practices

Taking for granted that a smooth-running flow through the involved organizations is beneficial for the acute brain injury patients' rehabilitation process, we have identified some constraining dynamics that need attention. Perhaps most troublingly, the sick organ, the brain, and the neurosurgical and ensuing neuro-anaesthesiological treatment seem to have undergone a dramatic decline during the rehabilitation process. According to Album et al. (2017), the brain is, along with the heart, an organ associated with most prestige among medical professionals and specialities. From a relational perspective (see also Table 11.1), we observed all the prestigious attributes attached to the acute stage of neurorehabilitation (institution A): artefacts supporting life-saving (helicopter, medico-technical equipment, everything must yield at the escalator to allow the medical staff to act) and the ward is staffed with the

HCPs, even as they produce new tasks and, in doing so, expand their jurisdiction, feel inadequate and frustrated by their experience of practising tasks of patient transfer. The economic and symbolic resources expended at the acute care stage contrast significantly to those spent at the final institution prior to discharge. In this way, the uneven resources spread over the trajectory of the rehabilitation process reduce the quality and likelihood of a coherent rehabilitation, which clearly does not benefit patients. Therefore, future discussions should consider the extent to which efforts expended during the acute stage match the outcome when patients reach the stable stage of their rehabilitation; in other words, saved lives must be lived.

References

Abbott, A. (1988). *The system of professions – An essay on the division of expert labor*. Chicago: University of Chicago Press.

Abbott, A. (2005). Linked ecologies – States and universities as environments for professions. *Sociological Theory, 23*, 245–274.

Album, D., Johannessen, L. E., & Rasmussen, E. B. (2017). Stability and change in disease prestige: A comparative analysis of three surveys spanning a quarter of a century. *Social Science & Medicine, 180*, 45–51.

Andersen, K. K., Dalton, S. O., Steding-Jessen, M., & Olsen, T. S. (2014). Socioeconomic position and survival after a stroke in Denmark, 2003 to 2012: Nationwide hospital-based study. *Stroke, 45*(12), 3556–3560. https://doi.org/10.1161/STROKEAHA.114.007046.

Anke, A., Andelic, N., Skandsen, T., Knoph, R., Ader, T., Manskow, U., et al. (2015). Functional recovery and life satisfaction in the first year after severe traumatic brain injury: A prospective multicenter study of a Norwegian national cohort. *Journal of Head Trauma Rehabilitation, 30*(4), E38–E49. https://doi.org/10.1097/HTR.0000000000000080.

Bambra, C. (2012). Social inequalities in health: The Nordic welfare state in comparative context. In J. Kvist, J. Fritzell, B. Hvinden, & O. Kangas (Eds.), *Changing social equality: The Nordic welfare model in the 21st century* (pp. 143–164). Bristol: Policy Press.

Bossen, C., Danholt, P., & Klausen, M. (2016). Diagnoser som styringshybrider Diagnoserelaterede grupper i sundhedsvæsenet. *Tidsskrift for Forskning i Sygdom og Samfund, 13*(25). https://doi.org/10.7146/tfss.v13i25.24995.

Bourdieu, P. (1990). *The logic of practice*. Stanford: Stanford University Press.

Bourdieu, P. (1994). De tre former for teoretisk viden (M. Nørholm & K. A. Petersen, Trans.). In S. Callewaert, P. Bourdieu, M. Munk, M. Nørholm, & K. A. Petersen (Eds.), *Pierre Bourdieu: Centrale tekster indenfor sociologi og kulturteori* (pp. 72–108). Copenhagen: Akademisk. Original work published as: Bourdieu, P. (1973). The three forms of theoretical knowledge. *Social Science Information, 12*(1), 53–80.

Bourdieu, P. (1997). *Af praktiske grunde: omkring teorien om menneskelig handlen* [Practical reason: On the theory of action]. Copenhagen: Hans Reitzels.

Bourdieu, P. (2000a). *Homo academicus* (Reprint). Stanford: Stanford University Press.

Bourdieu, P. (2000b). *Pascalian meditations*. Oxford: Polity Press.

Bourdieu, P. (2002). *Distinction – A social critique of the judgement of taste*. London: Routledge.

Bourdieu, P., & Passeron, J. C. (2000). *Reproduction in education, society and culture* (New ed.). London: Sage.

Devaux, M., & de Looper, M. (2012). *Income-related inequalities in health service utilisation in 19 OECD countries, 2008–2009* (OECD health working papers, No. 58). Paris: OECD Publishing. https://doi.org/10.1787/5k95xd6stnxt-en.

Eikemo, T. A., Bambra, C., Joyce, K., & Dahl, E. (2008). Welfare state regimes and income-related health inequalities: A comparison of 23 European countries. *The European Journal of Public Health, 18*(6), 593–559.

Engberg, A. W., Liebach, A., & Nordenbo, A. (2006). Centralized rehabilitation after severe traumatic brain injury – A population-based study. *Acta Neurologica Scandinavica, 113*(3), 178–184.

Guldager, R. (2018). *Inequality in neurorehabilitation: Different practices among patients and relatives during rehabilitation after stroke and severe traumatic brain injury: A qualitative study*. Doctoral dissertation, Aalborg Universitetsforlag.

Hammersley, M., & Atkinson, P. (2007). *Ethnography: Principles in practice*. London: Routledge.

Husted, H., Jensen, C. M., Solgaard, S., & Kehlet, H. (2012). Reduced length of stay following hip and knee arthroplasty in Denmark 2000–2009: From research to implementation. *Archives of Orthopaedic and Trauma Surgery, 132*(1), 101–104. https://doi.org/10.1007/s00402-011-1396-0.

Kamper-Jørgensen, F., & Rasmussen, J. G. (2008). Ulighed i behandling [Inequality in healthcare]. In F. Diderichsen, J. G. Rasmussen, & N. Döllner (Eds.), *Den tunge ende: sandheden om ulighederne og uretfærdighederne i den danske sundhed: debatbog* (pp. 27–45). Copenhagen: Dagens Medicin Bøger.

Larsen, K., Cutchin, M. P., & Harsløf, I. (2013). Health capital: New health risks and personal investments in the body in the context of changing Nordic welfare states. In I. Harsløf & R. Ulmestig (Eds.), *Changing social risks and social policy responses in the Nordic welfare states* (pp. 165–188). London: Palgrave Macmillan.

Mackenbach, J. P., Stirbu, I., Roskam, A.-J. R., Schaap, M. M., Menvielle, G., Leinsalu, M., & Kunst, A. E. (2008). Socioeconomic inequalities in health in 22 European countries. *New England Journal of Medicine, 358*(23), 2468–2481.

National Board of Health. (2011). *Hjerneskaderehabilitering – en medicinsk teknologivurdering* [Brain injury rehabilitation – A medical technology assessment]. Copenhagen: National Board of Health.

Reay, D. (1998). 'Always knowing' and 'never being sure': Familial and institutional habituses and higher education choice. *Journal of Education Policy, 13*(4), 519–529.

Walford, G. (2009). For ethnography. *Ethnography and Education, 4*(3), 271–282.

Willis, K., Collyer, F., Lewis, S., Gabe, J., Flaherty, I., & Calnan, M. (2016). Knowledge matters: Producing and using knowledge to navigate healthcare systems. *Health Sociology Review, 25*(2), 202–216. https://doi.org/10.1080/1 4461242.2016.1170624.

World Medical Association. (2018). *Declaration of Helsinki – Ethical principles for medical research involving human subjects.* https://www.wma.net/policies-post/wma-declaration-of-helsinki-ethical-principles-for-medical-research-involving-human-subjects. Accessed 4 July 2018.

12

Rehabilitation as a Curricular Construction

Per Koren Solvang and Marte Feiring

12.1 Introduction

Rehabilitation is a contested interdisciplinary practice. In some academic networks, influences from social science and disability activism are perceptibly on the rise; in other networks, a strong commitment to clinical trials for improving functioning holds the leading epistemological position. A few studies have addressed the difficulty in defining rehabilitation (Feiring and Solvang 2013; Reinhardt et al. 2007; Solvang et al. 2017; Whyte 2008). How it is framed for emerging professionals enrolled in training programmes is important in terms of the development of rehabilitation as a professional practice. Despite this importance, though, a question seldom addressed in the literature is how rehabilitation is understood within higher education. A few contributions do exist. For example, Stucki and Celio (2007) outlined a framework for the development of academic programmes in human functioning and rehabilitation. Their aim was to stimulate reflections on the development of research training

P. K. Solvang (✉) • M. Feiring
Department of Physiotherapy, Oslo Metropolitan University, Oslo, Norway
e-mail: persol@oslomet.no; mafei@oslomet.no

© The Author(s) 2019
I. Harsløf et al. (eds.), *New Dynamics of Disability and Rehabilitation*,
https://doi.org/10.1007/978-981-13-7346-6_12

programmes. Similarly, Whyte (2005) addressed the need for training academic researchers and considered which areas of competence are rendered relevant. However, neither of these prior contributions addressed how rehabilitation is actually understood in the development of curricula, in relation to both programmes that qualify for practice and those that qualify for research careers. This lacuna prompts the following research question and focus of this chapter: How is the scholarly profile outlined in programmes in which rehabilitation constitutes a core component? The knowledge gained in answering this question will deepen our understanding of the epistemological patterns in the field of rehabilitation.

Rehabilitation is a composite set of practices constructed by a wide set of actors. National and transnational professionals and governmental organizations are important agents; patient organizations play a role as well. A recent contribution to the multidimensional and interdisciplinary understanding of rehabilitation outlines a matrix of actors positioned on different levels of the social structure (Solvang et al. 2017); the three types of actors in this model are service users, professionals, and governmental authorities. Expanding on this model, we suggest considering educators as a fourth type of actor, at the intersection between professionals and governmental authorities (see Table 12.1).

This chapter focuses on the educators' meso-level activities—those captured in cell (7) of Table 12.1. Educators working at universities and university colleges teach rehabilitation. This teaching is situated inside a wide variety of study programmes, such as physiotherapy, occupational therapy, social work, and nursing, to name a few (Stucki and Celio 2007). According to most definitions of the term, rehabilitation is depicted as an interdisciplinary endeavour (Albrecht 2015). How this interdisciplinarity is composed will vary, partly because of the epistemological struggles in the field of rehabilitation and partly through the institutional settings that offer study programmes addressing rehabilitation. To deepen existing knowledge about how the interdisciplinary practices of rehabilitation are understood in educational settings, this chapter will present a study of programmes that include 'rehabilitation' in their title.

Table 12.1 presents an analytical model identifying three intersectional levels of society (i.e., micro, meso, and macro) and four different agents

Table 12.1 Matrix of key agents and levels of society in rehabilitation

Levels	Agents			
	Individuals experiencing disabilities	Clinical professionals	Educators	Governmental authorities
Micro	(1) Making life-world decisions relevant to rehabilitation	(2) Improving clients' level of functioning, participation, and well-being	(3) Teaching and assisting students in learning	(4) Governing citizens by expecting active care for own health and a strong work ethic
Meso	(5) Acting as service user representatives	(6) Organizing hospitals, local rehabilitation units, and rehabilitation chains	(7) Designing curricula and developing scholarly profiles	(8) Promoting efficient, accessible, and high-quality services
Macro	(9) Associations acting as advisory bodies and pressure groups	(10) Professional associations negotiating jurisdiction	(11) Contributing to the development of educational policies	(12) Securing democratic foundation of policy formation and just distribution of services

Adapted and extended from Solvang et al. (2017, p. 1985)

(service users, professionals, educators, and governmental authorities) who also interact with one another. Rehabilitation is a cross-field in which agents and institutions pursue their interests and ambitions at various levels of society, together shaping rehabilitation both as an area of research and scholarly knowledge and as a clinical practice. Table 12.1 identifies 12 intersections between different types of agents and levels of societal organization, in order to situate curricular work in the broader scope of rehabilitation as a social practice. While not exhaustive, each cell of the model identifies what are regarded as core examples of the issues important to rehabilitation. The role of an educator at a university is typically combined with that of a researcher (even if some educators only have a minor proportion of their position assigned to research), and, in this respect, they are also impacting the practice through their research dissemination. The educators are working within regulatory frameworks set by governmental authorities. The level of regulation differs, from strong in Scandinavia, with its predominantly state-owned universities and colleges, to weaker in the United States, which has a large proportion of private educational institutions (Bleiklie and Kogan 2007).

The chapter will analyse the curricula of key rehabilitation programmes in higher education in the Scandinavian countries, the United Kingdom, and Germany. The overall framework is the sociological study of knowledge—particularly the 'Mode 2' concept developed by Gibbons et al. (1994). This perspective highlights the emergence of inter- and transdisciplinarity and the involvement of users (patients and relatives) in knowledge production. As a more specific theoretical lens, Bourdieu's concept of cultural capital in the study of higher education will also be applied (Bourdieu 1988). The empirical design includes all present study programmes in rehabilitation at the graduate and postgraduate level. Curricula, reading lists, scholarly profiles of key teachers, and the nature of institutions/departments compose the key data collected. The textual information is then evaluated by applying a theory-driven content analysis. The subsequent discussion addresses differences and similarities between the countries studied regarding the scholarly profile of the respective programmes, with special attention paid to transdisciplinarity.

12.2   Analytical Perspectives

The revision of the International Classification of Functioning, Disability and Health (ICF) by the World Health Organization (WHO) in 2001 had a significant impact on the understanding of disability and rehabilitation in health and social services provision (World Health Organization 2001). The social model of disability was, to a certain degree, implemented (Bickenbach et al. 1999), instigating what has since been labelled both a 'social turn' (Solvang 2012) and a 'paradigm shift' (Reinhardt 2011) in rehabilitation. From being a medically dominated practice, rehabilitation has developed in such a way that psychology and sociology are no longer on the outskirts of the field but at its very heart. Thus, there is a medical- and pedagogical-dominated 'before' and a psychology- and social science-oriented 'now'. A specific interdisciplinary understanding of rehabilitation has been constructed by the ICF model development coordinated by the WHO, but this conceptualization is contested because of the variety of perspectives involved (Albrecht 2015). Hence, rehabilitation can be seen as a contested field of scholarship and practice that takes many forms. One perspective relies on predominantly health science-orientated conceptions, highlighting functioning as the outcome of interest (Stucki et al. 2018). This approach is echoed by the WHO, which defines rehabilitation as 'a set of interventions designed to optimize functioning and reduce disability in individuals with health conditions in interaction with their environment' (World Health Organization 2017, p. 1). The definition is followed up by a recommendation to organize rehabilitation as part of the health sector. Another scholarly position applies models that open up rehabilitation to perspectives from critical disability studies. In this latter group of models, all aspects of human existence, from the physical to the psychological (including social, relational, and indeed existential), are included (Gibson 2016; McPherson et al. 2015). Following this type of approach, the relevance of organizing rehabilitation as part of the health sector is not so obvious, and the governmental bodies of social services and education could equally well be possible sites for the organization of rehabilitation services. Both scholarly positions are interdisciplinary, but they apply different combinations of knowledge types in their framing of rehabilitation.

Bourdieu's theoretical concept of 'cultural capital' lends itself as a sensitizing device with which to understand the struggles of knowledge in defining rehabilitation. Cultural capital is embodied in the form of mental dispositions within which scholarly orientations, definitions, and professional competences can become subsumed; and in objectified and institutionalized forms, such as course books, instruments, and technologies, as well as educational programmes and formal qualification requirements (Bourdieu 1986). The cultural capital concept provides a framework in which to set our study's ambition to ascertain how rehabilitation is represented in educational programmes. In turn, their scholarly profile will influence which forms of knowledge and approaches are legitimate to draw upon in the actual rehabilitation practice.

According to a perspective from the sociology of knowledge, there has been a trend for the production of knowledge to migrate from autonomous universities to hybrid institutions where user steering plays a large role (Gibbons et al. 1994; Nowotny et al. 2001). This tendency is seen as a move from 'Mode 1' to 'Mode 2', following which the archetypical Mode 1 institutions—the universities—now reflect the Mode 2 society, by interacting more strongly with their surroundings. These developments set the scene for the growth of study programmes in rehabilitation that are prone to combinations with other specialties, such as geriatrics, and applications to certain social sectors, such as inclusion in working lives.

Analysing academic institutions, Bourdieu (1988) identified two opposing hierarchies, one based on social networks and economic capital (the 'heteronomous hierarchy') and the other on cultural forms such as scientific knowledge and autonomous research (the 'autonomous hierarchy'). Rehabilitation seems to correspond to a heteronomous hierarchy, because, at an institutional level, it has many intersections with other specialties, such as pedagogics, social work, and sociology, as well as towards governmental health policies and disability activism (Feiring and Solvang 2013). Furthermore, in recent years, the educational system has also migrated towards Mode 2. Students are not only expected to seek wisdom but also to qualify for competences required in the labour market. Universities try to compete for the students and design study programmes intended to attract prospective applicants. Through these processes, a diverse set of interdisciplinary study programmes is developed, reflecting a scholarly development typical of Mode 2 by promoting combinations that are attractive to prospective students pursuing a career as part of their working lives. The emergence of part-time programmes serving students seeking further education adds to the trends actualizing Mode 2.

These trends in higher education are part of the overall shift labelled by the sociology of knowledge as a change from Mode 1 to Mode 2. The production of knowledge migrates from autonomous universities to hybrid institutions where knowledge interests voiced by practitioners play a large role (Gibbons et al. 1994; Nowotny et al. 2001). Such processes are disputed by, for example, university boards highly influenced by representatives of private companies (Greenhalgh and Wieringa 2011). Nonetheless, these trends are increasingly setting the scene for the development of study programmes in rehabilitation that are inclined towards combinations with other specialties, such as geriatrics, and applications to certain social sectors, such as 'work life inclusion'.

12.3   Methodological Approach

The understanding of the curricular work in this study is based on texts published on university websites. These texts are situated in an institutional context. They take the form they do to accomplish a specific task (Mik-Meyer 2005), with the task of the texts at hand being to provide information to prospective students, and, in some cases, to employers assigning employees permission to enrol in a part-time study programme. These texts are also prone to being framed by university guidelines for presentation, typically highlighting the educational institution as innovative and attuned to the demands of working life.

Three geographical areas were strategically chosen for the study that echo the Northern European perspective of this book. Germany and the United Kingdom are leading countries in Europe in the health and social sciences, while Scandinavia represents important innovations in rehabilitation, introducing a version of the social model of disability at an early stage (Tøssebro 2004). As the aim of the present study is to highlight the role of educational institutions in rehabilitation—and not to provide a complete picture of how educational institutions work with rehabilitation—the use of three strategic geographical areas should not be considered a limitation of the study's design. On the contrary, a small number of cases such as this allows for an in-depth focus on the variety of conceptualizations of rehabilitation that can be found.

The selection of educational studies followed two requirements: (1) 'rehabilitation' had to be part of the name of the programme, but not necessarily the sole designator; (2) the programme had to be directed towards working with humans.[1] Both bachelor's and master's programmes

---

[1] Bachelor of Science degrees in animal rehabilitation offered by four British colleges and universities were excluded from the study programmes selected for analysis because they did not deal with humans. However, recent advances in disability studies have been giving attention to the intersection between animality and disability. This is not about using references to animals derogatively

are included, as well as PhD programmes. The key method for finding study programmes was through advanced Google searches. The search terms 'rehabilitation' and 'university' were put into the search engine and the search was restricted to one country at a time. Common terms in the local languages were applied as well. The pages of matches were combed through until no new study programmes appeared. The listing typically had only study programmes on the first 10–20 web pages retrieved. Eventually, new study programmes stopped being uncovered. For the UK-based searches, this took place around retrieved page 100; and for the Scandinavian countries-based searches, around retrieved page 30. Additional information was collected by contacting programme heads who were willing to set aside time to engage in e-mail correspondence. This information was restricted to reading lists. We cannot be certain that our list of study programmes is complete; some programmes may have slipped under our radar, but there is no indication that a high number of them will have done so.

The analysis was conducted through an open reading of all studies as presented on the websites. As a second stage, the texts were read as representations of rehabilitation and as representations of organizing higher education. Three categories emerged out of this reading. First, the countries are an organizing framework in the way that national profiles emerge. Second, the health–social science continuum emerged as an important framework for analysis. Third, study organization is clearly important. There is one body of studies that comprises on-campus bachelor's-level studies, and another that incorporates postgraduate programmes, offered both as on-campus full-time programmes and off-campus part-time programmes.

---

when giving negative evaluations of disabled people (Carlson 2009); from the post-humanist perspective, the intersection between disability and animality is infused with positive values. One much-cited example is that of Temple Grandin, a US professor of animal science and consultant to the livestock industry, who considers her ability to understand animal needs to be closely related to herself being on the autism spectrum (Wolfe 2010). The post-humanist perspective decentres the human and ascribes heightened status to animals, and, following this line of thought, animal rehabilitation may deserve a place in the study of the curricular construction of rehabilitation. Indeed, the animal rehabilitation programmes also use concepts such as 'rehabilitation' and 'nursing', and, through the rehabilitative approach, they somewhat humanise animals. Nonetheless, the programmes are institutionally framed by the veterinary sciences.

Table 12.2 Study programmes with 'rehabilitation' in their title in the Scandinavian countries, Germany, and the United Kingdom, distributed by educational level

	Scandinavia	Germany	United Kingdom
BSc	1	3	17
MSc	6	6	11
Total	7	9	28

12.4 Results

An overview of the number of study programmes is given in Table 12.2. If we take into consideration the number of inhabitants in the countries, Scandinavia (11 million) and the United Kingdom (65 million) offer a comparable number of study programmes. With its 82 million inhabitants, Germany has the smallest representation of study programmes in relative terms. Furthermore, using the programme title as our instrument for identifying programmes, we infer that rehabilitation is far more prevalent in the curricula in Scandinavian and UK universities and colleges, compared to those in Germany. Most of the 17 BSc programmes identified in the United Kingdom concern sport rehabilitation, a branch of physiotherapy that in many UK universities is organized in the form of a designated study programme. If we set these aside, the Scandinavian countries stand out as having the strongest focus on rehabilitation when measuring by programme name, and hold the number relative to the size of the country.

When we look at the key disciplines involved in the composition of rehabilitation as a university degree, three clusters emerge. The first is a cluster of programmes closely attuned to physiotherapy. Here, there are a large number of British universities providing BSc degrees in sports rehabilitation. In addition, there are several Master of Science programmes in which rehabilitation is situated within physiotherapy and orthopaedics, and many of these only admit certified physiotherapists. Second, there is cluster of programmes that aim at interdisciplinarity. Even if they are located within departments of health, the physiotherapy and health aspects are downplayed to the advantage of psychology and social science. Students enrol of these programmes from several professional backgrounds. Most of the Scandinavian programmes are situated in this cluster. Third, there is a cluster of programmes that situate rehabilitation within counselling and educational sciences. These are typically located at departments of special education in Germany. In sum, the curricular understanding of rehabilitation is framed by clusters within which the nodes are physiotherapy, interdisciplinarity, and educational sciences. In the following subsections, we take a closer look at each of them.

12.4.1 Physiotherapy

The BSc sports rehabilitation programmes are based in United Kingdom, but one MSc programme is offered at a German university. There are a total of 17 such programmes. They are typically offered together with BSc programmes in physiotherapy. In this way, they represent a specialization track in physiotherapy, and apply the concept of rehabilitation in a process of framing what characterizes the role of physiotherapy in sport. They of course feature a strong component of musculoskeletal themes, as well as skills in advising the individual. Most degree programmes make visible a biopsychosocial approach wherein the physical body is understood in the context of psychosocial approaches.

The physiotherapy-dominated MSc programmes have a strong focus on the functioning of the body. Courses typically address questions about anatomy, musculoskeletal functioning, ergonomics, and biomechanics. Exercise and training are also key parts of the courses offered. The programmes are situated in health departments. Subjects related to the organization of the rehabilitation process are also part of the curriculum. These typically focus on principles of evidence-based medicine, clinical governance, and, to some degree, skills in interpersonal communication.

There are also a variety of specialization programmes, such as cancer rehabilitation and cardiovascular rehabilitation. Some of these are situated in physiotherapy departments and have a strong focus on exercising and giving advice to clients in a process of rehabilitation. Other programmes are situated in technical faculties, such as programmes for visual rehabilitation and those for amputation and prosthetic management.

12.4.2 Interdisciplinarity

The interdisciplinary cluster of study programmes is not fully removed from physiotherapy. Several are situated in physiotherapy departments. However, they are open for all health BSc degrees and to a variety of social work and educational science BSc programmes. Accordingly, they create an interdisciplinary arena, as expressed by Oxford Brookes University in the following statement from its website:

> It provides you with the opportunity to challenge and critically evaluate your multi-professional and uni-professional clinical expertise in order to respond to the current and future needs of rehabilitation. You will have opportunities to work with practitioners from different professions, different patient and client groups, and a variety of countries – providing diverse views of rehabilitation.

Several of the courses offered in the interdisciplinary cluster of studies are leaning towards psychology, sociology, and even critical disability studies. The influence from social science and disability activism on rehabilitation is at its most pronounced among Canada- and Oceania-based scholars (Gibson 2016; Hammell 2006; McPherson et al. 2015). Disability studies has been picked up by two of the programmes—the ones at University of Southern Denmark and Oslo Metropolitan University, where the writings of the Canadian and Oceanian scholars hold a prominent position on the reading lists.

The interdisciplinarity is characterized by what seems to be an ambition to build programmes that combine the clinical trial-dominated paradigm and the paradigm strongly influenced by critical disability studies. One example is the programme at University of Southern Denmark, where the rehabilitation paradigm mirrors the disability studies approach, while courses on ideal trajectories and economics represent the clinical approach. This multiparadigmatic approach is reflected in the reading list, too, where both McPherson et al.'s (2015) *Re-thinking Rehabilitation* book and Derek Wade's row of editorials in *Clinical Rehabilitation* *(Wade 2015) is obligatory.

In Scandinavia, a salutogenic health promotion focus features strongly in several study programmes. In Sweden, for example, both identified programmes are oriented towards working life rehabilitation: 'When you study Health and Rehabilitation in Work Life, you will learn to promote health, prevent ill health, and engage in rehabilitation in the best way possible' [our translation]. Thus, rehabilitation is framed as an integrative part of a broader understanding of health, well-being, and participation. This approach corresponds with the policy trend discussed by Anne-Stine B. Røberg in Chap. 6 of this volume in which prevention tends to give more attention than rehabilitation in white papers and governmental strategy documents. It is also worth noting that both Swedish programmes are directed towards work life inclusion. In effect, in Sweden, as a programme name designator, 'rehabilitation' seems to be restricted to knowledge building and professional practice in working lives.

12.4.3   Educational Sciences

The cluster of programmes that situates rehabilitation within counselling and educational sciences is currently only found in Germany, and three of the programmes we identified even present themselves as being closely interrelated. The Humboldt University of Berlin states on its web pages:

> Besides Cologne and Dortmund is the Department for Rehabilitation Sciences at the Humboldt University of Berlin, offering a wide-reaching rehabilitation education from the pre-school phase through to work life inclusion and into the assistance offered to chronically ill, disabled, and old people.

They apply a life course approach and voice a multidisciplinary perspective by highlighting a knowledge base grounded in medicine, psychology, sociology, and educational sciences, as well as law and professionalization. Issues such as disability studies, communication, and language are commonly featured. One much-used course book is edited by Baumann et al. (2010) and titled *Rehapädagogik, Rehamedizin, Mensch*. It presents an interdisciplinary fusion between medicine and educational sciences; the child is understood as being socially situated, building on perspectives from interpretative sociology, and as acting in challenging environments, building on psychological concepts such as resilience and salutogenesis.

Pedagogics is the main reference point for this cluster of study programmes. The competence building has a goal of supporting disabled individuals within social service and health systems. Students develop an ability to plan diagnostic processes and follow them up. Knowledge about the legal system and institutional frameworks for rehabilitation is also a key goal. The entry requirement to the master's programmes is a bachelor's degree in educational sciences. The programmes are situated in departments of education at faculties of social science and humanities. As stated in the quotation above, the programmes at the Humboldt University of Berlin not only belong to the Department of Rehabilitation Sciences but also adhere to the educational framework by being situated in a discourse of rehabilitation pedagogics. The German group of rehabilitation studies also comprises programmes for the deaf and hard-of-hearing rehabilitation pedagogics. The programme at the Ludwig Maximillian University of Munich is categorized as language and cultural sciences, and there is even a specialization in sign language interpretation—indeed a far-reaching concept of rehabilitation.

12.4.4   Programme Structure and Pedagogics

Most of the UK and Scandinavian universities are offering the MSc programmes as part of a plethora of further education provision. Nearly all of them offer a part-time schedule, some of them so flexible that students can work their way through the programme in their own time on campus programmes. If they end up not doing the full degree, the courses taken will nonetheless qualify them for further education certificates. Additionally, as already noted, one body of studies comprises on-campus bachelor's degree studies, and the other encompasses postgraduate programmes offered as on-campus full-time courses or off-campus part-time ones.

All MSc programmes have a form of research assignment or thesis to be completed. At several of the British universities, the programme is organized along two lines, and the students must choose which to pursue: either they make an original contribution to research or they conduct a systematic review. The courses in methods are also divided according to these two styles of knowledge building. Within this, the systematic review is seen as an integral part of what are considered relevant skills for rehabilitation. This is in line with other health programmes as well, and may be seen as reflecting a trend in which systematic reviews are given high recognition in the health sciences.

Overall, the ICF seems to be the best candidate for a common ground within the wide variety of rehabilitation study programmes, as, in most of the programmes, the ICF is in some way referred to as a subject in relation to which the student will have their competences strengthened.

12.5   Discussion

Three patterns have emerged from our analysis. In the United Kingdom, a health science-based approach with physiotherapy as a dominating scholarly force is evident. In Germany, rehabilitation as a branch of the educational sciences is well established. Finally, in the Scandinavian countries, approaches giving a position to the social sciences hold a strong position. It is important to note that these geographically framed patterns are not without exceptions. Health science-dominated programmes are found in both Scandinavia and Germany too, and at least one programme leaning towards the social sciences is to be found in the United Kingdom. There are medical, educational, and social aspects of rehabilitation in all countries. Moreover, the three national practices have complex historical roots. Taking a longer time perspective, pedagogical–psychological approaches, with parallels to those currently found in Germany, were predominant in Norway prior to World War II, while a medical–physical approach with similarities to that found in the United Kingdom, dominated in Denmark after World War II (Feiring 2009, 2016).

These findings should be considered in light of three perspectives, which are themselves based on the observation that, when analysing education sensitized by the concept of cultural capital, rehabilitation is framed by interdisciplinarity, as well as actively meeting user expectations characteristic of the Mode 2 phase in knowledge production. Thus, first, rehabilitation is used in many combinations with other subjects, mirroring a pattern wherein the understanding of rehabilitation seems to be attuned to work life demands, presumably in order to attract students. Second, rehabilitation is to varying degrees understood as representing a holistic perspective and applying the social model of disability. Third, the ICF emerges as a unifying point of reference in the study programmes in terms of the way they are presented. This particular finding may add to the scholarly discussion concerning the ICF as a boundary object for clinical rehabilitation and disability research.

In diverse ways, the programmes are attuned to the demands of working lives. First, the MSc programmes in the United Kingdom and Scandinavia are designed to attract part-time students who combine their studies with their working life roles (predominantly physiotherapists, but other professionals as well). The combination seems to lay the ground for a close interaction between work life demands and curricular offerings. One example is the thesis that can be written in close conjecture with knowledge interest from the occupational position held. Second, the full-time programmes at bachelor's level—typically, the Swedish work life inclusion programmes and the German educational counselling ones— have a strong focus on national legislation and institutional frameworks for rehabilitation. In particular, the organization of the MSc programmes opens up opportunities for interaction with practice, strongly underlining the Mode 2 framework for science and knowledge production.

It is possible to draw a dividing line between the primarily health sciences programmes and the holistic and interdisciplinary programmes. In curricular settings, the rehabilitation concept is used to denote musculoskeletal treatment and exercise programmes, typically in sports rehabilitation, and to designate broad approaches to rehabilitation incorporating disability studies as well as counselling in social work and educational science frameworks. Physiotherapy seems to dominate the health science programmes. This leaves us with the question of what has happened to the position of occupational therapy in rehabilitation. In the curricular setting, it seems that occupational therapy may be part of the qualification for interdisciplinary MSc programmes, conceivably through developing in a more holistic direction when it comes to rehabilitation than seems to be the case with physiotherapy.

The ICF is an important tool for the active and visible rehabilitation research groups in Europe, situated in a nexus between the Swiss Paraplegic Centre (in Nottwil), the University of Lucerne (also in Switzerland), and the German Institute of Medical Documentation and Information (in Cologne). It has also been suggested by sociologists and others in the field of disability studies as a boundary object. According to these scholars, disability needs to be understood as a complex interaction between characteristics of the individual, characteristics of society, and what takes place in the professional support system (Bickenbach 2012; Imrie 2004; Shakespeare 2006). Despite the fact that it acknowledges complexity, however, the ICF is contested. For example, Gibson (2016) has argued that its two main problems are that, first, it reproduces the distinction of 'normal' versus 'abnormal', and, second, the concept of impairment is seen as a biological fact and not as a phenomenon that changes over time. Nonetheless, the ICF maintains its position as an institutional framework important for the development of rehabilitation as an interdisciplinary practice in which critical disability studies are part of the mix. This position is confirmed by the curricula for programmes in rehabilitation from the three studied areas of Northern Europe.

In the introduction to this chapter, we outlined a paradigm shift in rehabilitation, and we now posit that two scholarly clusters have picked up on this paradigm shift, in different ways. The ICF nexus situated in Europe has introduced some elements of the social model of disability. The rethinking group with a foothold in Canada has taken on board a wider set of elements from the social model and the way it is developed in critical disability studies, challenging normalization as a goal for rehabilitation. In the study programmes, the milder version of the paradigm shift is dominating. In the model geared towards improvement in functioning, represented by the British programmes, the frequent mention of the ICF in the learning outcomes reflects the reforms in understanding rehabilitation depicted by the ICF. The model strongly inspired by critical disability studies can be found in some of the study programmes in Scandinavia and in the German cluster of counselling programmes institutionally framed by education. However, there are only a small number of these programmes, and the educational framing of the German programmes causes them to be strongly influenced by learning psychology traditions. In sum, the programmes represent important trends in the development of rehabilitation as an inter- and transdisciplinary field of practice, where the ICF model of rehabilitation is predominant.

Study programmes are run by educators who are active as researchers. Hence, as teachers, they keep up to date on recent developments in their scholarly field of practice and implement these developments in various ways in the study programmes. In our study's setting, students will encounter important trends in rehabilitation—but what will be the impact on the practice of rehabilitation? Unfortunately, the current study's findings offer no data that shed light in respect of this particular question. However, when studying programme profiles, this query about impact needs to be addressed. What are the implications for practice when a scholarly profile of programmes in rehabilitation has a certain design? One way to approach this question would be to point out the high number of programmes that offer rehabilitation as a form of secondary education for students well established in their working lives. This group of students is likely to be able to implement the perspectives to which they are introduced through a position of more authority than students graduating at the bachelor's-degree level and taking up a position as a rehabilitation professional for the first time. This may be part of a general implication of the Mode 2 framework whereby knowledge production is closely attuned to the institutions of clinical practice. The academic scholarship of Mode 1 is still flourishing, but is increasingly integrated with the level of professional practice.

12.6 Conclusion

When we sought out programmes using 'rehabilitation' in their name, three outlined clusters emerged. There seems to be rather different national traditions in the curricular application of rehabilitation. Sports physiotherapy courses are framed within rehabilitation, mostly in the United Kingdom, as well as within a diverse set of health science programmes. Counselling programmes epistemologically grounded in educational sciences frame rehabilitation in Germany. In Scandinavia, interdisciplinary approaches are a clear trend, with an epistemological grounding not far from the German counselling programmes and a couple of the British programmes.

These findings tell us how rehabilitation is applied as a designator in three geographical areas in Northern Europe. Any future international overview should include other parts of the world, as well as further European countries, and it would be especially important to include Canada, the United States, and Australia, which are all leading countries in respect to rehabilitation research. An even more comprehensive overview would have been gained by including rehabilitation courses in programmes that do not feature 'rehabilitation' in the programme name. Despite these limitations, however, the epistemological diversities and geographical differences in the curricular construction of rehabilitation found through the present analysis should prove useful when applied to rethinking rehabilitation as a policy and a practice.

References

Albrecht, G. (2015). Rehabilitation. In R. Adams, B. Reiss, & D. Serlin (Eds.), *Keywords for disability studies* (pp. 148–151). New York: New York University Press.

Baumann, M., Schmitz, C., & Zieger, A. (Eds.). (2010). *Rehapädagogik, Rehamedizin, Mensch: Einführung in den interdisziplinären Dialog humanwissenschaftlicher Theorie- und Praxisfelder.* Hohengehren: Schneider.

Bickenbach, J. E. (2012). *Ethics, law and policy.* Los Angeles: Sage.

Bickenbach, J. E., Chatterji, S., Badley, E. M., & Ustun, T. B. (1999). Models of disablement, universalism and the international classification of impairments, disabilities and handicaps. *Social Science & Medicine, 48*(9), 1173–1187.

Bleiklie, I., & Kogan, M. (2007). Organization and governance of universities. *Higher Education Policy, 20*(4), 477–493.

Bourdieu, P. (1986). The forms of capital. In J. G. Richardson (Ed.), *Handbook of theory and research for the sociology of education* (pp. 241–258). New York: Greenwood Press.

Bourdieu, P. (1988). *Homo academicus*. Cambridge, UK: Polity Press.

Carlson, L. (2009). Philosophers of intellectual disability: A taxonomy. *Metaphilosophy, 40*(3–4), 552–566.

Feiring, M. (2009). *Sources of social reforms, 1870–1970: The rise of a Norwegian normalisation regime*. Doctoral dissertation, University of Oslo.

Feiring, M. (2016). Fra revalidering til rehabilitering – en dansk begrepshistorie [From 'revalidering' to rehabilitation – A Danish conceptual history]. *Tidsskrift for professionsstudier, 24*, 86–97.

Feiring, M., & Solvang, P. K. (2013). Rehabilitering – et grensefelt mellom medisin og samfunn [Rehabilitation – A boundary area between medicine and society]. *Praktiske Grunde, 7*(1–2), 73–84.

Gibbons, M., Limoges, C., Nowotny, H., Schwartzman, S., & Trow, M. (1994). *The new production of knowledge: The dynamics of science and research in contemporary societies*. London: Sage.

Gibson, B. E. (2016). *Rehabilitation. A post-critical approach*. Boca Raton: CRC Press.

Greenhalgh, T., & Wieringa, S. (2011). Is it time to drop the 'knowledge translation' metaphor? A critical literature review. *Journal of the Royal Society of Medicine, 104*, 501–509.

Hammell, K. W. (2006). *Perspectives on disability and rehabilitation: Contesting assumptions, challenging practice*. New York: Churchill Livingstone/Elsevier.

Imrie, R. (2004). Demystifying disability: A review of the international classification of functioning, disability and health. *Sociology of Health & Illness, 26*(3), 287–305.

McPherson, K., Gibson, B., & Leplège, A. (Eds.). (2015). *Rethinking rehabilitation: Theory and practice*. London: CRC Press.

Mik-Meyer, N. (2005). Dokumenter i en interaksjonistisk begrepsramme [Documents in an interactionist framework]. In M. Järvinen & N. Mik-Meyer (Eds.), *Kvalitative metoder i et interaksjonistisk perspektiv* [Qualitative methods in an interactionist perspective] (pp. 193–214). Copenhagen: Hans Reitzels.

Nowotny, H., Scott, P., & Gibbons, M. (2001). *Re-thinking science: Knowledge and the public in an age of uncertainty*. Cambridge, UK: Polity.

Reinhardt, J. D. (2011). ICF, theories, paradigms and scientific revolution. Re: Towards a unifying theory of rehabilitation. *Journal of Rehabilitation Medicine, 43*(3), 271–273.

Reinhardt, J., Hofer, P., Arenz, S., & Stucki, G. (2007). Organizing human functioning and rehabilitation research into distinct scientific fields. Part III: Scientific journals. *Journal of Rehabilitation Medicine, 39*(4), 308–322.

Shakespeare, T. (2006). *Disability rights and wrongs*. London: Routledge.

Solvang, P. K. (2012). Et faglig kryssfelt [A scholarly cross-section]. In P. K. Solvang & Å. Slettebø (Eds.), *Rehabilitering: individuelle prosesser, fagutvikling og samordning av tjenester* [Rehabilitation: Individual processes, professional development and service coordination] (pp. 15–34). Oslo: Gyldendal Akademisk.

Solvang, P. K., Hanisch, H., & Reinhardt, J. D. (2017). The rehabilitation research matrix: Producing knowledge at micro, meso and macro levels. *Disability and Rehabilitation, 39*(19), 1983–1989.

Stucki, G., & Celio, M. (2007). Developing human functioning and rehabilitation research. Part II: Interdisciplinary university centers and national and regional collaboration networks. *Journal of Rehabilitation Medicine, 39*(4), 334–342.

Stucki, G., Bickenbach, J., Gutenbrunner, C., & Melvin, J. (2018). Rehabilitation: The key health strategy of the 21st century. *Journal of Rehabilitation Medicine, 50*(4), 309–316.

Tøssebro, J. (2004). Introduction to the special issue: Understanding disability. *Scandinavian Journal of Disability Research, 6*(1), 3–7.

Wade, D. (2015). Rehabilitation – A new approach. Overview and part one: The problems. *Clinical Rehabilitation, 29*(11), 1041–1050.

Whyte, J. (2005). Training and retention of rehabilitation researchers. *American Journal of Physical Medicine & Rehabilitation, 84*(12), 969–975.

Whyte, J. (2008). A grand unified theory of rehabilitation (we wish!): The 57th John Stanley Coulter memorial lecture. *Archives of Physical Medicine and Rehabilitation, 89*(2), 203–209.

Wolfe, C. (2010). *What is posthumanism?* Minneapolis: University of Minnesota Press.

World Health Organization. (2001). *International classification of functioning, disability and health*. Geneva: World Health Organization. https://www.who.int/classifications/icf/en/. Accessed 26 Nov 2018.

World Health Organization. (2017). *Rehabilitation in health systems*. Geneva: World Health Organization.

13

Interdisciplinarity and Rehabilitation Research

Jerome Bickenbach and Berth Danermark

13.1 Introduction

Greene and Loscalzo (2017) have recently issued a plea for 'putting the patient back together' by pointing out the residual reductivism in the new science of 'network medicine'. Echoing calls from social scientists, and following decades of work on the social determinants of health, they argue that we must not be seduced by genetic or molecular reductionism but should rather shape our health science research in terms of a 'biosocial approach to medicine' (Greene and Loscalzo 2017, p. 2493). Their plea in the influential *New England Journal of Medicine* we take to be another manifestation of an accelerating interest across the health sciences in the

J. Bickenbach (✉)
Swiss Paraplegic Research, Nottwil, Switzerland
e-mail: jerome.bickenbach@paraplegie.ch

B. Danermark
The Swedish Institute for Disability Research, School of Health Sciences,
Örebro University, Örebro, Sweden
e-mail: berth.danermark@oru.se

© The Author(s) 2019   **293**
I. Harsløf et al. (eds.), *New Dynamics of Disability and Rehabilitation*,
https://doi.org/10.1007/978-981-13-7346-6_13

promotion of interdisciplinary research to ensure a fully integrative, and person-centred, approach to healthcare and health science research.

For several decades, major health research funders, such as the US National Institutes of Health (NIH) and the European Commission, have made multidisciplinary research-capacity building a funding priority (National Institutes of Health 2001). As a plea for cooperation among diverse scientific disciplines and for more collaborative research between biological and social sciences, these calls were reminders of the perils of professional insularity, overspecialization, and a breakdown in communication in health research and clinical practice, as well as, more theoretically, of the kind of reductivism that Greene and Loscalzo have more recently warned us about (Institute of Medicine 2001). Since then, however, the message from these health research funders, as well as theorists of scientific research, has moved beyond mere collaboration across disciplines, or multidisciplinarity, to the more paradigm-shifting sustained plea for further interdisciplinary health research.

One of the more elegiac calls for interdisciplinarity can be found in a US National Academies report from 2004, which describes it as:

> … one of the most productive and inspiring of human pursuits – one that provides a format for conversations and connections that lead to new knowledge… [and has] delivered much already and promises more: a sustainable environment, healthier and more prosperous lives, new discoveries and technologies to inspire young minds, and a deeper understanding of our place in space and time. (National Academy of Sciences, National Academy of Engineering, and Institute of Medicine 2004, p. 16)

Interdisciplinary health research is seen as pluralistic in method and focus and well suited, the report argues, to the complexity of salient research questions in health science.

The literature on interdisciplinary health research published since the National Academies report, however, has not always been consistent in what is meant by interdisciplinarity, or how it differs from multidisciplinarity. Scott and Hofmeyer (2007) noted that while multidisciplinary research merely 'connects' researchers, interdisciplinary research 'coordinates' them (see also Choi and Pak 2006). More systematically, Wagner et al. 2011 (p. 16; relying on earlier work by Stokols et al. 2008) have provided the following characterization:

> Interdisciplinary approaches integrate separate disciplinary data, methods, tools, concepts, and theories in order to create a holistic view or common understanding of a complex issue, question, or problem. The critical indicators of interdisciplinarity in research include evidence that the integrative synthesis is different from, and greater than, the sum of its parts.

The key word in this quote is 'integrate', for that appears to be at the core of interdisciplinarity, and the single most significant difference between it and multidisciplinarity.

Case studies of successful interdisciplinarity in health sciences invariably focus on, and stress the importance of, an integrative linkage between the biomedical sciences and the social sciences. This is argued to be more than a reluctant collaboration, with techniques and methods of one field being used in another; it should, rather, be seen as a true 'melding of disciplines'. This melding results in, and is characterized by, what is often said to be the key emergent property of such research; namely, that its outcomes are unique and not what could have been produced by the component disciplines separately. In short, the whole is greater than the sum of its parts (Rowe 2008). The hugely influential social determinants of health literature and the research agenda are viewed as the preeminent examples of the biosocial interdisciplinary success story—both in the way they have navigated the vagaries of the politics of science funding and as an intellectual achievement in re-understanding the complexity of the biological, social, economic, cultural, and psychological determinants of health outcomes (Marmot 2008; Marmot and Wilkinson 1999).

What is, to some extent, surprising in this substantial literature on interdisciplinarity in the health sciences is the lack of discussion concerning rehabilitation. This is surprising because it is widely agreed that rehabilitation, more than any other area of healthcare, is best provided—indeed, can only be successfully provided—by interdisciplinary health teams, comprising the full range of medical specialists: physical and rehabilitation medicine physicians; physical, occupational and speech therapists; rehabilitation psychologists; rehabilitation nurses; social workers, and others (Barnes and Ward 2005; DeLisa 2005; European Physical and Rehabilitation Medicine Bodies Alliance 2018; Neumann et al. 2010). More importantly, in rehabilitation practice, teamwork is not merely multi-professional, in the sense that practitioners representing different health professions treat patients *seriatim*, in sequence, or according to some overall treatment plan; rather, interdisciplinary rehabilitation teams try to *integrate* their diverse knowledge and practice bases—identifying connections between biological, psychological, and social determinants in order to come up with an integrated intervention strategy (Danermark 2017).

This is the received view of the character of rehabilitation practice within the rehabilitation professions. The fact that this view does not carry over to the research domain speaks more to the perceived state of rehabilitation research than anything else. Although empirical data on this point is sparse to non-existent, the common perception is that rehabilitation research is generally sidelined and underfunded, perhaps because of the equally common perception that rehabilitation research lacks the methodological rigour seen in other areas of health research. Organizers of the recently created Cochrane Collaboration on Rehabilitation[1] acknowledged early on that, 'For many years, rehabilitation medicine has been considered an unscientific discipline, due to the lack of good quality research and reliable data and tools … it is often considered a less noble topic than more important disciplines' (Negrini et al. 2016). What is typically meant by such remarks is that randomized controlled trial research designs are not as common in rehabilitation research as elsewhere.

It is, however, surprising that rehabilitation research is not immediately seen as a clear case of interdisciplinarity in health research. Because of the often-intense competition for research funding, rehabilitation scientists will naturally respond to the fact that disciplinary health research tends to be prioritized. Moreover, despite the claims of the NIH and other advocates, the theoretical foundations of interdisciplinary health research

---

[1] Cochrane formally approved the establishment of the Cochrane Rehabilitation Field on 22 October 2016 (see https://rehabilitation.cochrane.org/about-us).

have not been well thought through, especially with regard to innovative methodologies that are themselves emergent—that is, methods that could not have been derived by single disciplines on their own, but require interdisciplinary integration. In general, in the health sciences, we lack research tools for knowledge integration, despite the burgeoning literature on integrated care models.

This chapter is partially a response to these shortcomings. Our interest here is not historical, nor do we claim that multidisciplinarity can be historically traced to when rehabilitation emerged as a healthcare strategy (see, e.g., Caracheo et al. 2018). Instead, we focus exclusively on research and make the case for why rehabilitation research at all levels (clinical, public health, and health systems research) would benefit from the promise of interdisciplinarity. Along the way, we underwrite the intuition that the aim of any rehabilitation therapist should be to 'put the patient back together'. In addition, and in response to the lack of theoretical foundations for interdisciplinary health research, we want to make the more theoretical argument that rehabilitation as a health strategy is conceptually best served by research that strives to achieve the emergent potential of interdisciplinarity described above. This will require a diversion into the underlying model found in the World Health Organization's (WHO) International Classification of Functioning, Disability and Health (ICF) (World Health Organization 2001). We conclude this chapter by mentioning challenges to the prospects of truly interdisciplinary rehabilitation research.

13.2 Rehabilitation and the Promise of Interdisciplinarity

Since at least 1978, when the Declaration of Alma-Ata was made, promotion, prevention, cure, and rehabilitation have been acknowledged to be the primary healthcare strategies for clinical care and population health (World Health Organization 1978). Health promotion aims to optimize people's intrinsic resilience against health risks; prevention is intended to reduce the occurrence of diseases, injuries, and other health problems by targeting risk factors; and the curative strategy focuses on eliminating, or at least managing, disease processes. But what of rehabilitation? What are its aims and objectives? Only recently has it been possible to characterize the aims and objectives of rehabilitation intervention in a manner that clarifies why rehabilitation is a distinct health strategy.

Consider the example of rehabilitation for traumatic brain injury (TBI). In 1998, the NIH held a Consensus Development Conference on Rehabilitation of Persons with Traumatic Brain Injury, at which the panel recommended that TBI patients receive an individualized rehabilitation programme based upon the patient's strengths and capacities, and that rehabilitation services should be modified over time in order to adapt to the patient's changing needs (National Institutes of Health 1998). The panel also recommended that moderately to severely injured patients receive rehabilitation treatment that draws on and integrates the skills of many rehabilitation specialists, who, together, would provide individually tailored treatment programmes for physical therapy, occupational therapy, speech and language therapy, physiatry (physical medicine), psychology and psychiatry, and social support. The goal of rehabilitation is to optimize the patient's ability to function at home and in society, and this may require both enhancing the patient's intrinsic capacity and introducing environmental modifications that make everyday activities easier to perform (National Institutes of Health 1998).

Despite such statements, however, rehabilitation practitioners and researchers have not always been as clear about the objective of their health strategy as their more biomedical or public health colleagues. Often, rehabilitation professionals, especially physical and rehabilitation physicians, see themselves as mixing strategies in order to address the health needs of the 'whole patient'. When pressed, though, they acknowledge that rehabilitation does not so much aim at preventing, curing, reversing, or undoing the damage caused by disease or injury as trying to restore functioning, ameliorating the impact of biomedical damage, or minimizing the effects—disease sequelae or secondary conditions—of the underlying health condition (Meyer et al. 2011). Thus, rehabilitation *reduces* the impact of health conditions—as well as of natural processes such as ageing that inevitably involve a decline of functional capacity, often across distinct domains (the phenomena of multi-morbidity). Rehabilitation, it is also said, improves 'quality of life'—although this is a somewhat redundant assertion since quality of life has been conceptualized and related instruments designed not to capture life satisfaction or some other subjective assessment but rather levels of functional capacity in various domains.

Two other aspects of the practice of rehabilitation seem to stand out. First, although acute rehabilitation serves the temporary needs of patients' post-injury or post-medical intervention (especially invasive interventions like surgery), most patients have permanent or chronic health problems that require ongoing rehabilitation across the continuum of care. It is not an accident that rehabilitation came into its own as a health specialty as a response to the injuries that war veterans brought home with them, such as loss of limbs and other permanent mobility or sensory problems (Caracheo et al. 2018). Indeed, the very term 'rehabilitation', at least in the United States after World War I, originally meant the practice of making it easier for soldiers to return to their homes and workplaces, and the practice was restricted to that group of patients. Only several decades later was rehabilitation made universally available.

Second, as mentioned, rehabilitation was always claimed to be a 'whole-person' health strategy. Rehabilitation professionals might focus on specific body parts and facilitate the performance of specific actions, but ultimately their objective is to find ways to get the person back on their feet and participating in major life activities, as the outcome of the consensus conference on TBI makes clear (National Institutes of Health 1998). Moreover, it was recognized very early on in the development of rehabilitation that practitioners could not really make sense of this objective unless they had a clear idea of what the patient's own aims and objectives were—what kind of life they wanted for themselves after they were rehabilitated (Fox 1917).

These two factors undoubtedly spurred the need to augment the profession of physical and rehabilitation medicine with discrete and more practically focused therapies—physical, occupational, speech, psychological, educational, and vocational. These therapists concentrated on central functioning domains: mobility, communication, activities of daily living, school, and work. Serving the interests of the whole person—

recognizing the configuration, demands, and expectations of the home, employment, and community contexts of the patient—helped broaden the repertoire of therapeutic activities. Some therapists focused on optimizing the basic body functions of the patient, training the patient to accommodate, or work around, permanent loss of function. Others provided assistive devices that augmented or replaced lost or deteriorated body functions and structures; and yet others sought ways to modify the patient's home or work environment to accommodate his or her lost or decreased level of functioning in order to optimize patient performance in these environments.

But these therapeutic responses—and the sub-professions that carried them out—served the single objective of optimizing the ability of the patient to participate in major life activities. In practical terms, having this singular objective led to the characteristic model of rehabilitation practice—namely, the interdisciplinary team approach.

In sum, these intuitive characteristics of the nature and core objective of rehabilitation practice were enough to distinguish this healthcare strategy from the others. These features of the practice, moreover, also helped to create a professional self-image that set rehabilitation practitioners—especially the therapists—apart from the more biomedically focused, disease-oriented health practitioners (see, on this point, Serrett 1985; Dreeben-Irimia 2007). It also shaped the rehabilitation research agenda, and the kinds of methodologies that were employed. That said, the theoretical foundations for these intuitions were inchoate and rarely expressed in clear and operational language. It was only with the advent of the unifying concept of 'functioning' denoting the underlying essence of the health experience that rehabilitation could begin to clarify its focus.

13.2.1   Functioning and the ICF

The World Health Organization's (WHO) endorsement of the ICF in 2001 can be seen to represent a true 'paradigm shift' in how we understand health and disability—not to mention how we understand rehabilitation (Stucki 2016; World Health Organization 2001). Central to the ICF—

both as an international standard health classification and as a conceptual model of disability—is the notion of 'functioning'. Although rehabilitation literature has long used terms such as 'functional limitation' and 'functional loss', with the ICF, the WHO formalized the concept, using the term 'functioning' as a technical term denoting the myriad of ways the human body and mind function and the things that people do in their lives, from the simplest and most fundamental actions to, increasingly, behaviours, actions, and social roles.

The ICF was intended by the WHO as a companion classification to the ICD—International Statistical Classification of Diseases and Related Health Problems, now in its 11th edition (World Health Organization 2018)—with more or less the same aim; namely, to provide an internationally comparable standard language for describing health. Unlike the ICD, which focuses on diseases and health problems (as well as determinants and causes), the ICF set out domains of functioning at the bodily, personal, and societal levels. More recently, the WHO has added a third classification to its family of health bulletins; namely, the International Classification of Health Interventions (or ICHI).

Although the ICF is a robust epidemiological standard with a wide range of practical applications, it is its conceptual underpinnings that promise to have far-reaching consequences for health research. The ICF represents the culmination of conceptual developments regarding the nature of health and disability that go back several decades. With respect to the highly politicized and contentious notion of disability, the debates between the 'medical model' and the 'social model' that waged during the 1970s and 1980s more or less resolved themselves into a broader consensus by the time the ICF was in development at the end of the 1990s (see Bickenbach 2012). Since then, there has been a general consensus that, when someone experiences a problem with functioning directly linked to their health state (rather than, e.g., their level of income, social status, gender, or race), the underlying determinants include aspects of that person's underlying health state (the diseases, injuries, and other health problems they have, or the impact of ageing) as well as the overall context or environment in which the person lives and acts. This interactive 'person and environment' construct, now the standard view, was always implicit in rehabilitation practice. In some ways, the ICF merely brought to the wider health and social science communities the understanding of disability that rehabilitation had presumed for a hundred years.

Conceptually, the person–environment model of functioning and disability, in order to do the kind of scientific work asked of it, very much depends on a conceptual distinction between two perspectives or constructs of human experience, which are called, in the ICF, 'capacity' and 'performance'. 'Capacity' is a theoretical construct (statistically, a latent trait) that in practice typically presumes or embodies a clinical inference based on information about the underlying health conditions and clinical observations of how people carry out activities, given the impairments associated with underlying health problems. Capacity constitutes the intrinsic health state of a person, independent of the effect of features of their environment. It comprises all physiological, psychological functions, and anatomical structures of the body, and, by virtue of these functions in various combinations, results in the 'capacity' of the person to perform all human activities, from the very simple to the very complex. A person's capacity is (theoretically) independent of all aspects of external environmental determinants that may facilitate or hinder the actual execution of these activities.

'Performance', by contrast, is not an abstract construct so much as the full, factual description of what the individual actually does. The performance in real life of any human action always depends on features of the person's environment (i.e., what human action takes place). Environment here is understood very broadly to include the physical environment as well as the human-built, attitudinal, interpersonal, social, political, and cultural environment. Environmental factors—from climate to social attitudes—leave their mark on all of the things human beings do and, by extension, the complex social roles they perform (spouse, father, student, employee, and so on).

Importantly, environmental factors do not constitute a neutral, background context of action, but are constituent of the nature of the action. Environmental factors may make it harder to perform activities (e.g., poor air quality, inaccessible and non-accommodating physical environments, or stigma and discrimination, and social exclusion) or make it easier to perform activities (e.g., assistive technology, accessible buildings, supportive attitudes, and social arrangements). In either case, performance is the outcome of interactions between capacity and the environment. In other words, capacity and environmental factors are two sets of determinants of the existence or extent of performance. When performance in a functioning domain is chronically suboptimal (in terms of a threshold that ICF intentionally does not specify, but leaves to researchers and other ICF users to provide), the result is a disability in that domain.

Given that the same level of capacity to execute an action can be positively or negatively affected by environmental factors, the notion of disability—or decrement of functioning in a domain—possesses two important characteristics. First, disability is a continuous not a dichotomous notion: having a disability is a matter of more or less, not yes or no. Second, since maximal capacity of functioning in any domain is statistically unlikely, certainly across the lifespan, it is fair to say that disability is a near-universal phenomenon: everyone will have, or will develop as they age, disabilities of some level of severity in some domain. More realistically speaking, human beings as they age will invariably develop significant disabilities in several domains.

The ICF constructs of capacity and performance, and the general conceptual features of functioning, have been used to draw a heuristic distinction that assists in the task of operationalizing health in a manner that makes sense of the underlying nature and objective of rehabilitation (Stucki et al. 2017, 2018): capacity can be linked to purely *biological health*, while performance captures the actual manifestation of the experience of health in our lives—what might be called the *experience of lived health*. Although this was not the WHO's intent in developing the ICF, it is also possible to find in the inherent model of the ICF a distinction between health in a narrow 'under the skin' or purely biomedical sense, and health in a broader, more whole-person-focused 'lived health' sense.

These two dimensions of health are intimately linked, since lived health only makes sense in light of biological health, and biological health is an abstraction unless it is manifested in the lived experience of health in actual people in real-life circumstances. Significantly, implicit in both dimensions of health is the key ICF concept of functioning. Functioning not only links the two dimensions of health together, conceptually, but also provides the categories and relationships necessary to operationalize both dimensions. Epidemiologically speaking, finally, to fully understand the phenomena of health and to collect data relevant to the entire health experience, it is essential to view functioning, after mortality and morbidity, as the third indicator of health.

13.2.2   ICF and Rehabilitation: The Source of Interdisciplinarity

The conceptual essentials of the ICF—and, in particular, the constructs of capacity and performance—provide the tools for a theoretically robust conceptualization of rehabilitation that captures the intuitions of rehabilitation practitioners and researchers. Although the ICF is a generic classification, designed for a multitude of applications, derived instrumentation has been developed for specific applications. With respect to the TBI, for example, core sets—specifically, a comprehensive core set of 139 ICF categories and a brief core set of 32 categories—have been created by means of a robust methodology, for clinical and research applications (Laxe et al. 2013).

Bringing together some recent formulations, rehabilitation itself can be characterized as the health strategy that applies and interdisciplinarily integrates a variety of scientific disciplines and technologies to optimize a person's capacity to build on and strengthen their resources, and to provide a facilitating environment to enhance a person's performance in the interaction with the environment over the course of a health condition and along the continuum of care. In short, rehabilitation is the health strategy that enables people with health conditions experiencing or likely to experience disability to achieve and maintain optimal functioning (Gutenbrunner et al. 2011; Meyer et al. 2011, 2014; Stucki and Melvin 2007).

This theoretical account of rehabilitation as a health strategy underscores the intuitive view that the primary objective of rehabilitation interventions is to optimize functioning to enhance performance for individuals with compromised functioning in one or several domains. Few practitioners would describe as their therapeutic aim to 'optimize intrinsic biological health and to translate that capacity into performance in interaction with the environment' (Stucki 2016, p. 489). Yet, in less abstract language, they would recognize a therapeutic objective described as, say, 'extending upper-arm range motion to enhance wheelchair use'. The point is that the rehabilitation focus is not the underlying disease or injury as such but the impact of it on a person's life and the actual performance of activities. Rehabilitation, in other words, focuses on the lived experience of health rather than merely biological health.

What does this picture of rehabilitation practice tell us about rehabilitation research? The key insight from the ICF is that the lived experience of health is not reducible to a biomedical state, as this experience is fundamentally interactional: with the possible exception of states of pain or other forms of discomfort, the nature, quality, and extent of the impact of an impairment of body function or structure depend on features of the person's environment—whether the environment facilitates the performance of an activity or further hinders it. An assistive device like a wheelchair makes it possible for a person with mobility impairments associated with lower-body paralysis to be mobile, while a broken pavement or other environmental obstacles will hinder mobility despite the wheelchair. Rehabilitation research, minimally, must mirror this interaction. Better understanding of impairments associated with paralysis helps to improve movement capacity, and a better understanding of engineering in the design of an assistive product helps to improve performance. A focus on the whole person, in the actual context in which he or she lives and acts, mandates research that calls on the resources of very different disciplines. But, as the focus of rehabilitation is the interactive outcomes of the person and their environment, the mode of research must take into account this interaction and the emergent outcomes it yields. Yet, this is just the perspective of interdisciplinarity.

The ICF model has been used as a template for categorizing the wide range of scientific and humanistic disciplines that contribute to interdisciplinary health sciences. This ranges from research supporting clinical practice and services that address the needs of individuals, to research addressing the social provision of supports and services designed to meet those needs (Stucki et al. 2016). Biological disciplines focus on the study of the human body and pathology—addressing the issue of intrinsic health capacity and the perspective of biological health. Clinical disciplines focus on prerequisites for the provision of health and health-related care and supports—addressing the issue of the performance and the lived experience of health. And, finally, socio-humanistic disciplines address the contours and requirements of an effective societal response to health needs for health systems and their components (de Savigny and Adam 2009). Rehabilitation research naturally taps into all three categories of health science research: the biological and clinical, to address rehabilitation contribution to meeting the needs of persons; and disciplines from health economics and information sciences to systems analysis and implementation science, to provide the scientific support for the societal response to these needs.

This ICF-based categorization of health and health-related scientific disciplines canvasses the range of potential interdisciplinary rehabilitation research, and examples could easily be found in the rehabilitation research literature that exemplifies a vast range of permutations of biological, clinical, and health systems research.

13.3   The Challenge of Interdisciplinary Rehabilitation Research

Making the case for the promise of interdisciplinarity in rehabilitation research does not, unfortunately, mean that the promise can be easily fulfilled. Proponents of interdisciplinarity in health research generally face a challenge that affects the prospects of interdisciplinarity in general, and impacts rehabilitation research in particular. The challenge is brought about by the conceit that interdisciplinary research, more than a mere merging of health research disciplines and methodologies, is a *synergetic integration* that transcends disciplinary boundaries yielding scientific novelty—the emergent property already noted in which the whole is greater than its parts (Holland 2014; Rowe 2008). Sceptics argue that interdisciplinarity only makes sense when conducted between closely related disciplines, such as biology and chemistry, but is implausible or frankly impossible when very different and nonadjacent disciplines—say, genetics and sociology or geriatrics, demography, and economics science—are brought together for synergetic collaboration. Is rehabilitation research a counterexample to that scepticism?

Standard multidisciplinary health research addresses complex health phenomena by dividing them into component parts investigated separately by different disciplines. Biomedical sciences provide the knowledge base aspects of the health experience that are fundamentally biological and physiological, while behavioural and social determinants of health seem better served by the social sciences. Yet advocates of interdisciplinarity insist that 'the tools of individual disciplines, whether they be biologic, physiologic, psychologic, or sociologic, are no longer adequate by themselves to fully address the complex problems that we are facing' (Rowe 2008, p. 3). This is because inevitably one of disciplines will assume priority and insist that only its basic concepts and theories are capable of explaining the phenomena in question. For example, in research into geriatric 'frailty', it has been argued that the phenomena must a priori be taken to be entirely biological, and proposed behavioural or social determinants have absolutely no explanatory importance for understanding ageing (Fried et al. 2001).

One of the attractive features of interdisciplinary research in health is that it has the potential of avoiding the traps of oversimplification and reductionism (Rowe 2008). In the comment that opens this chapter, Greene and Loscalzo (2017) pointed to the hyperbole surrounding the Human Genome Project that encouraged the scientific community to believe in a future in which genomic variation would, reductivistically, inform health scientists about disease susceptibility and open the door to 'precision medicine'. Actually, the Human Genome Project taught a very different lesson about human disease; namely, that disease processes are almost infinitely variable and depend on complex environmental interactions (Greene and Loscalzo 2017). Network medicine, or some other set of complex methodologies designed to map out manifold interactions and fully recognize the significance of both biological and social determinants of diseases, is the only future for the health science. Only a truly interdisciplinary response can respond to the need of 'putting the patient back together again'.

A close reading of Greene and Loscalzo's call for action, however, makes it clear that their 'biosocial' approach never gets beyond the realm of biological health and leaves the domain of the lived experience of health more or less untouched. This omission suggests that the general scepticism about and challenge for interdisciplinarity—melding diverse scientific perspectives on the experience of health with truly synergetic research outcomes—does pose a significantly greater challenge for interdisciplinary rehabilitation research than it does for other domains of health research.

Here again, the ICF and ICF-derived instrumentation such as core sets may provide, if not a guarantee of synergetic novelty, then at least an informational platform that makes the promise of interdisciplinarity more plausible. This is certainly the WHO's intent and one of the raison d'être of the ICF was to avoid the fragmented and reductivist, linear model of causation in reasoning and research about disability (Bickenbach et al. 1999). Nor does the ICF model posit causal relationships of any sort between the components of the model, leaving it open to interdisciplinary research to identify and substantiate what associations there are.

As an informational platform for interdisciplinary rehabilitation research, the ICF can support a holistic approach to health, both in terms of biological and the lived experience of health. The ICF offers a common language of health that can facilitate cross-disciplinary communication and understanding—something that advocates of interdisciplinary health research have agreed is essential.

13.4   Conclusion

The current interest in interdisciplinary health research, as a reaction to fragmented and reductivist health science, is welcome, for all the reasons that Greene and Loscalzo mention. Yet, it remains surprising that what is clearly the most fertile ground for the promise of interdisciplinarity—namely, rehabilitation research—is not used as a paradigm example. We have made the case that the practice of rehabilitation is holistic, person–environment interactive, focused on the lived experience of health, and characteristically carried out by interdisciplinary teams—all of which argues for the need for interdisciplinary research. We have also, using the resources of the ICF model of functioning, made the theoretical argument that, by its nature as a health strategy, rehabilitation is inherently interdisciplinary. Finally, we raised the challenge to interdisciplinary health research that its promise of providing synergistically integrated knowledge from different health and non-health disciplines is not feasible. To this challenge, which certainly applies to rehabilitation research, we have tried to make the case that the ICF was envisioned from the outset to provide both a model and an informational platform that is at least congenial to truly synergetic interdisciplinary research, characteristic of the kind of research that rehabilitation practice and rehabilitation science requires.

References

Barnes, M. P., & Ward, A. B. (2005). *Oxford handbook of rehabilitation medicine*. Oxford: Oxford University Press.

Bickenbach, J. E. (2012). *Ethics, law, and policy* (Disability: Key issues and future directions) (Vol. 4). Thousand Oaks: Sage.

Bickenbach, J. E., Chatterji, S., Badley, E. M., & Ustun, T. B. (1999). Models of disablement, universalism and the international classification of impairments, disabilities and handicaps. *Social Science & Medicine, 48*(9), 1173–1187.

Caracheo, A., Bickenbach, J., & Stucki, G. (2018). The emergence of the rehabilitative strategy: The driving forces in the United States of America. *American Journal of Physical Medicine & Rehabilitation, 97*(3), 222–228.

Choi, B. C. K., & Pak, A. W. P. (2006). Multidisciplinarity, interdisciplinarity and transdisciplinarity in health research, services, education and policy, 1: Definitions, objectives, and evidence of effectiveness. *Clinical and Investigative Medicine, 29*(6), 351–364.

Danermark, B. (2017). Interdisciplinary work in a critical realist perspective. In M. Kjørstad & M.-B. Solem (Eds.), *Critical realism for professionals* (pp. 38–56). London: Routledge.

De Savigny, D., & Adam, T. (2009). *Systems thinking for health systems strengthening*. Geneva: Alliance for Health Policy and System Research; World Health Organization.

DeLisa, J. A. (Ed.). (2005). *Physical medicine and rehabilitation: Principles and practice* (4th ed.). Philadelphia: Lippincott Williams & Wilkins.

Dreeben-Irimia, O. (2007). Development of the physical therapy profession. In O. Dreeben-Irimia (Ed.), *Introduction to physical therapy for physical therapist assistants* (pp. 3–22). Sudbury: Jones and Bartlett.

European Physical and Rehabilitation Medicine Bodies Alliance. (2018). White book on physical and rehabilitation medicine in Europe. *European Journal of Physical and Rehabilitation Medicine, 54*(2), 125–155.

Fox, F. (1917). *Physical remedies for disabled soldiers*. London: Bailliére, Tindale and Cox.

Fried, L. P., Tangen, C. M., Walston, J., Newman, A. B., Hirsch, C., Gottdiener, J., et al. (2001). Frailty in older adults: Evidence for a phenotype. *The Journals of Gerontology, Series A: Biological Sciences and Medical Sciences, 56*(3), M146–M156.

Greene, J. A., & Loscalzo, J. (2017). Putting the patient back together – Social medicine, network medicine, and the limits of reductivism. *New England Journal of Medicine, 377*(25), 2493–2499.

Gutenbrunner, C., Meyer, T., Melvin, J., & Stucki, G. (2011). Towards a conceptual description of physical and rehabilitation medicine. *Journal of Rehabilitation Medicine, 43*(9), 760–764.

Holland, G. (2014). *Integrating knowledge through interdisciplinary research: Problems of theory and practice*. London: Routledge.

Institute of Medicine. (2001). *Crossing the quality chasm: A new health system for the 21st century*. Washington, DC: National Academies Press.

Laxe, S., Zasler, N., Selb, M., Tate, R., Tormos, J. M., & Bernabeu, M. (2013). Development of the International Classification of Functioning, Disability and Health core sets for traumatic brain injury: An international consensus process. *Brain Injury, 27*, 379–387.

Marmot, M. (2008). Social resources and health. In P. Kessel, L. Rosenfield, & N. B. Anderson (Eds.), *Expanding the boundaries of health and social science: Case studies in interdisciplinary innovation* (pp. 292–321). Oxford: Oxford University Press.

Marmot, M. G., & Wilkinson, R. G. (Eds.). (1999). *Social determinants of health*. New York: Oxford University Press.

Meyer, T., Gutenbrunner, C., Bickenbach, J., Cieza, A., Melvin, J., & Stucki, G. (2011). Towards a conceptual description of rehabilitation as a health strategy. *Journal of Rehabilitation Medicine, 43*, 765–769.

Meyer, T., Gutenbrunner, C., Kiekens, C., Skempes, D., Melvin, J. L., Schedler, K., et al. (2014). ISPRM discussion paper: Proposing a conceptual description of health-related rehabilitation services. *Journal of Rehabilitation Medicine, 46,* 1–6.

National Academy of Sciences, National Academy of Engineering, & Institute of Medicine. (2004). *Facilitating interdisciplinary research.* Washington, DC: National Academies Press.

National Institutes of Health. (1998). *Rehabilitation of persons with traumatic brain injury.* NIH consensus statement online. National Institutes of Health. https://consensus.nih.gov/1998/1998traumaticbraininjury109html.htm. Accessed 29 Jan 2019.

National Institutes of Health. (2001). *The NIH common fund.* http://commonfund.nih.gov/interdisciplinary/overview.aspx. Accessed 29 Jan 2019.

Negrini, S., Kiekens, C., Levack, W., Grubisic, F., Gimigliano, F., Ilieva, E., & Thorsten, M. (2016). Cochrane physical and rehabilitation medicine: A new field to bridge between best evidence and the specific needs of our field. *Archives of Physical Medicine and Rehabilitation, 97*(8), 1226–1227.

Neumann, V., Gutenbrunner, C., Fialka-Moser, V., Christodoulou, N., Varela, E., Giustini, A., & Delarque, A. (2010). Interdisciplinary team working in physical and rehabilitation medicine. *Journal of Rehabilitation Medicine, 42*(1), 4–8.

Rowe, J. (2008). Introduction: Approaching interdisciplinary research. In P. Kessel, L. Rosenfield, & N. B. Anderson (Eds.), *Expanding the boundaries of health and social science: Case studies in interdisciplinary innovation* (pp. 3–9). Oxford: Oxford University Press.

Scott, C. M., & Hofmeyer, A. T. (2007). Acknowledging complexity: Critically analyzing context to understand interdisciplinary research. *Journal of Interprofessional Care, 21*(5), 491–501.

Serrett, K. D. (1985). *Philosophical and historical roots of occupational therapy.* Philadelphia: Haworth Press.

Stokols, D., Hall, K., Taylor, B., & Moser, R. P. (2008). The science of team science overview of the field and introduction to the supplement. *American Journal of Preventive Medicine, 35*(2S), S77–S89.

Stucki, G. (2016). Olle Höök Lectureship 2015: The World Health Organization's paradigm shift and implementation of the International Classification of Functioning, Disability and Health in rehabilitation. *Journal of Rehabilitation Medicine, 48,* 486–493.

Stucki, G., & Melvin, J. (2007). The International Classification of Functioning, Disability and Health: A unifying model for the conceptual description of physical and rehabilitation medicine. *Journal of Rehabilitation Medicine, 39*, 286–292.

Stucki, G., Rubinelli, S., Reinhardt, J. D., & Bickenbach, J. E. (2016). Towards a common understanding of the health sciences. *Gesundheitswesen, 78*(8), e78–e82.

Stucki, G., Bickenbach, J., & Melvin, J. (2017). Strengthening rehabilitation in health systems worldwide by integrating information on functioning in national health information systems. *American Journal of Physical Medicine & Rehabilitation, 96*(9), 677–681.

Stucki, G., Bickenbach, J., Gutenbrunner, C., & Melvin, J. (2018). Rehabilitation: The health strategy of the 21st century. *Journal of Rehabilitation Medicine, 50*(4), 309–316.

Wagner, C. S., Roessner, J. D., Bobb, K., Klein, J. T., Boyack, K. W., Keyton, J., et al. (2011). Approaches to understanding and measuring interdisciplinary scientific research (IDR): A review of the literature. *Journal of Informetrics, 5*(1), 14–26.

World Health Organization. (1978). Declaration of Alma-Ata. *WHO Chronicle, 32*(11), 428–430. http://www.who.int/publications/almaata_declaration_en.pdf?ua=1. Accessed 29 Jan 2019.

World Health Organization. (2001). *International Classification of Functioning, Disability and Health*. Geneva: World Health Organization. https://www.who.int/classifications/icf/en/. Accessed 29 Jan 2019.

World Health Organization. (2018). *International statistical classification of diseases and related health problems (ICD-11)*. http://www.who.int/classifications/icd/en/. Accessed 29 Jan 2019.

Index[1]

---

[1] Note: Page numbers followed by 'n' refer to notes.

© The Author(s) 2019
I. Harsløf et al. (eds.), *New Dynamics of Disability and Rehabilitation*,
https://doi.org/10.1007/978-981-13-7346-6

Printed by Printforce, the Netherlands